Forensic Aspects
of Neurodevelopmental
Disorders

Forensic Aspects of Neurodevelopmental Disorders

A Clinician's Guide

Edited by

Jane M. McCarthy
Sussex Partnership NHS Foundation Trust, UK and University of Auckland, New Zealand

Regi T. Alexander
Hertfordshire Partnership University NHS Foundation Trust and University of Hertfordshire, UK

Eddie Chaplin
Institute of Health and Social Care, London South Bank University, UK

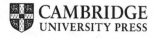

CAMBRIDGE
UNIVERSITY PRESS

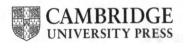

Shaftesbury Road, Cambridge CB2 8EA, United Kingdom

One Liberty Plaza, 20th Floor, New York, NY 10006, USA

477 Williamstown Road, Port Melbourne, VIC 3207, Australia

314–321, 3rd Floor, Plot 3, Splendor Forum, Jasola District Centre, New Delhi – 110025, India

103 Penang Road, #05–06/07, Visioncrest Commercial, Singapore 238467

Cambridge University Press is part of Cambridge University Press & Assessment, a department of the University of Cambridge.

We share the University's mission to contribute to society through the pursuit of education, learning and research at the highest international levels of excellence.

www.cambridge.org
Information on this title: www.cambridge.org/9781009360944

DOI: 10.1017/9781108955522

First published 2023

A catalogue record for this publication is available from the British Library.

A Cataloging-in-Publication data record for this book is available from the Library of Congress.

ISBN 978-1-009-36094-4 Paperback

About the Cover Page

Artbox London (www.artboxlondon.org) is a registered charity and social enterprise that runs art workshops, trips to galleries, puts on exhibitions and creates sales opportunities for people with learning disabilities and autism. Through exhibitions and an online presence, Artbox London aims to raise the visibility of people with learning disabilities and autism in our community and in the wider art world, improving attitudes towards this group. Artbox London curates and displays artists' work for exhibition. This brings art made by people with learning disabilities and autism into the mainstream, changing attitudes about what they can achieve. Work by Artbox London artists has previously appeared on the cover of the *British Journal of Psychiatry* and the *Oxford Textbook of Psychiatry of Intellectual Disability*. The cover of this book was created by Hisba, who is passionate about abstract art, and is continually finding new ways to experiment with shapes and materials. Architecture, art history, textiles and different cultures are among the most important themes in her art and these are continually referred to in her sketchbooks and outcomes. Her work includes geometric pieces based on combinations of triangles or of quadrilaterals, and pieces with fluid lines referencing Japanese woodblock prints.

Contents

Section 1: An Overview: Definitions, Epidemiology and Policy Issues

Section 2: Assessment and Therapeutic Approach

Contributors

Dr Jane M. McCarthy is a consultant psychiatrist at Sussex Partnership NHS Foundation Trust, Honorary Associate Professor in Psychological Medicine at University of Auckland, New Zealand and Visiting Senior Lecturer at the Department of Forensic and Neurodevelopmental Sciences, King's College London, UK. She has over 27 years of experience as a psychiatrist working in the UK and New Zealand with people with neurodevelopmental disorders presenting across forensic services, including prisons and courts. She has also held a number of national and international roles, including Clinical Advisor on Adults with Autism for the Department of Health, England.

Professor Regi T. Alexander is a consultant psychiatrist at Hertfordshire Partnership University NHS Foundation Trust and Visiting Professor at the University of Hertfordshire, UK. He has over 22 years of experience as a psychiatrist, with research interests focusing on the interface between neurodevelopmental disorders, psychiatric illnesses and offending behaviour. An author of over 100 publications, he was Associate Dean of the Royal College of Psychiatrists and is currently President of the Royal Society of Medicine's Intellectual Disability Forum, Editor of the *Oxford Textbook of Psychiatry of Intellectual Disability* and Convenor of RADiANT – a research network of NHS Trusts, academics, patients, family members and community leaders.

Professor Eddie Chaplin is Professor of Mental Health in Neurodevelopmental Conditions and Director of the Foundation for People with Learning Disabilities at the Institute of Health and Social Care, London

South Bank University, UK. His areas of interest include people with intellectual disability, autism and attention deficit hyperactivity disorder in the criminal justice system, and developing mental well-being training and peer mentoring schemes via co-production with people with intellectual disability and autism. He is currently Head of the Scientific Committee of the European Association of Mental Health and Intellectual Disabilities (EAMHID) and has edited the journals *Advances in Autism* and *Advances in Mental Health and Intellectual Disabilities.*

Salma Ali is a registered and chartered forensic psychologist, North London Forensic Service, Barnet, Enfield and Haringey Mental Health NHS Trust, London, UK.

Professor Clare S. Allely is Professor of Forensic Psychology, School of Health and Society, University of Salford, Manchester, UK and affiliate member of the Gillberg Neuropsychiatry Centre, Sahlgrenska Academy, University of Gothenburg, Gothenburg, Sweden.

Dr Zaid Al-Najjar is a general practitioner, NHS Practitioner Health, UK.

Dr Harinder Bains is Clinical Director, and a consultant psychiatrist, Elysium Healthcare, UK.

Dr Harm Boer is a consultant forensic psychiatrist for people with learning disability, Coventry and Warwickshire Partnership NHS Trust, Brooklands Hospital, Birmingham, UK.

Rt Hon Lord Bradley is Chair of Council University of Salford, Hon Special Advisor University of Manchester, Trustee Centre for Mental Health, Trustee Prison Reform Trust and Hon Fellow of the Royal College of Speech and Language Therapists.

Dr Eleanor Brewster is a consultant in psychiatry of learning disabilities, Medical Director for Scotland, Cygnet Health Care, Dundee and lecturer in Medical Ethics and Law School of Medicine, University of Dundee, Scotland.

Dr Penelope Brown is a consultant forensic psychiatrist and research fellow, South London and Maudsley NHS Foundation Trust, London, UK and Institute of Psychiatry, Psychology and Neuroscience, King's College London, UK.

Verity Chester is Research Associate and Network Manager, Research in Developmental Neuropsychiatry (RADiANT), Hertfordshire Partnership University NHS Foundation Trust and University of East Anglia, UK.

Dr Kelly Cocallis is a clinical psychologist, Northumbria Healthcare NHS Foundation Trust, Tyne and Wear, UK.

Professor Penny A. Cook is Professor of Public Health, School of Health and Society, University of Salford, UK.

Dr Ken Courtenay is a consultant psychiatrist in intellectual disability, Barnet, Enfield and Haringey Mental Health NHS Trust, London, UK.

Professor Prathiba Chitsabesan is a consultant child and adolescent psychiatrist, Pennine Care NHS Foundation Trust and Visiting Professor, University College London and Manchester Metropolitan University, UK.

Dr Mark David Chong is an associate professor in criminology and criminal justice studies, College of Arts, Society and Education, James Cook University, Australia.

Dr John Devapriam is Medical Director, Herefordshire and Worcestershire Health and Care NHS Trust, Worcester, UK.

Dr Jana de Villiers is a consultant psychiatrist, High Secure Forensic ID Service for Scotland and Northern Ireland and Forensic Network Clinical Lead for Intellectual Disability, Scotland, UK.

Dr Mhairi Duff is a consultant psychiatrist in forensic intellectual disability, Waitemata District Health Board, Auckland, New Zealand.

Dr Rachel Elvins is a consultant child and adolescent psychiatrist, Royal Manchester Children's Hospital and Honorary Senior Lecturer, University of Manchester, Manchester.

Professor Andrew Forrester is a professor of forensic psychiatry, Department of Psychological Medicine and Clinical Neurosciences, School of Medicine, Cardiff University, UK.

Dr Catherine Franklin is a senior research fellow and Director, Queensland Centre for Intellectual and Developmental Disability, Mater Research Institute–University of Queensland, Brisbane, Australia and psychiatrist and director, Mater Intellectual Disability and Autism Service, Mater Hospital Brisbane, Brisbane, Australia.

David Gilbert is a PhD student, School of Health and Society, University of Salford, UK.

Elizabeth Harris is a clinical psychologist, Department of Psychology, Royal Holloway University of London, UK.

Dr Søren Holst is a researcher and counsellor at the secured institution Kofoedsminde and Aalborg University, Department of Sociology and Social Work, Denmark.

Professor Nathan Hughes is Professor of Adolescent Health and Justice, Department of Sociological Studies, University of Sheffield, UK.

Dr Corey Lane is a clinical psychologist and an adjunct lecturer in criminology, College of Arts, Society and Education, James Cook University, Australia.

Professor Jessica Jones is Professor of Psychiatry and Psychology, Department of Psychiatry, Queen's University, Kingston, ON, Canada.

Dr Voula Marinos is a professor, Department of Child and Youth Studies and program director, Forensic Psychology and Criminal Justice Program, Brock University, St. Catharines, ON, Canada.

Dr Caryl Marshall is a consultant psychiatrist in intellectual disabilities, Oxleas NHS Foundation Trust, London, UK.

Dr Ryan McHugh is a consultant psychiatrist for adults with an intellectual disability, Western Health and Social Care Trust, Northern Ireland, UK.

Dr Iain McKinnon is a consultant psychiatrist and honorary clinical senior lecturer, Cumbria, Northumberland, Tyne and Wear NHS Foundation Trust, Northgate Hospital, Morpeth, UK and Institute of Population Health Sciences, Newcastle University, UK.

Dr Catrin Morrissey is a consultant forensic psychologist, Lincolnshire Partnership NHS Foundation Trust, UK.

Professor Raja Mukherjee is a consultant psychiatrist, National FASD Specialist Behaviour Clinic, Surrey and Borders Partnership NHS Foundation Trust and is Honorary Professor, School of Health and Society, University of Salford, UK.

Dr David Murphy is a chartered forensic and consultant clinical neuropsychologist at the Department of Psychology, Broadmoor High Secure Psychiatric Hospital, Crowthorne, Berkshire, UK.

Dr Bhathika Perera is a consultant psychiatrist, Barnet, Enfield and Haringey Mental Health NHS Trust, London, UK.

Dr Jane Radley is a consultant psychiatrist, St Andrews Healthcare, Northampton, UK.

The Hon Mr Justice Richard D. Schneider is Chair, Ontario Review Board, Toronto, ON, Canada.

Dr Matthew Slinger is a consultant forensic psychiatrist, West London Foundation NHS Trust, UK.

Dr Erik Søndenaa is an associate professor at the Norwegian University of Science and Technology, Department of Mental Health and St. Olavs University Hospital, Department of Brøset, Norway.

Dr Samir Srivastava is a consultant in forensic psychiatry, South London and Maudsley NHS Foundation Trust, Bethlem Royal Hospital, UK.

Dr Priyanka Tharian is a consultant psychiatrist, East London Foundation NHS Trust, London, UK.

Dr Maheera Tyler is a higher trainee in general adult psychiatry, Barnet, Enfield and Haringey Mental Health NHS Trust, London, UK.

Dr Louise Theodosiou is a consultant psychiatrist, Manchester University NHS Foundation Trust, Manchester, UK.

Dr Anto Varughese is a higher specialist trainee, Norfolk and Suffolk NHS Foundation Trust, UK.

Lisa Whittingham is a PhD candidate, Department of Child and Youth Studies, Brock University, St. Catharines, ON, Canada.

Professor Huw Williams is Professor of Clinical Neuropsychology and Co-Director of the Centre for Clinical Neuropsychology Research, School of Psychology, University of Exeter, UK.

Dr Kiriakos Xenitidis is a consultant psychiatrist in intellectual disability, East London NHS Foundation Trust, London, UK.

Professor Susan Young is Director of Psychology Services Limited, London, UK and the Department of Psychology, Reykjavik University, Iceland.

Foreword by the Rt Hon Lord Bradley

I would like to thank the editors for inviting me to write the foreword for this new handbook on *Forensic Aspects of Neurodevelopmental Disorders: A Clinician's Guide*.

It is the case that people with neurodevelopment conditions including autism spectrum disorder, attention deficit hyperactivity disorder and intellectual disability have similar characteristics to the majority of offenders with lower-level mental health needs and therefore, with effective risk management, could be better treated outside prison. People with neurodevelopmental conditions are likely to have a number of vulnerabilities, including high rates of coexisting mental health problems, and are often subject to similar disadvantages such as lack of employment, access to housing and family support, as others in the criminal justice system. Further, they may also exhibit behaviours likely to increase the complexity of their presentation, which act as destabilisers, for example substance use.

It is also the case that all too often hospital care or community services to support people with neurodevelopmental conditions is difficult to access outside specialist services, with many falling between the gaps in services, or caught by eligibility criteria geared more towards those without serious mental health problems. This can have further adverse effects, with clinicians working in specialist services making it clear that, without proper levels of support and appropriate interventions, the issues faced by individuals with neurodevelopmental conditions may inevitably escalate to crisis level before they come to the attention of health services or the criminal justice system, with the potential for more restrictive interventions and poorer outcomes.

Following my review of people with mental health problems or learning disabilities in the criminal justice system published in 2009 [1], research into the needs of people with neuro-development conditions has advanced significantly. However, the increasing awareness of what should be available to support this group has not always extended widely or deeply enough in all relevant services, with clinical staff often accepting that they are poorly prepared to meet their needs and advocate on their behalf. This lack of awareness at a service delivery level can mean that this group of people are not always considered a priority by commissioners when requests are presented to enhance current services or develop new initiatives. Additionally, while it is widely acknowledged that these groups are over-represented in the criminal justice system, exact numbers are difficult to quantify for a number of reasons, including the problems of identification using the current screening tools.

This lack of attention to, and poor understanding of, people with neurodevelopmental conditions is likely to impact negatively upon their experiences in the criminal justice system. With their support needs continuing to be missed, they may have difficulty understanding legal proceeding and court processes, limiting their ability to fully participate and engage meaningfully. This must be addressed to ensure equity and justice, by introducing a genuine multi-agency approach that does not just rely on guidance and reports but on agreed protocols and a clear delivery model for implementation. The recent evidence review of neurodiversity in the criminal justice system by the Joint Criminal Justice Inspectorate [2] identified several new initiatives which could make a huge difference in this area if provided universally.

Liaison and diversion services have now been rolled out across the country, which should enable early identification of people with neurodevelopmental conditions and the opportunity, where appropriate, to divert people away from the criminal justice system or support their needs within it. However, in a 10-year review of my report, it was still the case that for too many people are sentenced to prison without the identification of their needs and certainly without a comprehensive pre-sentence report on their vulnerabilities being available to the judiciary [3].

This handbook, therefore, is an important additional tool that will help to improve awareness of the complex issues faced by people with neurodevelopmental conditions, bringing together best practice informed by the latest research. The content has been designed as an easy reference book and is suitable for both specialists and non-specialists working with or supporting such an important group of people.

References

1. Department of Health. The Bradley Report: Lord Bradley's review of people with mental health problems or learning disabilities in the criminal justice system. Available at: https://lx.iriss.org.uk/sites/default/files/resources/The%20Bradley%20report.pdf.

2. Expectorate Criminal Justice Joint Inspection. *Neurodiversity in the Criminal Justice System a Review of Evidence*. London, 2021. Crown copyright.

3. Bradley RHL, Marriott C, Hughes S, Sobowale I, Dawson P, Gibbs P. Mental ill-health and fair criminal justice. *The Guardian* 2019, 21 June.

Terminology Used in the Book

The terms used across chapters have varied as a reflection of the diversity of authors working across different countries, using different diagnostic frameworks and depending on the context in which the term is being used or cited. Intellectual disability, learning disability, intellectual developmental disorder and developmental disabilities are all inter-changeable. Autism, autism spectrum disorder and autism spectrum condition are used interchangeably. Autistic is the preferred term used by neurodivergent people. Neurodevelopmental disorders and neurodevelopmental conditions are all also used interchangeably throughout the book.

Introduction

Jane M. McCarthy, Regi T. Alexander and Eddie Chaplin

What Are Neurodevelopmental Disorders?

Neurodevelopmental disorders have their onset in the developmental period and are lifelong. Within the *Diagnostic and Statistical Manual of Mental Disorders*, 5th edition: DSM-5 [1] they include intellectual disability (ID), attention deficit and hyperactivity disorder (ADHD), autism spectrum disorder (ASD), communication disorders, specific learning disorders and tic disorders. Neurodevelopmental disorders present with impairments across personal, social, academic or occupational functioning. The symptoms can include symptoms of excess such as hyperactivity as observed in ADHD or repetitive behaviours as seen in ASD as well as deficits such as cognitive impairment in those with ID or social impairment in those with ASD. All neurodevelopmental disorders share elements of social impairment, cognitive impairment and difficulties in emotional regulation. They are a heterogeneous group of conditions not only clinically but genetically, with a spectrum of presentations. Recent evidence points in the direction of genetic links between specific neurodevelopmental disorders such as ADHD and the wider group of neurodevelopmental disorders [2]. In addition, individuals with neurodevelopmental disorders share risks with other offenders for a number of psychosocial stressors such as social deprivation, early adversity, trauma, educational disengagement, rejection and bullying by peers as well a susceptibility to negative peer pressure when growing up [3].

From a biological perspective there is also a variation in the underlying pathology of neurodevelopmental disorders; for example, boys with ADHD have grey matter volume reduction in the right posterior cerebellum whereas boys with ASD have grey matter volume enlargement in the left middle temporal gyrus and superior temporal gyrus [4]. There are also recognised neurochemical differences between the disorders; for example, glutamate/gamma-aminobutyric acid (GABA) imbalance found in those with ASD [5] and catecholamine/dopamine imbalance in those with ADHD [6]. Cortical GABAergic interneurons are specified during the early formation of the brain within the ganglion eminences in which GABAergic interneurons develop so these cells are defined before they reach the developing cortex [7]. Such advances in neuroscience may one day lead to a better understanding of the origins of neurodevelopmental disorders. Even within one disorder such as ASD there is a significant challenge in delineating a specific dysregulated neurotransmitter system [8]. Other research at a biological level points to a pathway from genes to function involving various proteins and these common pathways include semantic plasticity/function, chromatin remodellers and the mammalian target of the rapamycin pathway. Further understanding of the mechanism behind these pathways will hopefully lead to targeted treatment approaches for individuals with neurodevelopmental disorders [9]. Research focusing on these semantic proteins may decipher the link between semantic signalling and the regulations of gene expression and protein synthesis to aid the identification of any shared pathogenic mechanisms across the neurodevelopmental disorders.

The Direction of Travel for Research on Neurodevelopmental Disorders

The *Lancet* Commission on the future of care and clinical research in autism concluded that research which had an immediate benefit for autistic people should be prioritised and that autistic people had similar needs to those with other neurodevelopmental disorders, so any advances for those with autism would benefit individuals with other neurodevelopmental conditions [10]. The research charity Autistica reported on research investment and research priorities in the UK between 2013 and 2016 [11]. It found there has been a relative lack of research producing evidence on the best ways for adult services to meet autistic people's day to day needs. There was a steady rise in investment for research into treatment and interventions, with a short rise in biology-based research from 2015 to 2016, which is reflected in the more recent published evidence. Investment in screening, diagnosis and service research peaked in 2014, which is most relevant to the current needs of autistic people in contact with the criminal justice system.

A recent special edition published by the *British Journal of Psychiatry* on neurodevelopmental disorders found that publications were mainly longitudinal cohort studies of large sample size, so increasing understanding of outcomes over time [12]. The recommended research priorities by the National Institute for Health and Care Excellence covering various neurodevelopmental disorders emphasises further work that looks at interventions, particularly psychological and pharmaceutical interventions in those with complex presentations [13]. The importance of early recognition of specific disorders, such as ADHD in females, for example, and the use of preventative interventions in girls with ADHD, may be key to improving long-term outcomes, such as high risk for self-harm [14]. The emphasis is on developing the evidence much more in children and young people with neurodevelopmental disorders and this is in keeping with previous work by Murphy et al., in 2018 [15]. This was a longitudinal study of individuals with ASD and ADHD in which significant unmet needs of those transitioning through adolescence and into young adult life was identified. A major contributor to unmet needs was the presence of associated mental health symptoms. Most of the young people were undiagnosed and so untreated by clinical services. The key finding was that the largest determinant of service provision was age and not the severity of symptoms. In essence, if the young person was identified early in life, this was more likely to ensure that they had their needs met. For example, in ADHD, each one-year increase in a young person's age reduces the odds of being seen by services by 38%.

Research focusing on forensic mental health services for neurodevelopmental disorders is limited worldwide, including in high-income countries [16]. A more focused and collaborative research agenda is required for forensic health services research, which must include those with neurodevelopmental disorders. Currently, research into neurodevelopmental disorders for those in contact with the criminal justice system is evolving but remains underdeveloped with a lack of parity in funding and academic capacity compared with general forensic services. Agreement exists amongst clinicians that universal screening should be in place across countries and jurisdictions [17], but due to a lack of research there is no consensus to inform an agreed international approach to screening and how the criminal justice and/or correctional systems respond to vulnerable defendants with neuro-developmental disorders. Saying this, there is a broad agreement by clinicians that defendants with neurodevelopmental disorders do require support through the legal process and during court proceedings. However, there is a divergence of disposable options across jurisdictions for those with neurodevelopmental disorders, which could range from being hospital focused to some form of mandated secure care or prison sentencing. Further evidence is required to understand this variation in practice and, as discussed below in relation to the recent sentencing guidelines for England and Wales, there is a lack of research, for example, on the relationship between sentencing and optimal outcomes for this group of defendants.

Policy and Neurodevelopmental Disorders

An editorial on mental healthcare highlights that the policy aim of the past 30 years of delivering high-quality healthcare across the criminal justice and correctional services in the least restricted environment, that is, an environment that enables a person with as much choice and self-direction as safely appropriate, has not been achieved for those with mental illness [18]. This needs to be acknowledged if we are to address the healthcare needs of those with neurodevelopmental disorders also in contact with the criminal justice system. The recent review of evidence on neurodiversity in the criminal justice system [19] for England and Wales looked at screening, support and training. This review found good evidence of local partnerships, but it was clear that such provision is patchy, uncoordinated and too little is being done to meet the needs of those with neurodivergent conditions. The main recommendation was that a coordinated and cross-government approach is required to improve outcomes for neurodivergent people within the criminal justice system. The review also accepted that there is no universally agreed definition of neurodiversity, but clearly that up to half of those entering prison may have some form of neurodivergent condition that impacts on the person's ability to engage with rehabilitation within a prison setting.

The national strategy covering England titled 'Autistic children, young people and adults: 2021 to 2026, policy paper' [20] has elevated the profile and needs of neurodivergent offenders within the chapter on improving support within the criminal and youth justice systems. The main emphasis of this strategy is to improve the experience of autistic people coming into contact with the criminal and youth justice systems by ensuring staff have a better understanding of autism and the needs of autistic people. Several areas were highlighted in which support can be improved, including ensuring adjustments that assist the autistic person to participate in sentencing and rehabilitation, alongside early identification so that appropriate supports can occur in a timely manner. It is recognised the current poor support results in autistic people having difficulty accessing health and social care services or even general support on leaving custody. As a result, National Health Service (NHS) England are rolling out a new service called RECONNECT to provide care after custody for people leaving prison who have ongoing health vulnerabilities, including autistic people. The service starts working with people before they leave prison to ensure those with recognised vulnerabilities are engaged with community-based health and care services on leaving prison.

Guidance from NHS England for health commissioners, providers and staff working in prison sets out a number of guiding principles for people with ID. These include a rights-based approach, person-centred care, early identification and appropriate support, an informed workforce and working in partnership with all types of health services and other agencies to develop a whole prison approach [21]. This guidance strongly recommends prisons employ a learning disability nurse or practitioner based within the primary or secondary prison health service, ensuring that the prisoner with ID has a care plan and annual health check.

From 1 October 2020, a new guideline for England and Wales on sentencing adults with mental disorders including those with developmental disorders and neurological impairments came into place [22]. The emphasis of the guidance is on community orders with treatment requirements but the research evidence on taking this approach is limited for defendants with mental and neurodevelopmental disorders [23]. The sentencing guideline also covers the subject of assessing culpability and the sentencer must consider whether, at the time of offence, the offender's impairment or disorder impacted on their ability to excise appropriate judgement, make rational choices and understand the nature and consequences of their actions. There must be sufficient connection between the impairment or disorder and the offending behaviour. The sentencer may consider expert evidence, which also includes expert assessment of those with neurodevelopmental disorders. Again, this is an area with little or no evidence on the impact of expert evidence of sentencing outcomes.

Fitness to plead is considered in Chapters 3, 8, 18 and 19 in those with neurodevelopmental conditions. The legal defence of 'insanity' relies on principles created by judges in case law, following the trial of Daniel M'Naghten in 1843 [24], where the law was stated as follows:

> the jurors ought to be told that in all cases that every man is presumed to be sane, and to possess a sufficient degree of reason to be responsible for his crimes, until the contrary is proved to their satisfaction; and that to establish a defence on the ground of insanity, it must be clearly proved that, at the time of the committing of the act, the party accused was labouring under such a defect of reason, from disease of the mind, as not to know the nature and quality of the act he was doing, or, if he did know it, that he did not know he was doing what was wrong.

For an insanity defence to be available, the criteria described above must be met. In a case where an accused person presents with a neurodevelopmental disorder and the possibility of an insanity defence has been raised, experts will be sought to provide evidence to the court [25]. In England and Wales, diminished responsibility is a partial defence to murder, initially set out in the Homicide Act 1957 and later amended by the Coroners and Justice Act 2009 [26]. This defence may be available to defendants with a neurodevelopmental condition but there is little reported in the literature [27]. Culpability is the degree to which a person can be held morally or legally responsible for the conduct and has been linked to the person's mental state at the time of the offence [28, 29]. Hallett [28] argues that psychiatrists should resist explicably commenting on culpability because, even if a mental disorder was considered in the context of culpability, it is an issue that is determined by the court. On the issue of insanity [28], Hallett recommends that psychiatrists are allowed to comment on the effect of a person's thought processes, which may affect their appreciation of wrongfulness, but the ultimate issue should be left to a jury. He [28] challenges McChesney and Doucet [30], who consider conditions such as ASD, ADHD and ID to impact on moral concerns. Hallett argues that to separate a lack of moral concern due to a neurodevelopmental disorder may be difficult to do from the defendant's own character. However, O'Sullivan [27] and Allely [31] argue that autistic defendants may have specific deficits that impact on their capacity to appreciate the potential of harm to others and that a non-guilty by reason of insanity plea can be considered in cases of violent behaviour among autistic individuals.

The evolving approach to policy and guidance for those with neurodevelopmental disorders in contact with the criminal justice system is occurring alongside advances in the understanding of genetic and biological basis of neurodevelopmental disorders. The purpose of the book is to bring together this latest evidence and understanding of neurodevelopmental disorders, describing the needs of offenders across the range of intellectual functioning. These include those with ASD, ADHD and other relevant developmental disorders, requiring assessment and treatment by professionals working across the criminal justice system and within forensic services.

Overview of the Book

The book is divided into three sections. The first section, which includes this chapter, provides an overview with an introduction to individual neurodevelopmental disorders and covers aetiology, prevalence, comorbid mental disorder and relevant policy to date.

The second section of the book focuses on the clinical aspects of the range of neurodevelopmental disorders including screening, assessment, diagnosis, risk assessments and therapeutic approaches.

The final section examines the pathways through the criminal justice system from police to court to disposal including probation services and addresses the specific aspect of fitness to plead or stand trial for those with neurodevelopmental disorders. This section also describes current relevant legislation within the UK as well as forensic services and pathways for those with neurodevelopmental disorders from a national and an international perspective.

Topics Covered in Section 1

This first chapter offers a summary of the book and serves to introduce the remaining chapters in Section 1 and the following sections.

Chapter 2 provides an overview and definition of neurodevelopmental disorders. The chapter provides a summary of the aetiology of neurodevelopmental disorders, particularly those conditions that present within forensic settings. This includes not only genetic factors but also social and environmental risk factors. Neurodevelopmental disorders that are commonly identified within forensic settings include fetal alcohol spectrum disorders (FASD), ADHD and ID.

Chapter 3 provides an overview of clinical practice relating to offenders with ID. It examines the 'offending journey' of people with ID whose behaviour reaches the threshold for criminal justice system involvement. This journey ranges from being accused of a crime, interactions with the police, decisions regarding prosecution and the processes involved in court cases. The chapter also reviews key research in this area, examining characteristics and the risk factors for offending in this population, along with models of treatment and treatment outcomes.

Chapter 4 is a critical overview of offenders with ADHD but acknowledges that undiagnosed or not correctly treated ADHD is associated with a range of adverse outcomes. Evidence from metanalyses confirms an increased prevalence of ADHD in the young and adult offender population, and the relationship between ADHD and criminal offending, particularly in terms of comorbidity and long-term consequences, is discussed. The chapter provides a framework for understanding the association between ADHD and criminal offending, such as the impact of impulsivity, lack of planning involved and the subsequent difficulties for a person with ADHD going through the criminal justice system.

Chapter 5 is an overview of offenders with ASD, which illustrates this diverse group. The chapter discusses the challenge of determining the prevalence of autistic individuals entering the criminal justice system and, in particular, the gaps in our knowledge around the presence of autistic women within the forensic system. The chapter also highlights the influence of the media in how autistic people are portrayed following significant criminal offences.

Chapter 6 describes the different types of offences associated with individuals with ASD and explores the different types of offences, including cybercrimes, violent and sexual offending. The chapter particularly looks at extreme examples of violent crime, such as mass shootings, and aims to increase our understanding of how individuals may exert warning signs in the weeks, months or years leading up to the attack. A detailed examination of different push and pull factors that may lead to autistic people engaging in terrorist behaviours is also discussed in the context of the core symptoms of ASD, such as a circumscribed interest, impaired social imagination or obsessionality.

Chapter 7 is an overview of young people with neurodevelopmental impairments. The authors provide key findings from relevant research, particularly when young people with neurodevelopmental impairments are exposed to social and environmental risks for offending. The chapter highlights a range of studies across international settings revealing a high instance of neurodevelopment impairments amongst young offenders in comparison to young people in the general population. Social environmental factors such as educational disengagement, peer-group influencers and parenting practices are considered as factors to increase the risk for offending behaviours. The authors emphasise the importance of early intervention through education and family support, early identification and a much more responsive criminal justice system to reduce the risk of ongoing offending behaviours.

Chapter 8 provides an overview of offenders with FASD. The first part of the chapter focuses on the process for assessment and diagnosis. The second part of the chapter looks at the prevalence of FASD in offenders, acknowledging that, because of the complexity of the diagnosis, FASD may not be commonly diagnosed, so making it difficult to ascertain good prevalence studies. The third part of the chapter focuses on the relationship between FASD and young offenders within the criminal justice system. The final part of the chapter looks at the ability of young offenders, particularly those with FASD, to defend themselves within the legal system and understand the processes, including the interviewing process. The authors provide recommendations on how to question individuals with neurodevelopmental disorders during legal proceedings, as professionals may overestimate a defendant's abilities and underestimate their needs, which may lead to poorly informed and detrimental decisions such as harsher sentencing.

Chapter 9 introduces the concept of subthreshold neurodevelopmental disorder, describing individuals who do not meet diagnostic criteria thresholds for any neurodevelopmental disorder. Recent research identifies that there is a group with neurodevelopmental difficulties in contact with the correctional system that may require specific support and early identification. This group has been found to have high levels of mental health needs and increased vulnerability for self-harm and suicide-related behaviours when compared to neurotypical offenders. The chapter also summarises currently available screening tools and the need for further studies that require a coordinated approach to understand this group with subthreshold difficulties, including an agreed common definition using a dimensional approach.

Chapter 10, examines comorbidity between mental disorders and neurodevelopmental conditions. Comorbidity between neurodevelopmental disorders is common but also comorbidity with other mental disorders. Although it is acknowledged that neurodevelopmental disorders commonly occur with psychiatric disorders, this seems to be a particular risk for those who are in contact with the criminal justice system. Those with autistic conditions may often present with conduct disorders, depression and psychotic disorders; whereas offenders with ADHD are more likely to present with mood disorders, substance use disorders, anxiety and personality disorders with the overlap between substance use and personality disorders being significant predictors of criminality. The importance of identifying the presence of comorbid psychiatric disorders, particularly substance use disorder, is highlighted.

Topics Covered in Section 2

Chapter 11 is on the assessment and treatment of ADHD in forensic settings. Evidence to date has found a high prevalence of ADHD in prisons and forensic populations but there is still a challenge in identifying this group. The chapter provides examples of potential screening tools used in forensic settings such as the Adult ADHD Self-Report Scale (ASRS) and the Barkley Adult ADHD rating scale. There is also guidance on diagnostic interview tools with an emphasis on using DSM-5 criteria and the need to consider the assessment of comorbid conditions such as severe mental illnesses or personality disorders. The authors provide an overview on treatment approaches including psychoeducation, use of non-pharmacological treatment as well as pharmacological treatment with both stimulants and non-stimulant medications. The treatment of comorbid mental disorders is equally important to achieve good outcomes for those offenders presenting with ADHD and to ensure management continues after release from prison or forensic settings.

Chapter 12 outlines assessment and therapeutic approaches within forensic settings for autistic adults. The authors highlight that many offenders entering forensic settings may have an established diagnosis, but many do not, and it is important to undertake a diagnostic assessment. The chapter covers the role of psychopathy in the context of offenders with ASD and while similarities have been drawn with features of psychopathy in those who offend, the evidence remains limited. The chapter also emphasises the importance of assessing for co-occurring mental illness as well as alcohol and illicit substance misuse. In terms of therapeutic approaches, the chapter covers psychological approaches, including adaptive cognitive behaviour therapy, leading to behavioural changes that increase the individual's ability to function rather than necessarily resulting in cognitive changes. The use of medication for comorbid symptoms such as irritability and aggression among those with ASD and the importance of treating co-occurring conditions such as ADHD or mood disorders is summarised. The importance of staff training and awareness across criminal justice systems, encouraging staff to work to the individual's strengths in an autistic-friendly environment, is highlighted. The issue of women offenders with ASD is recognised as an under-researched group, who may have different therapeutic needs – for example, requiring an approach that is more trauma focused.

Chapter 13 describes the assessment and therapeutic approaches to people with ID within forensic settings. The chapter emphasises that it is difficult to identify offenders with

ID within the criminal justice system and that the prevalence figures vary across the world depending on the type of approach or screening tool used. The importance of understanding that an assessment of a person with ID is not only a measure of cognitive function but must include adaptive functioning and other factors in the person's development, such as access to education or childhood trauma experiences. The chapter gives an overview of available screening tools including the Hayes Ability Screening Index and the Learning Disability Screening Questionnaire, describing the benefits and difficulties with each of the screening tools available. The importance of taking a rehabilitation approach to offenders with ID in developing their life and social skills alongside specific offender-related interventions, such as violence reduction programmes and programmes for sexual offenders, is emphasised. Interventions need to be adapted to the person's level of cognitive impairment and set around the individual's needs as well as their risk factors for offending behaviours. The authors also highlight the need for staff to also be aware of the environment and how they respond to the person in a therapeutic or criminal justice setting

Chapter 14 provides an approach to risk assessments in people with neurodevelopmental disorders. The chapter highlights that structured professional judgement risk-assessment tools are used essentially to develop a risk formulation, which needs to take into account the function of risk behaviours within the context of each neurodevelopmental condition. An overview of the evidence based on specific tools such as the HCR-20 is provided. Good practical advice is given on how to use the tool in the context of a person with ID: it is not the scoring of each item that helps the clinician; the strength of the tools lies in the rigorous gathering of evidence to inform a formulated-based approach to plan future risk management. There is less evidence around risk-assessment approaches in those with ASD and the chapter provides a detailed summary of the FARAS (a framework to aid risk assessment with offenders on the autistic spectrum) manual, which gives guidance to support risk assessment in offenders with ASD. The guidelines are organised through seven sections, each addressing a different facet of ASD including social imagination, obsessionality-type behaviours, social interaction and communication difficulties, cognitive style and sensory processing. In addition, details of a parallel tool for use in those diagnosed with ADHD, namely the Framework for the Assessment of Risk and Protection in Offenders with Attention Deficit Hyperactivity Disorder (FARAH), is described. As with the FARAS, this is not a risk-assessment tool but takes the form of comprehensive clinical guidelines for risk assessors to use alongside mainstream risk assessments such as the HCR-20 V3 as an aid to formulation The chapter provides two case studies using the HCR-20 in the context of a young person with ASD and a person with ID.

Chapter 15 covers the assessment and treatment of young offenders. Young offenders are a vulnerable group and, while in contact with the youth offending system, there is an opportunity to address unmet needs around health including neurodevelopmental impairments, education and the impact of adverse childhood events. The authors highlight the need to use recognised assessment tools such as AssetPlus, which provides an understanding of the strengths and needs of the young person, including their wider social circumstances, their educational needs and other health needs including a neurodisability assessment. AssetPlus is a dynamic tool, so it can be updated to monitor changes over time. It is also designed to work with the Comprehensive Health Assessment Tool and is available for use both in community and in custodial settings. There is a range of different models of healthcare delivery from the lone health practitioner model to an outreach consultative model for young offenders. An example is provided in which clinicians are based between a community youth offending service and a generic child and adolescent mental health service. The importance of supporting young offenders through the transition into adult services is highlighted by a case example. The youth justice system can be a final chance to engage a young person within the system and address any unmet needs such as substance abuse.

Topics Covered in Section 3

Chapter 16 describes the pathways through the criminal justice and correctional systems for individuals with neurodevelopmental disorders. These steps through the pathways may include screening at a police station, assessment by liaison and diversion services or interventions within a correctional setting. The pathway is not linear and there are many routes into and out of the pathway. A number of case studies are given on how, at critical points, the identification of a person with a neurodevelopmental disorder may lead to an intervention such as support to effectively participate in the court process. There remains a limited evidence base on what works, with the possible exception that screening is beneficial in identifying those with neurodevelopmental disorders early on in the pathway.

Chapter 17 describes the Mental Health Act and other relevant legislation in the UK in relation to people with neurodevelopmental disorders. The four countries of the UK are covered with a summary of relevant sections, including those within Part III of the Mental Health Act of England and Wales that relates to those who come before the courts in terms of their offending behaviours. The chapter also touches on the subjects of the Mental Capacity Act, including Deprivation of Liberty Safeguards and the future introduction of liberty protection safeguards. Relevant to the Scottish Mental Health Act, it discusses the recent review of legislation in Scotland and the debate regarding the inclusion of ID and ASD as a mental disorder.

Chapter 18 covers fitness to plead and the right to a fair trial. The authors consider the international approach to fitness to plead and suggest that, at times, it may not safeguard vulnerable defendants. Concepts such as decision-making capacity and effective participation are being recommended in England and Wales as a way to modernise fitness to plead. Comparisons are made on the approaches to the law and fitness to plead in other adversarial jurisdictions, such as the USA, Canada and Australia. The evidence supports the need to incorporate formal cognitive assessments when assessing fitness to stand trial or fitness to plead, to ensure that the specific cognitive functions of the individual are identified.

Chapter 19 also covers fitness to plead, with a specific focus on people with ID in relation to mental health and capacity legislation for England and Wales, including use of sections 35 and 36 of the Mental Health Act.

Chapter 20 offers an overview of community and inpatient hospital services in England with neurodevelopmental disorders. The policy in England has been driven by the uncovering of institutional abuse over the past decade, with the aim to support and treat most people in the community. The tier approach to delivery of services is outlined with Tier 4 including six categories of inpatient services. The development of Tier 3 community-based forensic services for people with neurodevelopmental disorders remains patchy and not universally available across the UK. The chapter outlines standards that services should adhere to when admitting a patient into forensic or secure services.

Chapter 21 is an overview of offenders with neurodevelopmental disorders covering four Nordic countries. The chapter provides an excellent overview of the practice, research and legislation in the Nordic countries of Denmark, Sweden, Norway and Finland. Each country has a slightly different defined threshold for considering a person criminally irresponsible; for example, the function of a person is set at a threshold of intelligence quotient (IQ) less than 70 in Denmark and Finland and at an IQ less than 55 in Norway. The treatment facilities and policy also vary between countries, which are highlighted in this chapter.

Chapter 22 provides an outline of the intersection of legal and forensic pathways for people with neurodevelopmental disorders in Ontario, Canada. In this chapter, there are two case studies that illustrate how legal and health services work for a person with developmental disabilities through the criminal justice system. The interface is with a number of services and programmes not only from health and the criminal justice system but the social care sector, including appropriate support within the community. The chapter emphasises that a person with a neurodevelopmental disorder, even though they might be similar to another offender, can have vastly different experiences and outcomes depending on a number of variables as they go through the criminal justice system, such as the discretion of multiple decision makers, the resources available and extra-legal factors such as support networks. The chapter advocates for therapeutic justice for this group of offenders and that appropriate rehabilitation be available for the individual to be safely moved through into the community.

Chapter 23 describes the Australasian perspective on the forensic needs of individuals with neurodevelopmental disorders. This chapter covers a vast geographical area of Australia, Aotearoa New Zealand, Papua New Guinea and the neighbouring islands of the Pacific. The countries of this region have long histories that pre-dated the British Colonisation in the late eighteenth century but the latter part of the history for Australia and Aotearoa New Zealand has been shaped by this influence on the current legislative and healthcare systems. The chapter provides details of healthcare in Australia and Aotearoa New Zealand, with particular emphasis on the legal frameworks and the development of mental healthcare systems for both countries. Understanding the cultural needs of the Indigenous people of Australia who are the First Nations Australians and the Māori people of Aotearoa New Zealand is very important in the context of the person's experiences of forensic services. The fundamental challenge facing Australia and Aotearoa New Zealand is the lack of capacity in the workforce in both mental health service and forensic services to deliver to this complex group of offenders with neurodevelopmental disorders. The chapter provides details on the legislation for the different states of Australia. One interesting aspect of legislation in relation to the recent debate in England, Wales and Scotland is that, in Aotearoa New Zealand, ID was removed from the Mental Health Act as a mental disorder. Specific legislation for people with ID who came to the courts, namely the Intellectual Disability Compulsory Care & Rehabilitation Act of 2003, was subsequently required.

Finally, Chapter 24 offers the editors an opportunity to reflect on the book and offer concluding comments.

Conclusion

This guide, primarily aimed at working clinicians and researchers is the first comprehensive text to examine offenders with neurodevelopmental disorders, their assessment, treatment, policy, pathways, legislation, clinical and offending characteristics, offering an international perspective. Previously, books have tended to focus on single conditions. By focusing across neurodevelopmental disorders, this work reveals commonly shared issues such as cognitive and social impairment can present differently between conditions and highlights the need for adequate screening and diagnosis.

References

1. American Psychiatric Association. *Diagnostic and Statistical Manual of Mental Disorders, 5th edition: DSM-5*. American Psychiatric Association, 2013.

2. Du Rietz E, Pettersson E, Brikell I, Ghirardi L, Chen Q, Hartman C, et al. Overlap between attention-deficit hyperactivity disorder and neurodevelopmental, externalising and internalising disorders: separating unique from general psychopathology effects. *British Journal of Psychiatry* 2021; 218(1): 35–42.

3. Murray J, Farrington DP. Risk factors for conduct disorder and delinquency: key findings from longitudinal studies. *Canadian Journal of Psychiatry* 2010; 55(10): 633–42.

4. Lim L, Chantiluke K, Cubillo A, Smith A, Simmons A, Mehta M, et al. Disorder-specific grey matter deficits in attention deficit hyperactivity disorder relative to autism spectrum disorder. *Psychological Medicine* 2015; 45(5): 965–76.

5. Horder J, Petrinovic MM, Mendez MA, Bruns A, Takumi T, Spooren W, et al. Glutamate and GABA in autism spectrum disorder: a translational magnetic resonance spectroscopy study in man and rodent models. *Translational Psychiatry* 2018; 8(1) :1–11.

6. Kooij JJS, Bijlenga D, Salerno L, Jaeschke R, Bitter I, Balazs J, et al. Updated European Consensus Statement on diagnosis and treatment of adult ADHD. *European Psychiatry* 2019 ;56: 14–34.

7. Shi Y, Wang M, Mi D, Lu T, Wang B, Dong H, et al. Mouse and human share conserved transcriptional programs for interneuron development. *Science* 2021; 374 (6573): eabj6641.

8. Marotta R, Risoleo MC, Messina G et al., (2020). The Neurochemistry of Autism. *Brain Sciences*, 10, 163.

9. Parenti I, Rabaneda LG, Schoen H, Novarino G. Neurodevelopmental disorders: from genetics to functional pathways. *Trends in Neurosciences* 2020; 43 (8): 608–21.

10. Lord C, Charman T, Havdahl A, Carbone P, Anagnostou E, Boyd B, et al. The *Lancet* Commission on the future of care and clinical research in autism. *Lancet* 2022; 399(10321): 271–334.

11. Autistica. A review of the research funding landscape in the United Kingdom. 2018. Available at: https://issuu.com/fitcreative .ltd.uk/docs/autistica-autism_research_funding_l/1.

12. Langdon PE, Alexander R, O'Hara J. Highlights of this issue. *British Journal of Psychiatry* 2021; 218(1): A3.

13. Alexander RT, Langdon PE, O'Hara J, Howell A, Lane T, Tharian R, et al. Psychiatry and neurodevelopmental disorders: experts by experience, clinical care and research. *British Journal of Psychiatry* 2021; 218(1): 1–3.

14. O'Grady SM, Hinshaw SP. Long-term outcomes of females with attention-deficit hyperactivity disorder: increased risk for self-harm. *British Journal of Psychiatry* 2021; 218(1): 4–6.

15. Murphy D, Glaser K, Hayward H, Eklund H, Cadman T, Findon J, et al. Crossing the divide: a longitudinal study of effective treatments for people with autism and attention deficit hyperactivity disorder across the lifespan. *Programme Grants Appl Res* 2018; 6(2).

16. Ryland H, Davies L, Kenny-Herbert J, Kingham M & Deshpande M. (2021). Advancing research in Forensic Mental Health Services in England. *Medicine, Science & the Law*, 1–5.

17. McCarthy J, Chaplin E, Hayes S, Søndenaa E, Chester V, Morrissey C, et al. Defendants with intellectual disability and autism spectrum conditions: the perspective of clinicians working across three jurisdictions.

Psychiatry, Psychology and Law 2021; 29 (5): 698–717.

18. Brooker C, Coid J. Mental health services are failing the criminal justice system. *BMJ* 2022: 376.

19. Criminal Justice Inspectorates. Neurodiversity in the criminal justice system. Available at: www.justiceinspecto rates.gov.uk.

20. HM Government. National strategy for autistic children, young people and adults: 2021 to 2026, policy paper. Available at: www.gov.uk/government/publications/nat ional-strategy-for-autistic-children-young -people-and-adults-2021-to-2026.

21. NHS England. *Meeting the healthcare needs of adults with a learning disability and autistic adults in prison.* Available at: www .england.nhs.uk/publication/meeting-the- healthcare-needs-of-adults-with-a-learning- disability-and-autistic-adults-in-prison/.

22. Sentencing Council. Sentencing offenders with mental disorders, developmental disorders, or neurological impairments. 2020. Available at: www.se ntencingcouncil.org.uk/overarching- guides/magistrates-court/item/senten cing-offenders-with-mental-disorders- developmental-disorders-or-neurological -impairments/.

23. Taylor PJ, Eastman N, Latham R, Holloway J. Sentencing offenders with mental disorders, developmental disorders or neurological impairments: what does the new Sentencing Council Guideline

24. *R* v. *M'Naghten* [1843] 8 ER 718; [1843] 10 Cl & F 200.

25. Baroff GS, Gunn M, Hayes S. Legal issues. In Lindsay WR, Taylor JL, Sturmey P, eds., *Offenders with Developmental Disabilities.* Wiley, 2004: 37–66.

26. Hallett N. Psychiatric evidence in diminished responsibility. *Journal of Criminal Law* 2018; 82(6): 442–56.

27. O'Sullivan OP. Autism spectrum disorder and criminal responsibility: historical perspectives, clinical challenges and broader considerations within the criminal justice system. *Irish Journal of Psychological Medicine* 2017; 35(4): 333–9.

28. Hallett N. To what extent should expert psychiatric witnesses comment on criminal culpability? *Medicine, Science and the Law* 2020; 60(1): 67–74.

29. Moore MS. Prima facie moral culpability. *Boston University Law Review* 1996; 76: 319.

30. McChesney D, Doucet M. Culpable ignorance and mental disorders. *Journal of Ethics and Social Philosophy* 2018; 14: 227.

31. Allely CS. Autism spectrum disorders in the criminal justice system: police interviewing, the courtroom and the prison environment. In *Recent Advances in Autism.* SM Group Open Access eBooks, 2016: 1–13.

Aetiology of Neurodevelopmental Disorders

Jana de Villiers

Introduction

Neurodevelopmental disorders is an umbrella term that incorporates a range of conditions characterised by some form of disruption to 'typical' brain development. These disorders begin in childhood and result in long-term impairments, in contrast to major mental illnesses that tend to have a remitting and relapsing course. This chapter considers the aetiology of neurodevelopmental disorders as relevant to forensic settings.

The World Health Organization's International Classification of Diseases 11th Revision (ICD-11) defines neurodevelopmental disorders as those that involve significant difficulties in the acquisition and execution of specific intellectual, motor, language or social functions with onset during the developmental period. The developmental period encompasses the period between birth and adulthood, with adulthood assumed to have been reached at age 18. Neurodevelopmental disorders causing significant levels of impairment are generally identified well before the end of adolescence, subsequently persisting into adulthood. Some development continues beyond the age of 18, with limited data on the long-term stability of diagnostic criteria for neurodevelopmental disorders that have less severe associated functional impairments. There is no significant divergence in classification of neurodevelopmental disorders between ICD-11 and the American Psychiatric Association's *Diagnostic and Statistical Manual of Mental Disorders*, 5th edition (DSM-5) [1].

Conditions included under this overarching category include intellectual disability (ID), autism spectrum disorder (ASD), attention deficit hyperactivity disorder (ADHD), tic disorders and specific learning disorders. Within the UK, learning disability (LD) is used synonymously with ID. Fetal alcohol spectrum disorders (FASD) are an additional type of neurodevelopmental disorder common in criminal justice settings, being one of the most common causes of preventable brain injury in children.

Neurodevelopmental disorders have a range of possible aetiologies. These include genetic variation (e.g., copy number variants (CNVs), single-gene disorders such as fragile X and chromosomal disorders such as trisomy 21) (see Figure 2.1), nutritional factors (e.g., iodine deficiency), infectious causes (e.g., intrauterine rubella or, more recently, Zika virus), metabolic disorders (e.g., hypothyroidism or phenylketonuria) and neurotoxic conditions (e.g., FASD). The interplay of these factors with additional social and environmental factors (including social attitudes towards disability, poverty, neglect and abuse in childhood) is particularly relevant when considering those with neurodevelopmental disorders who come into contact with criminal justice services.

Although described as distinct categories within the current classification systems (ICD-11 and DSM-5), in practice neurodevelopmental disorders frequently overlap in terms of

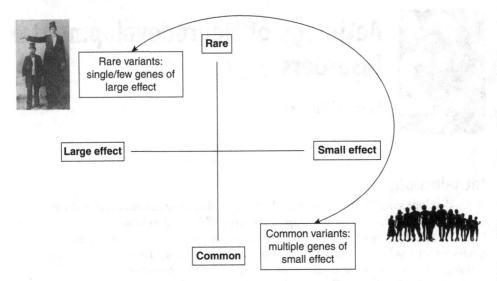

Figure 2.1 Genetic variation of neurodevelopmental disorders – from rare to common variants.

their core symptom domains and often co-occur [2]. Most neurodevelopmental disorders are diagnosed on the basis of observed behaviour as assessed by self-report, observer scales and/or clinician observation. This clustering of observed behaviours into diagnostic categories does not consider aetiology, an approach that is likely to require modification in future as underlying genetic and environmental factors are increasingly recognised.

Genetic Variation

Advances in genetic testing (particularly the development of genome-wide association technologies and large international collaborations) have led to significant progress in identifying genetic risk variants for major psychiatric conditions, including neurodevelopmental disorders. Karyotyping techniques have been in clinical use since the 1970s, and technology has advanced significantly with the development of high-resolution genome-wide chromosomal microarray analysis (CMA). CMA encompasses array comparative genomic hybridisation (CGH) and single-nucleotide polymorphism (SNP) arrays. Array CGH is able to identify clinically relevant CNVs in 15–20% of patients with unexplained intellectual disability [3]. More recently, whole exome sequencing has become available and affordable (see Figure 2.2), with the ability to identify further pathogenic genetic mutations.

CNVs are structural changes in chromosomes that result in deletions, duplications, inversions or translocations of large DNA segments (more than 1,000 DNA base pairs). Small benign CNVs are found in the genomes of healthy individuals but numerous pathogenic CNVs have now been identified as causing genomic disorders. Examples of genomic disorders include Prader–Willi and Angelman syndromes (deletions at 15q11–q13). CNVs are classed as pathogenic when there is a disruption of genes known to be important for neurodevelopmental functions such as neurotransmission.

CMA is recommended as the first-tier cytogenetic test for developmental delay/intellectual disability. Health economic studies provide evidence of the cost-effectiveness of CMA

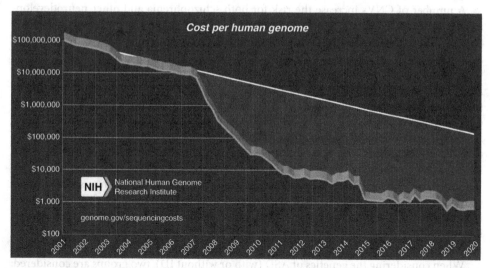

Figure 2.2 Cost per human genome. Courtesy: National Human Genome Research Institute (www.genome.gov).

as first tier in comparison to other testing strategies. However, CMA has significant limitations, including the inability to detect balanced translocations, single-gene disorders (such as fragile X) or low-level mosaicism.

Based on current levels of diagnostic yield following CMA, genetic testing is recommended for anyone presenting with ID or ASD. Standard baseline tests include array CGH, SNP arrays and additional testing for specific single-gene disorders (such as fragile X) associated with ID or ASD. Any additional testing needs to be considered on an individual basis depending on clinical features, in consultation with clinical geneticists. Exome sequencing is becoming increasingly available for clinical assessment, and may further improve diagnostic yield.

Identifying pathogenic CNVs or specific genetic syndromes in individuals with neurodevelopmental disorders, in particular ID and ASD, is important for a range of reasons. These include: ensuring that monitoring for known comorbidities is part of the ongoing management, providing information to the patient and family regarding prognosis and familial risk and raising awareness of increased rates of comorbid mental illness such as schizophrenia. For example, duplication at 16p11.2 increases the risk of ID and ASD, and is associated with a 14-fold increase in the risk of psychosis.

In people identified as having 22q11 deletion syndrome (formerly called DiGeorge syndrome or velocardiofacial syndrome), 30% will develop schizophrenia and 75% have cardiac abnormalities. A wide range of psychiatric and physical health issues is associated with 22q11 deletion syndrome, many of which have implications for assessment and treatment. Fifty per cent of people will have cognition within the 'normal' range, although planning and abstract reasoning are frequently impaired. Facial features are a poor guide to diagnosis, and the range of symptoms and signs varies considerably.

To date, clinical and research data on CNV syndromes have been largely focused on paediatric populations. However, key phenotypic features may only become apparent in adulthood as psychiatric disorders emerge.

A number of CNVs increase the risk for both schizophrenia and other neurodevelopmental disorders. Other CNV loci specifically increase the risk of ID, congenital malformation or ASD (but not schizophrenia). Cumulatively, pathogenic CNVs are found in approximately 7% of individuals with ID, congenital malformations or ASD, as compared to 2.5% in people with schizophrenia. Rates in control populations are much lower. Penetrance rates (the percentage of carriers that will develop the disorder) can differ significantly, depending on the CNV (10.4% for 15q11.2 deletions, 46.8% for 16p11.2 duplications and 100% for 22q11.2 deletion). Generally, penetrance rates are much higher for early neurodevelopmental disorders than for schizophrenia. Higher rates of CNVs are detected in individuals with both schizophrenia and ID, as compared to individuals with schizophrenia only [4].

For individuals with ID, increased rates of major mental illnesses such as schizophrenia or bipolar disorder, as well as a broad range of physical health comorbidities, have been identified. In contrast to the general population, multimorbidity did not increase with measures of neighbourhood deprivation, with findings similar in the most affluent and most deprived areas [5].

When considering the genetics of ASD (with or without ID), two groups are considered: 'simple' autism, and complex/syndromic autism. CMA provides an aetiology for 10% of people with ASD, with higher yields in the complex/syndromic group. The American College of Medical Genetics and Genomics published guidelines in 2013 for the clinical genetic evaluation of individuals with ASD [6].

The genetics of ADHD and tic disorders follow a similar pattern to that observed for ID and ASD: evidence for heritability largely attributable to CNVs, with rare genetic syndromes observed in some cases. This genetic liability is not specific to ADHD or tic disorders, conferring increased risk for a range of other disorders. Equally, ADHD is a common comorbidity in a number of rare genetic disorders [7]; see Figure 2.3.

Interestingly, a large Swedish cohort study from 2015 confirmed common genetic origins for common psychiatric disorders – but also for violent criminal convictions. This replicated findings from past twin, family and genomic studies. Impaired executive function, a feature of neurodevelopmental disorders, may be relevant to this finding and for the

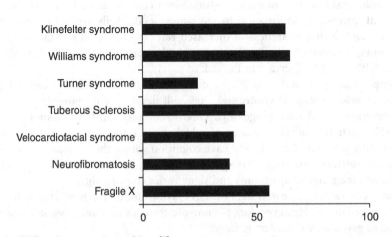

Figure 2.3 ADHD and rare genetic conditions [7].

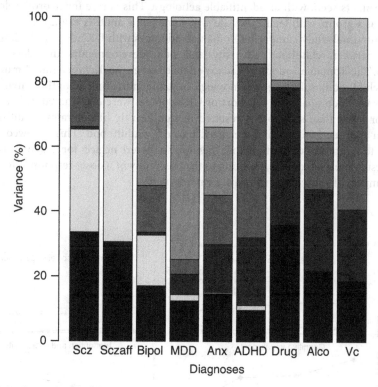

Figure 2.4 Psychiatric disorders share same genetic origin [8]. Variance attributable to genetic and non-shared environmental sources for each diagnosis. ADHD, attention deficit hyperactivity disorder; Alco, alcohol abuse; Anx, anxiety; Bipol, bipolar; Drug, drug abuse; MDD, major depressive disorder; Scz, schizophrenia; Sczaff, schizoaffective disorder; Vc, conviction of violent crimes

higher prevalence of neurodevelopmental disorders within criminal justice settings [8]; see Figure 2.4.

Neurodevelopmental disorders are common, with a significant proportion being caused by rare copy number and sequence variants. Genetic testing is an important component of clinical assessment of neurodevelopmental disorders, to ensure a full understanding of aetiological factors and potential comorbidities over the lifespan.

Social Factors

In addition to the genetic factors outlined above, adverse experiences during the developmental period have been demonstrated to have long-term impacts on a range of outcomes for those affected. Neglect and abuse in childhood can result in features that resemble those of other neurodevelopmental disorders (e.g., attachment disorder vs ASD) and can contribute to the development of later-onset mental disorders such as personality disorders. It can be challenging to differentiate between the effects of abuse and neglect and the effects of intrauterine exposure to alcohol, for example. A recent study indicates that the biological effects of prenatal alcohol exposure are distinct, and that the impairments seen cannot be attributed solely to adverse experiences in early life [9]. The neurobiology of FASD causes the impairments seen, with an identifiable aetiology. This is rare for neurodevelopmental disorders as a group, with fetal valproate syndrome being another example.

A longitudinal study comparing Romanian adoptees with UK adoptees highlighted the interplay between childhood adversity and neurodevelopmental disorders [10]; see Figure 2.5. The Romanian adoptees had experienced severe neglect for a time-limited period in early childhood, subsequently moving to stable nurturing adoptive environments. Outcomes when compared to a cohort of UK adoptees were determined. Of note, severe neglect for more than six months resulted in significantly higher rates of autism in the Romanian adoptee group, which persisted into early adulthood. This followed a similar trajectory to symptoms of inattention/hyperactivity. Severe neglect for less than six months did not result in elevated rates, pointing to the possibility of a dose–response effect and the positive impact of subsequent nurturing environments.

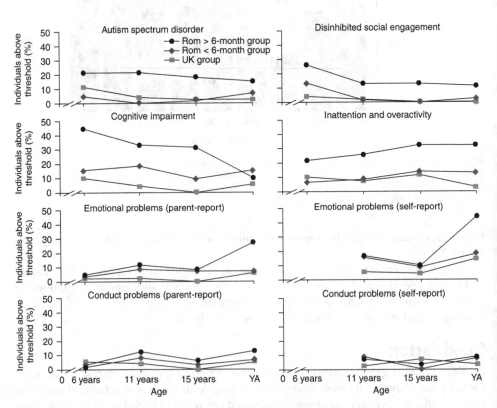

Figure 2.5 Developmental trajectories for neurodevelopmental disorders [10].

The effect on cognitive development was even more marked. At the time of adoption, just under half of the group who had experienced more than six months of severe neglect were considered to have cognitive impairment within the intellectual disability range. Once the children were placed in stimulating and nurturing environments, a gradual improvement in cognitive functioning was noted, such that by young adulthood the rate of cognitive impairment was the same as that within the control group. This highlights the complexity of assigning a diagnosis of a neurodevelopmental disorder to a child who has experienced extreme adversity. The presentation may change substantially if the child receives adequate care, with 'cognitive recovery' in a significant proportion being achievable. This is in contrast to children with neurodevelopmental disorders independent of early life experiences, with impairments being stable and persistent in a small proportion in all cohorts of this longitudinal study. It is also worth noting that a higher rate of 'emotional problems' emerge in mid-adolescence for the group who had lengthier experiences of extreme neglect in early life, a late manifestation of an adverse outcome.

Cognitive and skill development continues over the lifespan, although most rapidly during the developmental phase. In individual cases, this can present a challenge if detention under mental health legislation within secure forensic ID services is based on the criteria of 'learning disability' alone. Legal criteria require categorical diagnoses, with clinical practice sometimes being more complex, as illustrated by Case Study 2.1.

Neurodevelopmental disorders such as ID, ASD and ADHD are on a spectrum across the population, with no clear boundary on any measure when compared to the general population. Cut-off scores reflect standard deviation rather than categorical differences. Diagnostic criteria help to guide clinical decision making, with significant impairment in functioning due to the presenting features generally required to make a clinical diagnosis. Psychometric assessment tools attempt to identify factors that distinguish various groups. As noted above, there is considerable overlap between these factors among neurodevelopmental disorders. Cognitive assessment tools have additional limitations.

Case Study 2.1

An 18-year-old young man with mild learning disability is referred for admission to a low secure forensic ID service. He is in a secure childcare setting, with a lengthy history of physical violence and charges for two attempted rapes. His childhood experiences included well-documented severe physical abuse and neglect, prior to him being taken into care at age 9. Cognitive assessment at age 14 found him to function within the mild learning disability range. He is detained under mental health legislation (category of 'learning disability' as a mental disorder) for assessment. Following admission, he receives individual psychology sessions and a range of skill development interventions. However, episodes of aggression continue, with escalating levels of violence towards staff ultimately resulting in referral to medium secure services after a four-year period. On being assessed by medium secure services, the assessing team note his sophisticated use of language and independence in daily living skills. A re-assessment of his cognitive and adaptive functioning is requested. The cognitive assessment demonstrates that he now functions in the 'low average' range, and assessment of his adaptive functioning skills do not show any significant impairment. He therefore no longer meets the criteria for a diagnosis of ID, having improved his cognitive functioning and daily living skills over time. This means that he can no longer be detained under mental health legislation. His risk towards others (physical and sexual violence) remains unchanged.

In the UK, the fourth edition of the Wechsler Adult Intelligence Scale (WAIS-IV) (standardised for the UK population) is most widely used when assessing cognitive functioning. Clinicians need to be aware that this tool largely does not assess frontal-lobe functioning, and therefore significant impairment in executive functioning may not be identified. This is particularly relevant for disorders where general cognition may not fall within the intellectual disability range (defined as two standard deviations below the mean for the population), such as FASD or approximately half of people with 22q11 deletion syndrome. The functional impairment associated with impaired executive functioning may not be identified if cognitive assessment is limited to assessment using WAIS-IV.

The social context within which cognitive assessments are undertaken affect the outcome. Structured assessment tools need to be standardised for the population in which they are used. There is also robust evidence that changes at a population level impact on the scores obtained. The Flynn effect [11], the well-documented rise in IQ scores over time observed globally, appears to be largely due to modern environments improving attainment on IQ tests at a population level. IQ scores are an imperfect measure of 'intelligence'. Unless re-normed regularly in a given population, the prevalence of diagnoses that rely on IQ scores (such as ID) fluctuates based on population-wide trends and their interactions with assessment tools.

The implications for clinical practice include awareness of the limitations of structured assessment tools, and the need to comprehensively assess individuals across multiple domains. A comprehensive neurodevelopmental assessment generally includes a detailed developmental history, multidisciplinary assessment (to consider biological, psychological and social factors) and an assessment of adaptive functioning. A full assessment ensures a detailed understanding of underlying impairments and the context within which they impact on the individual. Interventions and supports can then be provided on an individualised basis.

Environmental Factors

In addition to the genetic and social factors outlined above, environmental risk factors for neurodevelopmental disorders have been identified. Exposure to infective or toxic agents in the prenatal period and early childhood can significantly affect development, particularly if these occur at sensitive time windows during the development of the nervous system. The developing fetus is especially vulnerable due to many substances easily crossing the placenta and the fetal blood–brain barrier. Many substances are lipophilic and accumulate in maternal adipose tissue and/or breast milk. Young children have higher energy demands, with evidence of higher ingestion of certain substances, which may be compounded by behaviours such as crawling or playing on the ground.

Some environmental factors are associated with distinct presentations, such as FASD. Other substances increase the risk more broadly, leading to impairments of cognition and behaviour. FASD describe a range of physical, cognitive, neurological and behavioural impairments that result from prenatal exposure to alcohol. Extensive animal and human research have demonstrated that alcohol is a powerful teratogenic substance in humans. FASD are now recognised to be one of the most common causes of preventable brain injury in children. It appears to be over-represented in the criminal justice system, although evidence for a singular profile within these settings is lacking. Individuals within criminal justice settings, particularly those with disabilities, commonly have additional psychopathology, early life adversity and histories of violence. Complex presentations are the norm, highlighting the need for individualised approaches to assessment and treatment [12].

Exposure (either prenatally or in early childhood) to a range of other substances has been associated with autism and ADHD; see Figure 2.6. These include polychlorinated biphenyls (PCBs), methylmercury (MeHg) and lead. These substances are directly toxic to the developing nervous system, including in the postnatal period.

Maternal use of medication has been associated with specific syndromes in subsequent offspring. Thalidomide is a well-known example, resulting in characteristic limb abnormalities. Fetal valproate syndrome encompasses craniofacial anomalies, neural tube defects and limb abnormalities. Strict prescribing guidelines for women of childbearing age are in place in the UK to reduce the risk of prenatal exposure to valproate.

Prior to widespread immunisation, congenital rubella was recognised as causing an increase in the prevalence of intellectual impairment and autism in affected children. Longer-term follow-up indicated that a significant proportion of individuals subsequently developed non-affective psychosis in early adulthood. A similar increase in prevalence of schizophrenia in offspring was noted following influenza in the first or second trimester. A 2010 Danish study noted an increase in diagnosis of autism in children of mothers who had either a viral or bacterial infection during the first two

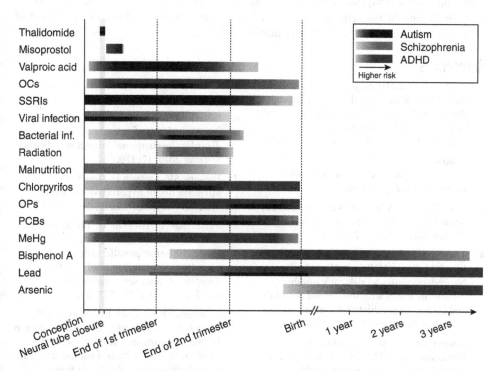

Figure 2.6 Sensitive time windows for exposure to environmental toxicants and susceptibility to neurodevelopmental disorders. Increases in opacity are used to indicate the period of the highest risk, with different shadings representing different neurodevelopmental disorders. These sensitive time windows are estimated based on findings from both epidemiological and experimental research. OCs, oral corticosteroids; OPs, organic pollutants; SSRIs, selective serotonin reuptake inhibitors. (Reproduced with permission from Elsevier [13].)

trimesters of pregnancy. It is postulated that activation of cytokines as part of the immune response affects neurodevelopment, resulting in an increased risk of a range of neurodevelopmental disorders in children born of mothers who experienced infection during pregnancy. At present it is unknown whether any effect will be seen from the coronavirus (COVID-19) pandemic.

These environmental factors appear to cause the effects on neurodevelopment via common pathways: oxidative stress, immune system dysregulation, hormone disruption and effects on neurotransmitters. The impacts are greatest during key periods of neurodevelopment, and in particular in the period between conception and birth [13].

Conclusion

Neurodevelopmental disorders are common in the criminal justice system. This may at least be partly accounted for by common features of neurodevelopmental disorders such as impaired executive functioning skills and poor impulse control. The aetiology of these disorders includes genetic, social and environmental factors. These factors interact to lead to unique clinical profiles and a range of functional abilities. Neurodevelopmental disorders can impact on the ability to effectively participate in legal proceedings, can impair the ability to cope in custodial settings and can limit the effectiveness of treatment programmes if impairments have not been recognised. These disorders share common aetiological pathways and have overlapping clinical presentations. Comprehensive individualised assessment, including of underlying aetiological factors, contributes to clinical formulation of offending behaviour and to effective treatment approaches.

References

1. Reed GM, First MB, Kogan CS, Hyman SE, Gureje O, Gaebel W, et al. Innovations and changes in the ICD-11 classification of mental, behavioural and neurodevelopmental disorders. *World Psychiatry* 2019; 18(1): 3–19.

2. Thapar A, Cooper M, Ruttern M. Neurodevelopmental disorders. *Lancet Psychiatry* 2017; 4: 339–46.

3. Kirov G, Rees E, Walters J. What a psychiatrist needs to know about copy number variants. *BJPsych Advances* 2015; 21: 157–63.

4. Thygesen JH, Wolfe K, McQuillin A, Viñas-Jornet M, Baena N, Brison N, et al. Neurodevelopmental risk copy number variants in adults with intellectual disability and comorbid psychiatric disorders. *British Journal of Psychiatry* 2018; 212: 287–94.

5. Cooper SA, McLean G, Guthrie B, McConnachie A, Mercer S, Sullivan F, et al. Multiple physical and mental health comorbidity in adults with intellectual disabilities: population-based cross-sectional analysis. *BMC Family Practice* 2015; 16: 110.

6. Schaefer GB, Mendelsohn NJ. Clinical genetics aspects of autism spectrum disorder. *International Journal of Molecular Sciences* 2016; 17: 180.

7. Faraone SV, Larsson H. Genetics of attention deficit hyperactivity disorder. *Molecular Psychiatry* 2019; 24: 562–75.

8. Pettersson E, Larsson H, Lichtenstein P. Common psychiatric disorders share the same genetic origin: a multivariate sibling study of the Swedish population. *Molelcular Psychiatry* 2016; 21: 717–21.

9. Mukherjee RAS, Cook PA, Norgate SH, Price AD. Neurodevelopmental outcomes in individuals with fetal alcohol spectrum disorder (FASD) with and without exposure to neglect: clinical cohort data from a national FASD diagnostic clinic. *Alcohol* 2019; 76: 23–28.

10. Sonuga-Barke EJS, Kennedy M, Kumsta R, Knights N, Golm D, Rutter M, et al. Child-to-adult neurodevelopmental and mental health trajectories after early life deprivation: the young adult follow-up of the longitudinal English and Romanian adoptees study. *Lancet* 2017; 389: 1539–48.

11. Trahan LH, Stuebing KK, Hiscock MK, Fletcher JM. The Flynn effect: a meta-analysis. *Psychol Bull* 2014; 140: 1332–60.

12. Flannigan K, Pei J, Stewart M, Johnson A. Fetal alcohol spectrum disorder and the criminal justice system: a systematic literature review. *International Journal of Law and Psychiatry* 2017; 57: 42–52.

13. Heyer DB, Meredith RM. Environmental toxicology: sensitive periods of development and neurodevelopmental disorders. *Neurotoxicology* 2017; 58: 23–41.

Overview of Offenders with Intellectual Disability

Verity Chester, Priyanka Tharian, Matthew Slinger, Anto Varughese and Regi T. Alexander

The Offending Journey

Challenging and Offending Behaviour

How an individual with intellectual disability (ID) is categorised as an offender is less straightforward than in the general population. This is because the dividing line between 'challenging behaviour' and 'offending behaviour' is often blurred in this group [1]. Challenging behaviour is defined as behaviour 'of such an intensity, frequency or duration as to threaten the quality of life and/or the physical safety of the individual or others and is likely to lead to responses that are restrictive, aversive or result in exclusion' [2]. Not all challenging behaviour gets characterised as offending, and that distinction can therefore depend on a combination of offence factors, patient factors and system factors. Offence factors include the seriousness of the act, visibility of the act, pattern of repetition or escalation, etc. Patient factors include the degree of ID, visibility of the disability, presence of mental illness and personality disorder comorbidity, etc. System factors include the availability of supportive specialist services, court diversion schemes, advocacy from family members, nature of coverage in the media, the values or attitudes of key professionals, etc. Thus, the decision of whether a person with ID and a particular kind of challenging behaviour is characterised as being an offender or not can sometimes appear to be rather arbitrary. Further, under the law in England and Wales, a crime is defined by two components: actus reus (the act of crime) and mens rea (the intent to commit that crime). Intent can be difficult to elicit in people with ID, due to communication difficulties. This can make ascertaining legal responsibility particularly problematic [3].

Risk Factors for Offending and Population Characteristics

Patients treated within forensic ID services are predominantly male [4], and are typically from significantly disadvantaged psychosocial backgrounds [5]. Histories of emotional, physical and sexual abuse are common. While patients are approximately 30 years of age on admission, it has been highlighted that violent or antisocial behaviour is first observed in childhood or adolescence for the majority of inpatients [6].

The level of ID is usually in the borderline to mild range, with an occasional patient with difficulties classified as moderate. Patients are diagnostically complex, with multiple diagnoses (including major mental illness, personality disorders, autism spectrum disorder (ASD), attention deficit hyperactivity disorder and substance use disorders) [5, 7]. Mental health presentations can be atypical in those with ID, with primary and secondary diagnoses overshadowing other clinically relevant symptoms, such as difficulties differentiating or diagnosing both autism and psychosis in this population [8]. Rates of self-injury are very high, with approximately 80% of inpatients having a history [5].

Winter et al. [9] examined factors predisposing to suspected offending by adults with ID. These authors reported the relevance of factors such as losing contact with their father, forensic contact of family members, past homelessness, illicit drug/alcohol use/dependence, experiencing an excess of recent life events, behavioural problems at school, truancy, childhood police contact and contact with probation services. A recent study has also highlighted the potential role of traumatic brain injury as a risk factor for offending in those with ID, with rates at a similar level as the general prison population [10]. Indeed, risk-assessment tools that have not been specifically developed for those with ID, which are based on an extensive evidence base investigating risk factors in the general offending population, have been demonstrated to be of equal or superior validity regard to predicting future offending [11, 12].

Prevalence

Just as in the general population, where the criminal offences recorded in official statistics provide only limited information about the incidence and prevalence of illegal behaviours, offending behaviour can be under-reported in those with ID [13]. Family and paid carers of people with ID can be less likely to involve the police when an offence is committed [14]. The availability of specialist community ID forensic teams who can respond to incidents can also affect whether behaviour reaches the attention of police [15]. The ID teams provide interventions and manage risk in the community setting, avoiding the need for further processing by the criminal justice system. Behaviour is often managed within community/ inpatient mental health or ID services until it reaches a threshold that is unmanageable within such settings. The individual is then referred to forensic services known as an 'upwards referral'. When a person has moderate to severe ID, unless the crime is very serious, they are unlikely to be dealt with through the criminal justice system. In those with mild ID, however, there are still challenges often requiring specialist evaluation to determine their understanding of the offence [16].

Police Involvement

Studies have suggested that between 5% and 9% of suspects seen at police stations have ID [17]. In the UK, several cases involving miscarriages of justice have shown that suspects with ID are disadvantaged when interviewed by the police, because they may 'without knowing or wishing to do so, be particularly prone in certain circumstances to provide information which is unreliable, misleading or self-incriminating' [18]. Therefore, safeguards must be put in place and the Code of Practice sets out a specific process at police stations: being cautioned first, then informed verbally by the custody officer of the rights to obtain legal advice and to have someone informed of the arrest, followed by a written leaflet (the 'Notice to Detained Persons') reiterating and expanding upon the information already given verbally. Finally, the right to have a copy of the custody record is also explained [19].

People with ID are more prone to suggestibility, confabulation, compliance and false confessions [20–23]. Therefore, they have a right to have an appropriate adult at the police interview, in addition to their legal representative. This safeguard is to support them in communication during questioning, observe whether the police are acting with respect for the detainee's rights and to ensure the detainee understands these. However, there are several potential problems in this process. Screening for ID is not well established in police stations [24]. Even when screening systems are in place, some people with ID remain unidentified [25]. The appropriate adult may not be trained to facilitate communication between the police and a person with ID [21]. There are also circumstances where there is significant police dissatisfaction with the support given by an appropriate adult during the interview [26]. Liaison and diversion schemes at the police station can ensure appropriate assessment and links with services at the court, but their availability varies geographically [27].

Courts

If an offender with a suspected ID is arrested by the police and charged with an offence, they will be taken to a magistrates' court [28]. Where an alleged offence is non-indictable or triable either way (i.e., in a magistrates' court or Crown Court) the alleged offence may progress no further. A magistrates' trial is commenced by a summons sent to the defendant, whereas a Crown Court trial is preceded by a charge. At the commencement of a Crown Court trial, the defendant hears the charge, and is asked to plead either guilty or not guilty. It is possible for the defendant's barrister to claim that their client is unfit to plead at this stage [29].

At trial, ID may be relevant when assessing whether the defendant has mens rea for the offence, regarding fitness to plead [29, 30] or the defence of insanity [29] and for the provision of courtroom support. Ascertaining mens rea in a case involving a person with ID can be a core part of serious cases involving murder, rape and violence against the person. It involves the defendant intending the consequence of their act or recognising the risk and taking it [29].

Fitness to plead is an important consideration in defendants with ID. The main criteria used in determining fitness to plead are capacity to plead with understanding, ability to follow the proceedings, being able to challenge a juror, ability to question the evidence and ability to instruct counsel. The defendant's fitness to plead is decided by the judge, usually on the basis of reports from psychiatry or medical practitioners and does not require a jury [17]. If fitness to plead is present, the judge can provide further support for the defendant but, if absent, the case may proceed on a 'trial of facts'.

For there to be a defence of insanity, the disease of the mind must cause the defendant to have a 'defect of reason'. If it is determined that the defendant is guilty by reason of insanity, the judge can use a range of sentencing options including hospital, guardianship, supervision and treatment, or absolute discharge orders [31]. If the defendant has ID, experts will be sought to provide evidence to the court in each individual case. 'Diminished responsibility' is a defence that can only be used when charged with murder; if successful, the conviction is reduced from murder to manslaughter [32]. ID can also be stated as the basis of diminished responsibility [31]. However, the burden of proof in both these cases is on the defendant and must be proven on the balance of probabilities and not beyond reasonable doubt. It is important to note that psychiatric defence differs between countries and examples of these differences can be seen in McCarthy et al. [33].

Sentencing

The first sentencing decision takes place when a defendant appears in court for the first time, and concerns whether to offer bail or to remand in custody [17]. Sentencing also marks the final stage of the criminal justice process. The Criminal Justice Act 2003 [34] sets out the objectives of sentencing: punishment of offenders; reduction of crime (including reduction by deterrence); reform and rehabilitation of offenders; protection of the public; and making of reparation by offenders to persons affected by their offences. The court requests access to information on a defendant's needs at the pre-sentence stage, to inform the sentencing decision through a pre-sentence report prepared by a probation officer. This should include information pertaining to any mental health conditions, which would enable the court to decide on an appropriate disposal or outcome for the defendant [27]. With patients who have ASD, with or without ID, it has been suggested that the courts may misinterpret certain behaviours as lack of empathy and thus sentence them more harshly [35].

Courtroom support arrangements for those with ID, and other developmental disorders such as ASD, support the principle of justice by ensuring the defendant has the right to a fair trial, by avoiding miscarriages of justice and limiting the need for an appeal. The arrangement of support within the court is dependent on accurately identifying defendants with ID. The Nacro report [36] noted that most court diversion schemes were focused on offenders with mental illness and that there were only three schemes in England and Wales that had either ID practitioners or links with ID services. The Bradley report [27] recognised the problems resulting from these limited schemes and the non-recognition of ID at the court stage. The report recommends that the probation service and the judiciary should receive mental health and ID awareness training [16].

A registered intermediary is sometimes employed to support defendants with ID [21]. They are impartial, not working for the prosecution or the defence. The registered intermediary's role was introduced to facilitate communication between the police, the courts and vulnerable witnesses, for example those with ID. They can assist the police in communicating with witnesses at the investigation stage, take part in pre-trial meetings and court familiarisation visits and assist in communication with the witness at trial. Access to such an intermediary, however, is not currently a legal right across England and Wales.

Models of Treatment

The Legal Structure

Few of the programmes designed to address recidivism within prison or probation services are modified to make them accessible for people with ID [17]. This means that people with ID who receive custodial or non-custodial sentences often have a lack of equity, not just in access to remedial programmes but also in long-term prognosis and outcomes. This is precisely why this group requires diversion to access treatment and achieve rehabilitation through health services, whether based in hospitals or in the community.

Under the Mental Health Act in England and Wales, 'learning disability' (or ID) is named as a mental disorder if it is associated with abnormally aggressive behaviour or seriously irresponsible conduct. Although there is currently a proposal to remove ID from the remit of the Mental Health Act, Part III of the Act (i.e., the part that refers to the courts and criminal disposals) is not earmarked for change [37]. This means that the option for someone with ID to be diverted away from prisons to hospitals or the community for treatment and rehabilitation will remain the predominant model.

The following factors determine whether a community disposal is appropriate: nature of the current offence, history of previous offending, the presence of mental illness, personality disorders, comorbid substance misuse, capacity to consent, the need for public protection, issues of vulnerability in prison settings, availability of adapted treatment programmes, etc. In England and Wales, a person with ID can be treated in the community via a guardianship order or a supervision and treatment order. This route has been shown to manage risk and avert the need for expensive secure hospital admission. The full range of sentencing or diversion options available within the criminal justice system has been described earlier [16] and is examined in some detail in chapter 17 of this book.

Forensic Hospitals

Forensic psychiatry services have grown and become more complex in structures, processes and pathways [38]. In the UK, there are forensic hospital beds at three levels of security – high, medium and low. Treatment options in hospital under the Mental Health Act can involve hospital orders to either specialist forensic ID hospitals or, occasionally, mainstream forensic psychiatry facilities. When electing to transfer or remand an individual to hospital, the individual's antecedents, presentation and (alleged) offence governs the level of security in the hospital they are sent to, for example, a general psychiatric hospital vs a forensic hospital. In the UK, forensic hospitals are commissioned differently and attract higher funding than their general psychiatric counterparts, typically resulting in a better provision and availability of specialist psychologists, social workers and occupational therapists together with a medical and nursing team with higher staff-patient ratios. In theory, this allows time and expertise for a thorough assessment for people with ID and other developmental disorders. Treatment outcomes from these services are described later in this chapter.

Forensic Community ID Teams

While hospital-based services have been well developed in the UK, community forensic ID teams are still in their relatively early stages. Published literature in this area is limited to service descriptions and initial service evaluations that are limited to single services [15, 39, 40]; see also Chapter 13.

Treatment Programmes

One of the persistent criticisms of the treatment model within forensic settings has been a lack of definition. Chapter 13 describes a four-phase approach to treatments with phase 1 involving the interface with the courts and criminal justice system, phase 2 being the acute treatment and alleviation of distress, phase 3 being rehabilitation and phase 4 reintegration. Chapter 14 describes the methods of risk assessment and management that are quite central to the treatment plans. Both Chapters 13 and 14 describe in some detail the various assessment tools that are used in the assessment and treatment process. Assessing and treating a patient is a collaborative effort between a multidisciplinary treating team and the patient. The 10-point treatment plan described by Alexander et al. [5] (see Table 3.1) covers phases 2, 3 and 4 and offers a useful framework for the assessment, treatment and rehabilitation of individuals with ID and offending behaviours, whether in a hospital or community settings.

Measuring healthcare outcomes is paramount for evaluating the effectiveness of various treatment options to provide the best patient care. This has become particularly relevant following the Winterbourne View abuse scandal, after which an agenda to care for people

Table 3.1 The 10-point treatment programme

A multi-axial diagnostic assessment	Covers the degree of intellectual disability, cause of intellectual disability, pervasive developmental disorders, other developmental disabilities, mental illnesses, substance misuse or dependence, personality disorders, physical disorders, trauma and other psychosocial disadvantages, types of behavioural problems
A psychological formulation	Developed collaboratively with the patient.
A behaviour support plan	Incorporating positive behaviour support principles
Risk assessment and management plans	Using actuarial and structured clinical judgement tools
Pharmacotherapy	Targeting both comorbid mental illnesses and the predominant symptom clusters that are problematic. Physical conditions are treated with input from primary and secondary care.
Individual and group psychotherapy	Guided by the psychological formulation and will include motivational work, supportive therapy, social skills training, assertiveness training, management of emotions, addressing comorbidities like substance misuse or issues like bereavement, etc.
Offence-specific, individual and group psychotherapies	Particularly those targeting anger and interpersonal violence, sexual offending, fire setting, etc.
Education, skills acquisition, and occupational/ vocational rehabilitation	Providing a structured, predictable and rehabilitation-focused programme of daily activity
Community participation	Providing rehabilitation and reintegration through a system of graded escorted, shadowed and unescorted leave periods.
Discharge and community transition.	Rehabilitation and reintegration into the community

with ID within mainstream psychiatric services, as well as provide good quality of care in the community rather than be kept unnecessarily in hospitals or other restrictive environments, was recommended [41]. The Winterbourne View review also highlighted concerns over inappropriate care models, lack of personalised care plans allowing the patient to stay within easy reach of their families and poor care standards, all of which underline why measuring outcomes are vital in this population.

A systematic review involving 60 studies extracted data on outcome domains in people with ID who had involvement with forensic services [42]. In consultation with patients and family members, the authors formulated a framework to examine treatment effectiveness, patient safety and patient, and carer experience. Table 3.2 summarises the key outcome

Table 3.2 Framework of outcome domains (reproduced from Morrissey et al., 2017 [42])

Effectiveness

Discharge outcome/direction of care pathway

Delayed discharge/current placement appropriateness

Readmission (i.e., readmitted to hospital or prison)

Length of hospital stay

Adaptive functioning

Clinical symptom severity/treatment needs: patient rated

Clinical symptom severity/treatment needs: clinician rated

Recovery/engagement/progress on treatment goals: clinician rated

Recovery/engagement/progress on treatment goals: patient/carer rated

Re offending (i.e., charges/convictions) on discharge

Offending-like behaviour (no criminal justice system involvement) on discharge

Incidents (violence/self-harm) (in care setting)

Risk-assessment measures

Security need (i.e., physical/procedural/escort/leave)

Patient safety

Premature death/suicide

Physical health

Medication (i.e., PRN usage/exceeding BNF limits/side effects patient rating)

Restrictive practices (restraint)

Restrictive practices (seclusion/segregation)

Victimisation/safeguarding

Patient/carer experience

Patient experience: involvement in care

Patient experience: satisfaction/complaints

Quality of life: patient rated

Therapeutic climate

Access to work/meaningful activity (where appropriate)

Level of support/involvement in community/social network (post discharge)

Carer experience: communication with services/involvement in care

domains identified. Notwithstanding its limitations, this evidence base suggests that treatment within specialised services delivers good treatment outcomes.

It can be difficult to measure outcomes in a forensic ID setting due to numerous factors. First, the views of the healthcare professionals, patients and carers may vary as carers and patients may look at the quality-of-service provision and their experience of receiving the service as well as the clinical outcome, but healthcare professionals may only focus on the clinical outcome. In any case, even the outcome variables that have been used have question marks against their reliability and validity. Secondly, conventional methods of measuring long-term outcomes by examining reconviction or reoffending rates may not be appropriate for this group, a point made with clarity in one of the first outcome studies in this area that showed that, while reconviction rates were low at around 10%, the rate of 'offending-like behaviours' was well over the 50% mark [43]. Thirdly, many of the outcome studies so far are either from single sites or from the same country. This may not reflect the potential differences between different geographic areas within a country as well as internationally.

Finally, most studies looked at the cohort of patients who were discharged successfully from the hospital and hence did not account for those who continued as inpatients for long periods. Interestingly, one of the few large-scale studies using a countrywide stratified random sample of long-stay patients in medium and high secure settings found that those with ID were not disproportionately higher in comparison to those without ID (44). This suggests that while there is indeed a sub-group of patients in forensic settings who stay for long periods of time, there may be factors mediating that which go beyond the presence of ID. There is an urgent need to explore the other clinical, risk and socio-demographic variables that mediate treatment outcomes for this vulnerable group.   •

References

1. Douds F, Bantwal A. The 'forensicisation' of challenging behaviour: the perils of people with learning disabilities and severe challenging behaviours being viewed as 'forensic' patients. *Journal of Intellectual Disabilities and Offending Behaviour* 2011; 2 (3): 110.

2. Royal College of Psychiatrists and British Psychological Society and Royal College of Speech and Language Therapists. Challenging behaviour: a unified approach (CR144). 2007. Available at: www.rcpsych.ac.uk/docs/default-source/improving-care/better-mh-policy/col lege-reports/college-report-cr144.pdf? sfvrsn=73e437e8_2.

3. Blackburn R. *The Psychology of Criminal Conduct.* John Wiley & Sons, 1993.

4. Chester V, Alexander RT, Lindsay WR. Women with intellectual disabilities and forensic involvement. In *The Wiley Handbook on Offenders with Intellectual and Developmental Disabilities.* John Wiley & Sons, 2018: 328–45.

5. Alexander RT, Hiremath A, Chester V, Green FN, Gunaratna IJ, Hoare S. Evaluation of treatment outcomes from a medium secure unit for people with intellectual disability. *Advances in Mental Health and Intellectual Disabilities* 2011; 5 (1): 22–32.

6. Chester V, Wells H, Lovell M, Melvin C, Tromans SJ. The prevention of offending behaviour by people with intellectual disabilities: a case for specialist childhood and adolescent early intervention. *Advances in Mental Health and Intellectual Disabilities* 2019; 13(5): 216–27.

7. Plant A, McDermott E, Chester V, Alexander RT. Substance misuse among offenders in a forensic intellectual disability service. *Journal of Learning Disabilities and Offending Behaviour* 2011; 2(3): 127.

8. Rai R, Tromans S, Kapugama C, Alexander RT, Chester V, Gunaratna I, et al. A phenomenological approach to diagnosing psychosis in autism spectrum disorder and intellectual disability: a case series. *Advances in Autism* 2018; 4(2): 39–48.

9. Winter N, Holland AJ, Collins S. Factors predisposing to suspected offending by adults with self-reported learning disabilities. *Psychological Medicine* 1997; 27 (3): 595–607.

10. Chester V, Painter G, Ryan L, Popple J, Chikodzi K, Alexander RT. Traumatic brain injury in a forensic intellectual disability population. *Psychology, Crime and Law* 2018; 24(4): 400–13.

11. Gray NS, Fitzgerald S, Taylor J, MacCulloch MJ, Snowden RJ. Predicting future reconviction in offenders with intellectual disabilities: the predictive efficacy of VRAG, PCL-SV, and the HCR-20. *Psychological Assessment* 2007; 19(4): 474–9.

12. Fitzgerald S, Gray NS, Alexander RT, Bagshaw R, Chesterman P, Huckle P, et al. Predicting institutional violence in offenders with intellectual disabilities: the predictive efficacy of the VRAG and the HCR-20. *Journal of Applied Research in Intellectual Disabilities* 2013; 26(5): 384–93.

13. Holland T, Clare ICH, Mukhopadhyay T. Prevalence of 'criminal offending' by men and women with intellectual disability and the characteristics of 'offenders': implications for research and service development. *Journal of Intellectual Disability Research* 2002; 46(s1): 6–20.

14. Lyall R, Kelly M. Specialist psychiatric beds for people with learning disability. *Psychiatric Bulletin* 2007; 31(8): 297–300.

15. Devapriam J, Alexander RT. Tiered model of learning disability forensic service provision. *Journal of Intellectual Disabilities and Offending Behaviour* 2012; 3(4): 175–85.

16. Royal College of Psychiatrists. Forensic care pathways for adults with intellectual disability involved with the criminal justice. 2014. Available at: www.rcpsych.ac.uk/docs/default-source/members/faculties/forensic-psychiatry/forensic-fr-id-04.pdf?sfvrsn=2fdf0def_2.

17. Talbot J. No one knows: offenders with learning disabilities and learning difficulties. *International Journal of Prisoner Health* 2009; 5(3): 141–52.

18. Police and Criminal Evidence Act 1985. Available at: www.legislation.gov.uk/ukpga/1984/60/contents.

19. Home Office. CODE C Revised: Code of Practice for the detention, treatment and questioning of persons by police officers. 2017. Available at: https://assets.publishing.service.gov.uk/government/uploads/system/uploads/attachment_data/file/903473/pace-code-c-2019.pdf.

20. Clare ICH, Gudjonsson GH. The vulnerability of suspects with intellectual disabilities during police interviews: a review and experimental study of decision-making. *Mental Handicap Research* 1995; 8(2): 110–28.

21. O'Mahony BM. The emerging role of the registered intermediary with the vulnerable witness and offender: facilitating communication with the police and members of the judiciary. *British Journal of Learning Disabilities* 2010; 38(3): 232–7.

22. Gudjonsson GH. The relationship of intelligence and memory to interrogative suggestibility: the importance of range effects. *British Journal of Clinical Psychology* 1988; 27(2): 185–7.

23. Gudjonsson GH, Clare ICH. The relationship between confabulation and intellectual ability, memory, interrogative suggestibility and acquiescence. *Personality and Individual Differences* 1995; 19(3): 333–8.

24. Boer H, Alexander R, Devapriam J, Torales J, Ng R, Castaldelli-Maia J, et al. Prisoner mental health care for people with intellectual disability. *International Journal of Culture and Mental Health* 2016; 9(4): 442–6.

25. Mckinnon I, Thorp J, Grubin D. Improving the detection of detainees with suspected intellectual disability in police custody. *Advances in Mental Health and Intellectual Disabilities* 2015; 9(4): 174–85.

26. Leggett J, Goodman W, Dinani S. People with learning disabilities' experiences of being interviewed by the police. *British Journal of Learning Disabilities* 2007; 35(3): 168–73.

27. Department of Health. The Bradley Report: Lord Bradley's review of people with mental health problems or learning disabilities in the criminal justice system. 2009. Available at: https://lx.iriss.org.uk/sites/default/files/resources/The%20Bradley%20report.pdf.

28. Chester V. People with intellectual and developmental disorders in the United Kingdom criminal justice system. *East Asian Archives of Psychiatry* 2018; 28(4): 150–8.

29. Taylor ILA. Fitness to plead and stand trial: the impact of mild intellectual disability. Doctoral thesis, University College London, 2011.

30. Rogers TP, Blackwood NJ, Farnham F, Pickup GJ, Watts MJ. Fitness to plead and competence to stand trial: a systematic review of the constructs and their application. *Journal of Forensic Psychiatry and Psychology* 2008; 19: 576–96.

31. Baroff GS, Gunn M, Hayes S. Legal issues. In Lindsay WR, Taylor JL, Sturmey P, eds., *Offenders with Developmental Disabilities*. John Wiley & Sons, 2004: 37–66.

32. Mental Health Act 1983. Available at: https://www.legislation.gov.uk/ukpga/1983/20/contents.

33. McCarthy J, Chaplin E, Hayes S, Søndenaa E, Chester V, Morrissey C, et al. Defendants with intellectual disability and autism spectrum conditions: the perspective of clinicians working across three jurisdictions. *Psychiatry, Psychology and Law* 2021; 29(5): 698–717.

34. Criminal Justice Act 2003. Available at: www.legislation.gov.uk/ukpga/2003/44/contents.

35. Archer N, Hurley EA. A justice system failing the autistic community. *Journal of Intellectual Disabilities and Offending Behaviour* 2013; 4(1): 53–9.

36. Nacro. Liaison and diversion for mentally disordered offenders. 2015. Available at: www.nacro.org.uk/wp-content/uploads/2015/05/Liaison-and-diversion-for-mentally-disordered-offenders.pdf.

37. Department of Health & Social Care. Consultation outcome: reforming the Mental Health Act. Available at: www.gov.uk/government/consultations/reforming-the-mental-health-act.

38. Benton C, Roy A. The first three years of a community forensic service for people with a learning disability. *British Journal of Forensic Practice* 2008; 10(2): 4–12.

39. Dinani S, Goodman W, Swift C, Treasure T. Providing forensic community services for people with learning disabilities. *Journal of Intellectual Disabilities and Offending Behaviour* 2010 Jan 1; 1(1): 58–63.

40. Lindsay WR, Steele L, Smith AHW, Quinn K, Allan R. A community forensic intellectual disability service: twelve year follow up of referrals, analysis of referral patterns and assessment of harm reduction. *Legal and Criminological Psychology* 2006; 11(1): 113–30.

41. Department of Health *Transforming Care: A national response to Winterbourne View Hospital Department of Health Review: Final Report.* Department of Health, 2012.

42. Morrissey C, Langdon PE, Geach N, Chester V, Ferriter M, Lindsay WR, et al. A systematic review and synthesis of outcome domains for use within forensic services for people with intellectual disabilities. *BJPsych Open* 2017 Jan; 3(1): 41–56.

43. Alexander RT, Crouch K, Halstead S, Piachaud J. Long-term outcome from a medium secure service for people with intellectual disability. *Journal of Intellectual Disability Research* 2006; 50(4): 305–15.

44. Chester V, Tromans S, Kapugama C, Alexander RT, Völlm B. Long-stay patients with and without intellectual disability in forensic psychiatric settings: comparison of characteristics and needs. *BJPsych Open* 2018; 4(04): 226–34.

Chapter 4

Overview of Offenders with Attention Deficit Hyperactivity Disorder

Susan Young, Kelly Cocallis, Corey Lane and Mark David Chong

Introduction

Attention deficit hyperactivity disorder (ADHD) is a neurodevelopmental disorder arising in childhood, which comprises a range of inattentive and/or hyperactive-impulsive symptoms and which significantly interferes with functioning or development in two or more settings [1]. The prevalence of ADHD in the general population worldwide is estimated to be approximately 5% for children/adolescents [2], and 2.5% for adults [3].

Over-Representation of ADHD in Criminal Justice Offender Populations

Empirical studies have highlighted the significant over-representation of individuals with ADHD in youth and adult offender populations. A meta-analysis of 42 studies revealed a prevalence rate of 25.5% in incarcerated populations, reflecting a 5-fold and 10-fold increase (for youths and adults, respectively) in the prevalence of ADHD comparative to the general population [4]. These findings are consistent with a meta-analysis of 102 studies that found a prevalence rate of 26.2% [5]. In a later meta-analysis of 27 relevant studies, Beaudry and colleagues [6] calculated a prevalence rate of 17.3% and 17.5% for male and female adolescents, respectively. While lower than previously reported prevalence estimates, this remains considerably higher than general population prevalence rates. Of note, Young and colleagues [4] found a significant difference in the prevalence estimates between screenings and clinical interviews, while Baggio and colleagues [5] found no significant difference. Nevertheless, to alleviate the individual and wider societal costs, early identification, prevention and intervention strategies have been advocated [7].

Gender Effects

Meta-analyses have revealed no significant differences in prevalence rates for gender [4, 5], contrasting epidemiological findings from general population studies. Various explanations have been proposed for this disparity. Some authors postulate that, compared to their male peers, female offenders may represent more serious cases, demonstrating higher rates of adverse childhood experiences and psychiatric disorders, including ADHD [8]. An alternative postulation is that this disparity may reflect systematic referral preferences and identification biases. A meta-analysis demonstrated that ADHD is more likely to be diagnosed in males than females by health services in the general population [9]. This is despite growing evidence that suggests ADHD symptoms are as common in females as males [10, 11].

ADHD has traditionally been perceived as a male childhood disorder. Females may demonstrate later onset of impairment and may work harder to compensate for or hide their symptoms in an effort to meet parent and/or teacher expectations. Collectively, this may result in fewer referrals of females to health professionals. One potential source of confusion may be that hyperactivity is commonly (and erroneously) ascribed a 'male' symptom and inattention a 'female' symptom. This bias may impede accurate diagnosis of ADHD in females who display hyperactivity, and males who do not demonstrate overt hyperactive behaviour [7]. It is noted, however, that the gender ratio of ADHD within the general population narrows as individuals transition from childhood to adulthood [12–15]. In adulthood, females have an increased tendency to seek help from health professionals compared to their male peers, which may result in a shift in referral patterns [16], perhaps providing support for the referral/identification bias supposition.

Cultural Effects

Large variations exist in the reported rates of ADHD in the criminal justice system population for different countries [4, 5]. Some authors propose that the variability in prevalence rates may be indicative of specific judicial practices that affect the criminal justice system pathway of an individual with ADHD (e.g., diversion). Where prison population rates are high in a country, it is thought that the mental health status of the prison population may be more representative of the general population, resulting in more modest prevalence rates comparative to countries with lower prison population rates [17].

In Westmoreland and colleagues' [18] examination of the characteristics of male and female offenders in the USA, offenders with ADHD were more likely to be White, which is consistent with US studies of non-criminal justice system populations. Some authors however argue that not all groups are equally likely to be identified (and receive treatment), hampering the interpretation of findings. Children from ethnic minorities have been reported to be diagnosed with ADHD at a lower rate than White children [19–21]. However, most research has focused on African American and Hispanic children in western societies (predominantly in the USA), with less known about identification disparities for children of other ethnicities, particularly in non-western societies.

The reasons for the reported disparity in identification and treatment of ADHD among ethnic groups are complex and have not been wholly elucidated. Recognised barriers are associated with the patient and family (e.g., lack of knowledge/awareness about ADHD, negative attitudes and beliefs of illness/social stigma and degree of trust toward services) and/or the health system (e.g., lower likelihood of referral by school professionals, language barriers, biases or cultural expectations of what constitutes 'normal behaviour' and access to the health system due to lower socio-economic status). Some barriers are likely to be prominent due to differing health systems. For example, in the UK there is free access to healthcare whereas in the USA healthcare is private, which may reduce access to diagnosis and treatment for those of lower socio-economic status. Additionally, the extent to which other factors may confound reported disparities are unclear. When standardised diagnostic procedures are followed, research indicates limited evidence for differences in ADHD rates across different groups [22].

Type of Offending

The most frequent offences committed by individuals with ADHD leading to arrest, conviction or incarceration are assault/violence, theft, property offences, substance-related crimes and possession of weapons [23, 24]. Studies suggest that the types of offences committed by individuals with ADHD may vary dependent on age [25]. Mohr-Jensen and colleagues [24] found that, except for murder, the rates for all recorded offences were significantly higher for individuals with ADHD as compared to their non-ADHD counterparts. In contrast, Erskine and colleagues [26] found that there was no difference between those with ADHD as compared to controls for substance-related arrests (odds ratio (OR) 1.69, 0.75–3.77) (despite significant ORs for illicit substance use, dependence and disorders). ADHD, however, was significantly related to violence-related arrests (OR 3.63, 2.31–5.70).

Onset of Delinquent and Offending Behaviours

While it is not suggested that ADHD is a 'causal' factor of crime, there is empirical evidence to suggest that ADHD increases the risk for rule-breaking and the occurrence of delinquent behaviour [25]. Studies have shown an earlier onset of criminality for those with ADHD when compared to their non-ADHD peers. Individuals with ADHD have been found to be younger at the time of their first arrest [27] and first conviction [28] than those without ADHD. Silva and colleagues [29] found that males with ADHD but not females with ADHD had an earlier onset of criminality compared to matched controls. In their logistic regression analysis of the US National Longitudinal Study of Adolescent Health data, Fletcher and Wolfe [30] found that those symptomatic of ADHD between the ages of 5 and 12 years old were much more likely to self-report criminal behaviour (e.g., stealing, selling drugs, robbery and/or burglary) when they were young adults than those asymptomatic of ADHD.

Other studies have likewise found that ADHD significantly increases the risk of a number of other criminal indices including arrests, convictions and incarceration rates. Erskine and colleagues [26] found that those with ADHD were approximately 2.5 times as likely to be arrested, twice as likely to receive a court conviction and 2.5 times more likely to be incarcerated than individuals without an ADHD diagnosis. Similarly, in their meta-analysis of longitudinal studies involving 15,442 individuals, Mohr-Jensen and Steinhausen [23] found that, when compared to non-ADHD peers, those with ADHD had nearly a 3.5 times greater likelihood of receiving a court conviction and nearly three times greater likelihood of being incarcerated.

Risk of Recidivism

Studies have demonstrated an elevated risk of recidivism for offenders with ADHD. In their 15-year follow-up study, Philipp-Wiegmann and colleagues [31] found offenders with ADHD had a higher rate of recidivism and quicker time of relapse (reoffended 2.5 times faster) than offenders without ADHD. This finding is in opposition to an earlier study by Grieger and Hosser [32] where ADHD did not predict reoffending. Silva and colleagues [29] reported an elevated risk of recidivism for male offenders with ADHD but not female offenders with ADHD.

Progress in Institutional Settings

ADHD has been associated with behavioural disturbance in police custody, prison and forensic mental health settings and these findings have clear resource implications [1]. Analysis of police custody records found that ADHD contributes significantly to the frequency of requests being made of staff [33]. In prison and mental health settings, records document a greater risk of critical incidents involving verbal aggression, damage to property and severe physical aggression [34–37]. These behaviours are likely to have implications for staffing and resources. They may impede progress within the institution, attract adjudications and/or convictions and prevent early release. The underlying mechanisms for this association are likely to be hyperactivity/impulsivity, emotional distress and dysregulation [34].

Association between ADHD and Criminal Offending

While there are empirical links for the association between ADHD and criminal and delinquent behaviour, this relationship is complicated by the high frequency of comorbid disorders found for offenders with ADHD. A meta-analysis of 18 studies found an increased risk of conduct disorders, substance use disorders, depression, anxiety and personality disorders for prisoners with ADHD compared to non-ADHD prisoners [38]. High prevalence rates of traumatic brain injury, intellectual disability, communication disorders, autism spectrum disorder and post-traumatic stress disorder have also been found in the ADHD offender population [39–43]. The effects of such comorbidity are considered of particular importance when the comorbid disorder is itself found to be strongly associated with criminogenic behaviour (see Retz and colleagues [25] for further information regarding the impact of comorbidity). These include oppositional defiant disorder, conduct disorder, antisocial personality disorder and substance use disorder. Some authors argue that there is no association between ADHD and criminal and delinquent behaviour when controlling for other externalising disorders, particularly conduct disorder [44, 45]. However, some studies have found an independent effect of ADHD [46–48]. Pratt and colleagues [49] concluded that while other factors may be more strongly associated with deviant/criminal behaviour, ADHD nevertheless presents a significant risk factor for delinquency and criminality. One complication for understanding the association is that ADHD shares many symptoms with externalising disorders. Consequently, not only will the potentiality for a misdiagnosis be ever-present, an optimal understanding of why ADHD is criminogenic may likewise be compromised.

Course of Criminality Over the Long Term

At present, little is known about the long-term course of criminality for offenders with ADHD. Some authors suggest that ADHD may be associated with a criminal career that begins early in life and continues through adulthood, referred to as 'life-course-persistent offenders' within Moffitt's [50] developmental taxonomy theory. This contrasts with 'adolescent-limited offenders' who engage in criminality in their adolescent years only. There are, however, few longitudinal studies and, of those that do exist, most have demonstrated short follow-up periods.

One of the extant longitudinal studies demonstrating the longest follow-up period found a decline in offending across age. In their 30-year prospective follow-up study of hyperactive boys with conduct problems, Satterfield and colleagues [45] found that arrest rates were highest in early adulthood (59% were 18–21 years old) and declined steadily with increasing age (32% were 27–32 years old and 16%, 36–38 years old). A mean age of desistance (i.e., no further arrests occurred) of 30.1 years old was found, with a small subgroup continuing to offend in late middle age. Only childhood variables were used as predictors in the study, and therefore the contribution of adulthood variables (e.g., whether ADHD symptomatology persisted in full clinical range, as partial remission or full remission) in explaining the finding is unclear. In another study, the number of ADHD symptoms in adulthood, along with the number of childhood ADHD symptoms and the severity of ADHD during teenage years, were all found to be predictors of lifetime engagement in crime [51]. Additionally, studies have reported declining rates of ADHD with age in offender populations. Accordingly, it is possible that the decline in criminality may correspond with the decline in ADHD symptomatology over the lifespan. Further longitudinal studies with long follow-up periods, examining both childhood and adulthood predictors (including the interplay of environmental factors), are necessary to understand the long-term effects of ADHD on criminal offending.

Frameworks for Understanding the Association between ADHD and Criminal Offending

Harpin and Young [52] offer a range of reasons as to why offenders with ADHD are vulnerable in the justice system. First, they often commit crimes impulsively or opportunistically; the lack of planning involved in the criminal endeavour also likely means that they are more easily detected and caught. Second, once arrested and processed by the justice system, youth and adults who have ADHD may be less emotionally and mentally equipped to handle the stress of being interviewed, interrogated or questioned by the police and/or barristers in court. A growing body of research has identified a high susceptibility for individuals with ADHD to make a false confession [53, 54]. Third, on leaving prison, offenders with ADHD may have limited support in the community to help them successfully reintegrate into society (e.g., poor access to housing and medical care). Thus, the risk of them reoffending for subsistence or consuming illicit drugs as a coping mechanism or to self-medicate is high.

A variety of psychological and conceptual/theoretical platforms exist upon which scholars, clinicians, criminal justice workers, lawyers and other stakeholders may leverage upon to better understand why ADHD increases the risk of criminal and delinquent behaviour. Contributory factors are considered in the following three frameworks.

General Theory of Crime

The general theory of crime is a criminological theory proposed by Gottfredson and Hirschi [55]. This is both a meta-theory, in that it purports to account for all criminal conduct and 'analogous' behaviours, as well as being highly reductionist in nature since it ascribes blame to just one factor – a lack of self-control. This inability to delay gratification causes, among other traits, impulsivity, callousness and risk-taking, thereby increasing the likelihood of hedonistic self-interested acts. The cause of this low self-control stems from poor parenting, and if parents cannot monitor, instil proper values and address deviant behaviour before the child reaches the age of 8–10 years old, it is unlikely that they will be able to develop the self-control needed to live a normative life. Pratt and colleagues [49] suggest that ADHD should be considered 'a potential source of this low self-control' and expand the theory to include not only social experiences (e.g., parental management) but also a biological/genetic origin.

Criminogenic Cognitions

This concept refers to problematic thought patterns (also known as criminal thinking) that precede criminal behaviour [56]. Such cognitions are a key part of Walters' [57] criminal lifestyle theory, a paradigm that argues that these criminal thinking styles (e.g., mollification, cut off, entitlement, power orientation, sentimentality, super optimism, cognitive indolence and discontinuity) are 'cognitive processes that induce a tendency to act in a criminal or antisocial manner' [56]. In order to determine which ADHD symptoms were related to criminogenic cognitions, Engelhardt and colleagues [56] examined 192 community-recruited adult participants and found that these criminal thinking styles were: (a) strongly linked to inattention; (b) moderately associated to impulsivity and impulsivity/emotional lability; and (c) not linked to hyperactivity.

Motivational versus Reactive Factors

Within the literature, violence-related offences have been categorised as reactive–impulsive versus proactive–predatory. There is evidence to suggest that individuals with ADHD typically engage in violent criminal acts that are reactive (reaction to a provocation or a conflict, driven by emotional dysregulation) rather than proactive (instrumental and premeditated). Retz and Rösler [58] propose a theoretical framework for understanding the relationship between ADHD and antisocial behaviour. Those with early-onset conduct disorder who go on to develop antisocial personality disorder are proposed to commit crimes due to impulsive aggression as a reaction to a situation, rather than premeditated–proactive aggression. An alternative pathway is for those without a comorbid conduct disorder, who commit offences associated with social problems and rule-breaking behaviours (e.g., traffic infractions), but the rate of general delinquency is not elevated. Within this framework, substance use disorders may be an important mediator of ADHD-related antisocial behaviour [59].

Economic Consequences of ADHD in Criminal Justice Offender Populations

ADHD confers significant costs not only to the individual but to wider society [60, 61]. ADHD-related criminal justice annual costs in Australia are estimated to be $215 million [62]. In the USA, costs associated with youth criminogenic behaviour are estimated to fall between US$50 million and US$170 million per year to the victim, and between US$2 billion and US$4 billion per year to society [30]. In the UK, Young and colleagues [63] identified that costs associated with behaviour-related problems and medical treatment in the Scottish prison system amounted to £590 greater per annum for individual prisoners with ADHD when compared to those without ADHD. When accounting for ADHD prison prevalence rates, they estimated the annual medical and behaviour-related cost for Scottish prison systems to be £11.7 million. Young and Cocallis [64] argue that appropriate provision of treatment for prisoners with ADHD would likely result in a highly beneficial rate of return for wider society. The same argument may be made for those with ADHD in the broader criminal justice system (e.g., probation and detained forensic settings). Support for the reduced costs associated with treating ADHD in criminal justice populations is provided by Freriks and colleagues [65]. Treatment cost-effectiveness was measured using the net monetary benefit (NMB), which represents the fiscal worth of reduced quality-adjusted life years less total treatment costs. It is worth noting that costs associated with serious delinquency were included in this analysis. Freriks and colleagues [65] found an NMB of US$95,449 for medication management, US$88,553 for behavioural treatment and US$90,536 for combined treatments.

System Barriers and a Way Forward

Individuals with ADHD are acknowledged to be disadvantaged within the criminal justice system due to their symptoms being unrecognised and/or misunderstood, resulting in the lack of a diagnosis and consequently appropriate treatment. An expert consensus report [7] has highlighted several related system barriers including inadequate awareness (both staff and offenders) of ADHD symptoms and treatments; lack of appropriate training; a lack of appropriate use of tools to screen and diagnose ADHD; a lack of appropriate use of multimodal interventions; a lack of care management and multi-agency liaison; and a lack of preparation for prison release. To address these barriers, recommendations were made to address limitations in three core areas: (i) identification and assessment; (ii) interventions and treatment; and (iii) care management and multi-agency liaison, with recognition that work needs to begin with identification.

Identification and Assessment

To effectively identify and accurately diagnose ADHD within correctional facilities, four key elements were deemed to be needed: (i) accessibility to medical records; (ii) training in clinical interview assessments for clinicians; (iii) training for correctional staff to recognise ADHD symptomology; and (iv) the availability of appropriate screening and diagnostic tools. The implementation of a two-tiered screening framework was considered best practice. Recommended tools for youths included the Swanson, Nolan and Pelham Teacher and Parent Rating Scale (SNAP-IV), the Conners' Comprehensive Behaviour Rating Scale (Conners' CBRS) and the ADHD Child Evaluation (ACE). For adults, the brief version of the Barkley Adult ADHD Rating Scale (B-BAARS), the Conners' Adult ADHD Diagnostic Interview for DSM-4 (CAADID); the Diagnostic Interview for ADHD in Adults (DIVA-2) and the ACE+ (ACE for Adults) are recommended.

Interventions and Treatment

Once diagnosed, multimodal interventions were recommended. Combining pharmacological (stimulant and non-stimulant medication) and non-pharmacological (psychoeducation, psychological interventions and psychosocial treatment programmes) approaches allows for the broad needs (e.g., psychological, behavioural and educational) of offenders with ADHD to be addressed. The use of ADHD medication is thought to have a by-effect on non-pharmacological interventions through the reduction of ADHD symptoms, thereby allowing for increased engagement and benefit.

Various studies support the efficacy of pharmacological interventions for ADHD in criminal justice offender populations. A seminal study conducted to assess the effectiveness of methylphenidate in 30 Swedish prisoners with ADHD found that the treatment significantly reduced the severity of ADHD symptoms as well as enhanced global functioning [66]. Using national registry data, Lichtenstein and colleagues [67] found criminal conviction rates reduced by 32% for males and 41% for females when treated with ADHD medication, as compared with non-medicated periods. Chang and colleagues [68] similarly found positive results in their study analysing the effects of a pharmacological stimulant treatment provided to participants post-prison release in Sweden. The dispensed psychostimulants resulted in individuals being 42.8% less likely to commit a violent offence during the medication period as compared to the non-medication period. In another national registry data study, Mohr-Jensen and colleagues [24] found conviction and incarceration rates reduced by 30–40% when individuals were medicated for ADHD, as compared to non-medicated periods. A significant positive association was observed for males but not females on incarceration risk. However, the authors acknowledged that this discrepancy may be due to insufficient power to detect between-group differences due to the small sample size of incarcerated females in the study.

Despite growing evidence of its efficacy and success [69], the use of stimulants for offenders is somewhat controversial due to the potential for misuse and diversion, and increasing the risk of malingering and drug-seeking behaviour [70–73]. To minimise risks, extended release or non-stimulant preparations may be considered due to their limited abuse potential.

Multimodal interventions that include psychological interventions in addition to medication have demonstrated stronger effect sizes [74, 75]. The Reasoning and Rehabilitation 2 ADHD (R&R2ADHD) cognitive–behavioural-therapy-based programme has demonstrated medium to large effect sizes in functional outcomes, including self-reported antisocial behaviour at post-treatment and three-months follow-up [76, 77]. In 2016–2019, the R&R2ADHD programme was the focus of a controlled evaluation in Denmark. At the end of the study there were significant reductions in ADHD symptoms, problems with social functioning, emotional control, depression, anxiety, and temperament. Improvements in quality of life and greater personal locus of control were also found. Excluding the emotional control outcome, these results were sustained at three months post-treatment, with further improvements found for quality of life and personal locus of control. Long-term consequences (at 6 and 12 months post-treatment) were additionally considered using matched controls drawn from Danish registers. Completion of R&R2ADHD was associated with increased employment and education rates and decreased use of cash benefits and social services. After six months, there was an increase in visits to the hospital emergency room. Emergency room contact may be considered a proxy for impulsive behaviour or alternatively may reflect increased self-care and personal locus of control. While the data were unable to directly explain which of the two hypotheses drove the result, it was presumed a positive consequence (i.e., increased self-care). Because these participants were not specifically referred for antisocial behaviour, the study demonstrates the broader applicability of the R&R2ADHD programme in other sectors (e.g., more generally in the community). R&R2ADHD has also been rolled out within the Danish prison service [78].

Care Management and Multi-Agency Liaison

Due to the complex presentation and needs of offenders with ADHD, assistance from a range of services may be required, both while the individual is incarcerated and following release. In England, those with complex needs are often eligible to receive a care programme approach (CPA), which encompasses a structured multi-professional care management plan to support the needs of the individual. Within this format, issues are addressed according to distinct domains and professionals/services are allocated accordingly. The expert consensus recommended that offenders with ADHD receive a CPA or comparable care management plan [7]. It was recommended that a medication plan is included as a core component. Utilising a CPA or comparable care management approach is envisaged to mitigate issues that may arise during transitional periods (e.g., movement within and between prisons).

While the expert consensus report was developed primarily with reference to the prison population in the UK, the report offers a framework that can be adapted to the broader criminal justice system population across countries worldwide.

Conclusion

This chapter provides a critical analysis of the relationship between criminal offending and ADHD. Of particular note is the consistent empirical finding that those with ADHD are significantly over-represented in youth and criminal justice offender populations. Many of these individuals are undiagnosed; their ADHD symptoms are either missed or misdiagnosed. A critical need exists across international jurisdictions for the development and systematic employment of approaches aimed at optimising the early identification and treatment of ADHD. The provision of psychoeducation and training of staff across the criminal justice system is likely to confer better economic outcomes for the justice system and better clinical and social outcomes for individuals with ADHD. Importantly these may have broader implications within society.

References

1. American Psychiatric Association. *Diagnostic and Statistical Manual of Mental Disorders*, 5th edition: DSM-5. American Psychiatric Association, 2013.

2. Polanczyk G, de Lima MS, Horta BL, Biederman J, Rohde LA. The worldwide prevalence of ADHD: a systematic review and metaregression analysis. *American Journal of Psychiatry* 2007; 164(6): 942–8.

3. Simon V, Czobor P, Bálint S, Mészáros Á, Bitter I. Prevalence and correlates of adult attention-deficit hyperactivity disorder: meta-analysis. *British Journal of Psychiatry* 2009; 194(3): 204–11.

4. Young S, Moss D, Sedgwick O, Fridman M, Hodgkins P. A meta-analysis of the prevalence of attention deficit hyperactivity disorder in incarcerated populations. *Psychological Medicine* 2015; 45(2): 247–58.

5. Baggio S, Fructuoso A, Guimaraes M, Fois E, Golay D, Heller P, et al. Prevalence of attention deficit hyperactivity disorder in detention settings: a systematic review and meta-analysis. *Frontiers in Psychiatry* 2018; 9: 331.

6. Beaudry G, Yu R, Långström N, Fazel S. An updated systematic review and meta-regression analysis: mental disorders among adolescents in juvenile detention and correctional facilities. *Journal of the American Academy of Child and Adolescent Psychiatry* 2021; 60(1): 46–60.

7. Young S, Gudjonsson G, Chitsabesan P, Colley B, Farrag E, Forrester A, et al. Identification and treatment of offenders with attention-deficit/hyperactivity disorder in the prison population: a practical approach based upon expert consensus. *BMC Psychiatry* 2018; 18(1): 281–9.

8. Turner D, Wolf AJ, Barra S, Müller M, Gregório Hertz P, Huss M, et al. The association between adverse childhood experiences and mental health problems in young offenders. *European Child and Adolescent Psychiatry* 2021; 30(8): 1195–207.

9. Willcutt EG. The Prevalence of DSM-IV attention-deficit/hyperactivity disorder: a meta-analytic review. *Neurotherapeutics* 2012; 9(3): 490–9.

10. Biederman J, Faraone SV, Monuteaux MC, Bober M, Cadogen E. Gender effects on attention-deficit/hyperactivity disorder in adults, revisited. *Biological Psychiatry* 2004; 55(7): 692–700.

11. Corbisiero S, Hartmann-Schorro R, Riecher-Rössler A, Stieglitz R. Screening for adult attention-deficit/hyperactivity disorder in a psychiatric outpatient population with specific focus on sex differences. *Frontiers in Psychiatry* 2017; 8 (115): 115.

12. Cortese S, Faraone SV, Bernardi S, Wang S, Blanco C. Gender differences in adult attention-deficit/hyperactivity disorder: results from the National Epidemiologic Survey on Alcohol and Related Conditions (NESARC). *Journal of Clinical Psychiatry* 2016; 77(4): 421.

13. de Zwaan M, Gruss B, Müller A, Graap H, Martin A, Glaesmer H, et al. The estimated prevalence and correlates of adult ADHD in a German community sample. *European Archives of Psychiatry and Clinical Neuroscience* 2012; 262(1): 79–86.

14. Moffitt TE, Houts R, Asherson P, Belsky DW, Corcoran DL, Hammerle M, et al. Is adult ADHD a childhood-onset neurodevelopmental disorder? Evidence from a four-decade longitudinal cohort study. *American Journal of Psychiatry* 2015; 172(10): 967–77.

15. Williamson D, Johnston C. Gender differences in adults with attention-deficit/hyperactivity disorder: a narrative review. *Clinical Psychology Review* 2015; 40: 15–27.

16. Bramham J, Murphy DG, Xenitidis K, Asherson P, Hopkin G, Young S. Adults with attention deficit hyperactivity disorder: an investigation of age-related differences in behavioural symptoms, neuropsychological function and co-morbidity. *Psychological Medicine* 2012; 42(10): 2225–34.

17. Mundt AP, Alvarado R, Fritsch R, Poblete C, Villagra C, Kastner S, et al. Prevalence rates of mental disorders in Chilean prisons. *PLOS One* 2013; 8(7): e69109.

18. Westmoreland P, Gunter T, Loveless P, Allen J, Sieleni B, Black DW. Attention deficit hyperactivity disorder in men and women newly committed to prison: clinical characteristics, psychiatric comorbidity, and quality of life. *International Journal of Offender Therapy and Comparative Criminology* 2010; 54(3): 361–77.

19. Chung W, Jiang SF, Paksarian D, Nikolaidis A, Castellanos FX, Merikangas KR, et al. Trends in the prevalence and incidence of attention-deficit/hyperactivity disorder among adults and children of different racial and ethnic groups. *JAMA Network Open* 2019; 2(11): e1914344.

20. Coker TR, Elliott MN, Toomey SL, Schwebel DC, Cuccaro P, Tortolero Emery S, et al. Racial and ethnic disparities in ADHD diagnosis and treatment. *Pediatrics* 2016; 138(3): e20160407.

21. Morgan PL, Staff J, Hillemeier MM, Farkas G, Maczuga S. Racial and ethnic disparities in ADHD diagnosis from kindergarten to eighth grade. *Pediatrics* 2013; 132(1): 85.

22. Polanczyk GV, Willcutt EG, Salum GA, Kieling C, Rohde LA. ADHD prevalence estimates across three decades: an updated systematic review and meta-regression analysis. *International Journal of Epidemiology* 2014; 43(2): 434–42.

23. Mohr-Jensen C, Steinhausen H. A meta-analysis and systematic review of the risks associated with childhood attention-deficit hyperactivity disorder on long-term outcome of arrests, convictions, and incarcerations. *Clinical Psychology Review* 2016; 48: 32–42.

24. Mohr-Jensen C, Müller Bisgaard C, Boldsen SK, Steinhausen H. Attention-deficit/hyperactivity disorder in childhood and adolescence and the risk of crime in young adulthood in a Danish nationwide study. *Journal of the American Academy of Child and Adolescent Psychiatry* 2019; 58 (4): 443–52.

25. Retz W, Ginsberg Y, Turner D, Barra S, Retz-Junginger P, Larsson H, et al. Attention-deficit/hyperactivity disorder (ADHD), antisociality and delinquent behavior over the lifespan. *Neuroscience and Biobehavioral Reviews* 2020; 120: 236–48.

26. Erskine HE, Norman RE, Ferrari AJ, Chan GCK, Copeland WE, Whiteford HA, et al. Long-term outcomes of attention-deficit/hyperactivity disorder and conduct disorder: a systematic review and meta-analysis. *Journal of the American Academy of Child and Adolescent Psychiatry* 2016; 55(10): 841–50.

27. De Sanctis VA, Newcorn JH, Halperin JM. A prospective look at substance use and criminal behavior in urban ADHD youth: what is the role of maltreatment history on outcome? *Attention Deficit and Hyperactivity Disorders* 2014; 6(2): 79–86.

28. Rösler M, Retz W, Retz-Junginger P, Hengesch G, Schneider M, Supprian T, et al. Prevalence of attention deficit/hyperactivity disorder (ADHD) and comorbid disorders in young male prison inmates. *European Archives of Psychiatry and Clinical Neuroscience* 2004; 254(6): 365–71.

29. Silva D, Colvin L, Glauert R, Bower C. Contact with the juvenile justice system in children treated with stimulant medication for attention deficit hyperactivity disorder: a population study. *Lancet Psychiatry* 2014; 1(4): 278–85.

30. Fletcher J, Wolfe B. Long-term consequences of childhood ADHD on criminal activities. *Journal of Mental Health Policy and Economics* 2009; 12(3): 119–38.

31. Philipp-Wiegmann F, Rösler M, Clasen O, Zinnow T, Retz-Junginger P, Retz W. ADHD modulates the course of delinquency: a 15-year follow-up study of young incarcerated man. *European Archives of Psychiatry and Clinical Neuroscience* 2018; 268(4): 391–9.

32. Grieger L, Hosser D. Attention deficit hyperactivity disorder does not predict criminal recidivism in young adult offenders: results from a prospective study. *International Journal of Law and Psychiatry* 2012; 35(1): 27–34.

33. Young S, Goodwin EJ, Sedgwick O, Gudjonsson GH. The effectiveness of police custody assessments in identifying suspects with intellectual disabilities and attention deficit hyperactivity disorder. *BMC Medicine* 2013; 11(1): 248.

34. González RA, Gudjonsson GH, Wells J, Young S. The role of emotional distress and ADHD on institutional behavioral disturbance and recidivism among offenders. *Journal of Attention Disorders* 2016; 20(4): 368–78.

35. Young S, Gudjonsson GH, Wells J, Asherson P, Theobald D, Oliver B, et al. Attention deficit hyperactivity disorder and critical incidents in a Scottish prison population. *Personality and Individual Differences* 2009; 46(3): 265–9.

36. Young S, Misch P, Collins P, Gudjonsson G. Predictors of institutional behavioural disturbance and offending in the community among young offenders. *Journal of Forensic Psychiatry and Psychology* 2011; 22(1): 72–86.

37. Young S, Gudjonsson G, Ball S, Lam J. Attention deficit hyperactivity disorder (ADHD) in personality disordered offenders and the association with disruptive behavioural problems. *Journal of Forensic Psychiatry and Psychology* 2003; 14: 491–505.

38. Young S, Sedgwick O, Fridman M, Gudjonsson G, Hodgkins P, Lantigua M, et al. Co-morbid psychiatric disorders among incarcerated ADHD populations: a meta-analysis. *Psychological Medicine* 2015; 45(12): 2499–510.

39. McCarthy J, Chaplin E, Underwood L, Forrester A, Hayward H, Sabet J, et al. Characteristics of prisoners with neurodevelopmental disorders and difficulties. *Journal of Intellectual Disability Research* 2016; 60(3): 201–6.

40. Young S, González RA, Fridman M, Hodgkins P, Kim K, Gudjonsson GH. Health-related quality of life in prisoners with attention-deficit hyperactivity disorder and head injury. *BMC Psychiatry* 2018; 18(1): 209.

41. Young S, González RA, Mullens H, Mutch L, Malet-Lambert I, Gudjonsson GH. Neurodevelopmental disorders in prison inmates: comorbidity and combined associations with psychiatric symptoms and behavioural disturbance. *Psychiatry Research* 2018; 261: 109–15.

42. Hughes N, Williams W, Chitsabesan P, Walesby R, Mounce L. Nobody made the connection: neurodisability in the youth justice system. 2012. Available at: http://psychology.exeter.ac.uk/docu ments/Nobody_made_the_connection_ Neurodevelopment%20Report_OCC_Oc tober2012.pdf.

43. Pérez-Pedrogo C, Martínez-Taboas A, Gonzélez RA, Caraballo JN, Albizu-García CE. Sex differences in traumatic events and psychiatric morbidity associated to probable posttraumatic stress disorder among Latino prisoners. *Psychiatry Research* 2018; 265: 208–14.

44. Mordre M, Groholt B, Kjelsberg E, Sandstad B, Myhre AM. The impact of ADHD and conduct disorder in childhood on adult delinquency: A 30 years follow-up study using official crime records. *BMC Psychiatry* 2011; 11(1): 57.

45. Satterfield JH, Faller KJ, Crinella FM, Schell AM, Swanson JM, Homer LD. A 30-year prospective follow-up study of hyperactive boys with conduct problems: adult criminality. *Journal of the American Academy of Child and Adolescent Psychiatry* 2007; 46(5): 601–10.

46. Lundström S, Forsman M, Larsson H, Kerekes N, Serlachius E, Långström N, et al. Childhood neurodevelopmental disorders and violent criminality: a sibling control study. *Journal of Autism and Developmental Disorders* 2014; 44(11): 2707–16.

47. Gunter TD, Arndt S, Riggins-Caspers K, Wenman G, Cadoret RJ. Adult outcomes of attention deficit hyperactivity disorder and conduct disorder: are the risks independent or additive? *Annals of Clinical Psychiatry* 2006; 18(4): 233–7.

48. Sibley MH, Pelham WE, Molina BSG, Gnagy EM, Waschbusch DA, Biswas A, et al. The delinquency outcomes of boys with ADHD with and without comorbidity. *Journal of Abnormal Child Psychology* 2011; 39(1): 21–32.

49. Pratt TC, Cullen FT, Blevins KR, Daigle L, Unnever JD. The relationship of attention deficit hyperactivity disorder to crime and delinquency: a meta-analysis. *International Journal of Police Science and Management* 2002; 4(4): 344–60.

50. Moffitt TE. Adolescence-limited and life-course-persistent antisocial behavior: a developmental taxonomy. *Psychological Review* 1993; 100(4): 674–701.

51. Barkley RA, Fischer M, Smallish L, Fletcher K. Young adult follow-up of hyperactive children: antisocial activities and drug use. *Journal of Child Psychology and Psychiatry* 2004; 45(2): 195–211.

52. Harpin V, Young S. The challenge of ADHD and youth offending. *Cutting Edge Psychiatry in Practice* 2012; 2: 138–43.

53. Gudjonsson GH, Sigurdsson JF, Sigfusdottir ID, Asgeirsdottir BB, González RA, Young S. A national epidemiological study investigating risk factors for police interrogation and false confession among juveniles and young persons. *Social Psychiatry and Psychiatric Epidemiology* 2016; 51(3): 359–67.

54. Gudjonsson GH. *The Psychology of False Confessions: Forty Years of Science and Practice*. John Wiley & Sons, 2018.

55. Gottfredson MR, Hirschi T. *A General Theory of Crime*. Stanford University Press, 1990.

56. Engelhardt PE, Nobes G, Pischedda S. The relationship between adult symptoms of attention-deficit/hyperactivity disorder and criminogenic cognitions. *Brain Sciences* 2019; 9(6): 128. Doi: 10.3390/ brainsci9060128.

57. Walters G. *The Criminal Lifestyle: Patterns of Serious Criminal Conduct*. SAGE Publications, 1990.

58. Retz W, Rösler M. The relation of ADHD and violent aggression: what can we learn from epidemiological and genetic studies? *International Journal of Law and Psychiatry* 2009; 32(4): 235–43.

59. Román-Ithier JC, González RA, Vélez-Pastrana MC, González-Tejera GM, Albizu-García CE. Attention deficit hyperactivity disorder symptoms, type of offending and recidivism in a prison population: the role of substance dependence. *Criminal Behaviour and Mental Health* 2017; 27(5): 443–456.

60. Lane CJ, Chong MD. A hard pill to swallow: the need to identify and treat ADHD to reduce sufferers' potential involvement in the criminal justice system. *James Cook University Law Review* 2019; 25: 119–36.

61. Daley D, Jacobsen RH, Lange AM, Sørensen A, Walldorf J. The economic burden of adult attention deficit hyperactivity disorder: a sibling comparison cost analysis. *European Psychiatry* 2019; 61: 41–8.

62. Deloitte Access Economics. The social and economic costs of ADHD in Australia: report prepared for the Australian ADHD Professionals Association. 2019. Available at: www2.deloitte.com/au/en/pages/eco nomics/articles/social-economic-costs-adhd-Australia.html.

63. Young S, González RA, Fridman M, Hodgkins P, Kim K, Gudjonsson GH. The economic consequences of attention-deficit hyperactivity disorder in the Scottish prison system. *BMC Psychiatry* 2018; 18(1): 210.

64. Young S, Cocallis KM. Attention deficit hyperactivity disorder (ADHD) in the prison system. *Current Psychiatry Reports* 2019; 21(6): 41–3.

65. Freriks RD, Mierau JO, van der Schans J, Groenman AP, Hoekstra PJ, Postma MJ, et al. Cost-effectiveness of treatments in children with attention-deficit/hyperactivity disorder: a continuous-time Markov modelling approach. *MDM Policy and Practice* 2019; 4(2): 2381468319867629.

66. Ginsberg Y, Lindefors N. Methylphenidate treatment of adult male prison inmates with attention-deficit hyperactivity disorder: randomised double-blind placebo-controlled trial with open-label extension. *British Journal of Psychiatry* 2012; 200(1): 68–73.

67. Lichtenstein P, Halldner L, Zetterqvist J, Sjölander A, Serlachius E, Fazel S, et al. Medication for attention deficit-hyperactivity disorder and criminality. *New England Journal of Medicine* 2012; 367(21): 2006–14.

68. Chang Z, Lichtenstein P, Långström N, Larsson H, Fazel S. Association between prescription of major psychotropic medications and violent reoffending after prison release. *JAMA* 2016; 316(17): 1798–807.

69. Konstenius M, Jayaram-Lindström N, Guterstam J, Beck O, Philips B, Franck J. Methylphenidate for attention deficit hyperactivity disorder and drug relapse in criminal offenders with substance dependence: a 24-week randomized placebo-controlled trial. *Addiction* 2014; 109 (3): 440–9.

70. Burns KA. Commentary: the top ten reasons to limit prescription of controlled substances in prisons. *Journal of the American Academy of Psychiatry and the Law* 2009; 37(1): 50.

71. Appelbaum KL. Attention deficit hyperactivity disorder in prison: a treatment protocol. *Journal of the American Academy of Psychiatry and the Law* 2009; 37(1): 45–9.

72. Hall RC, Myers WC. Challenges and limitations to treating ADHD in incarcerated populations. *Journal of the American Academy of Psychiatry and the Law* 2016; 44(2): 164–70.

73. Pilkinton PD, Pilkinton JC. Prescribing in prison: minimizing psychotropic drug diversion in correctional practice. *Journal of Correctional Health Care* 2014; 20(2): 95–104.

74. Shaw M, Hodgkins P, Caci H, Young S, Kahle J, Woods AG, et al. A systematic review and analysis of long-term outcomes in attention deficit hyperactivity disorder: effects of treatment and non-treatment. *BMC Medicine* 2012; 10: 99.

75. Arnold LE, Hodgkins P, Caci H, Kahle J, Young S. Effect of treatment modality on long-term outcomes in attention-deficit/hyperactivity disorder:

a systematic review. *PLOS One* 2015; 10 (2): e0116407.

76. Emilsson B, Gudjonsson G, Sigurdsson JF, Baldursson G, Einarsson E, Olafsdottir H, et al. Cognitive behaviour therapy in medication-treated adults with ADHD and persistent symptoms: a randomized controlled trial. *BMC Psychiatry* 2011; 11 (1): 116.

77. Young S, Emilsson B, Sigurdsson JF, Khondoker M, Philipp-Wiegmann F, Baldursson G, et al. A randomized controlled trial reporting functional outcomes of cognitive–behavioural therapy in medication-treated adults with ADHD and comorbid psychopathology. *European Archives of Psychiatry and Clinical Neuroscience* 2017; 267(3): 267–76.

78. Ramboll and The National Board of Social Services. Better help for young people and adults with ADHD and corresponding difficulties: final evaluation report. 2020. Available at: www.psychology-services.uk.com/danish-report-on-r-r2-adhd.htm.

Overview of Offenders with Autism Spectrum Disorder

David Murphy and Clare S. Allely

Introduction

Autism spectrum disorder (ASD) encompasses a range of neurodevelopmental disorders that are characterised by reciprocal social interaction and communication impairments and restricted repetitive behaviours [1]. The *Diagnostic and Statistical Manual of Mental Disorders*, 5th edition (DSM-5) [2] categorises two core domains of impairment in ASD (it was three core areas of impairment in the previous edition, published in 2000), which vary across individuals, symptoms and levels of severity: (1) 'persistent deficits in social communication and social interaction' and (2) 'restricted, repetitive patterns of behaviour, interests or activities' [2]. There is just a single category of ASD as the DSM-5 no longer distinguishes subtypes of ASD, such as autistic disorder and Asperger syndrome. Brugha and colleagues [3] estimated that the prevalence of ASD in adults living in the community in England was 9.8 per 1,000. Although not outlined in any of the diagnostic criteria, individuals with ASD also tend to have a specific thinking style characterised by a literal interpretation of information, a tendency to focus on details at the expense of appreciating the 'bigger picture' and an egocentric perspective where other views are not considered or appreciated. Sensory sensitivities are also very common, as are emotional regulation difficulties and comorbid mood or anxiety disorders, other neurodevelopmental disorders (such as attention deficit hyperactivity disorder) and psychiatric disorders.

Outcomes of individuals with ASD vary. While many individuals will go on to have successful careers and relationships, some do not, and for a range of reasons become involved in some form of offending resulting in contact with the criminal justice system. The prevalence and reasons for specific offence behaviours are explored in other chapters of this book but, overall, offending behaviour is typically associated with a combination of the difficulties associated with having ASD, within a specific set of social and environmental circumstances. The latter is often characterised by stresses and demands that fall beyond an individual's ability to deal with them, whether that be social naïvety (such as being used by more able peers or failing to recognise that an action or behaviour is against the law), poor emotional regulation skills and poor social communication skills, failing to appreciate the impact of behaviour on self and others, as well as perhaps becoming preoccupied with specific details at the expense of appreciating the bigger picture. For some, psychiatric comorbidity may also be a factor in offending such as those acting on delusional ideas or auditory hallucinations [4] as well as, for others, the presence of a personality disorder or psychopathy [5]. However, addressing the difficulties and needs of individuals with ASD within the criminal justice system remains variable and poorly understood.

Following an outline of the prevalence of individuals with ASD in the criminal justice system and some issues relevant to understanding the assessment of risk for offending, this chapter explores the role of the media in shaping public perception of ASD and offending, including potentially influencing views of culpability. The influence of government legislation in shaping services and meeting needs is also discussed.

How Many Individuals with ASD Enter the Criminal Justice System?

While there is no evidence to suggest that individuals with ASD are more likely to offend than individuals without ASD and may actually more likely be victims of a crime [6], clearly some individuals do engage in behaviours that result in contact with the criminal justice system. However, the presence of numerous methodological differences between studies, such as how an individual's ASD was determined (such as being based on a self-report questionnaire or a detailed diagnostic assessment), and many studies being completed in a single setting restrict any view on how many individuals with ASD come into contact with the criminal justice system. There is also the issue that an individual may be involved with the criminal justice system at an early stage, but go no further. For example, within the UK, some illustration of the number of individuals with ASD who come into contact with the criminal justice system comes from an examination of adults with ASD across 98 different services in South Wales [7]. Within these services, 126 individuals were identified, 33 of whom had offended or whose behaviour could have resulted in contact with the criminal justice system. Among these, seven were reported as not having been processed/arrested, five had been imprisoned, one had been hospitalised and three were reported as living in the community. Within the USA, a study of adolescents and young adults ($n = 11, 270$, with 920 having ASD) also found that, by the age of 21 years, 20% reported being stopped and questioned by the police, with 5% being arrested [8]. Both these studies suggest that, in terms of obtaining an estimate of how many individuals with ASD have contact with the criminal justice system as a result of some form of offending, there is the need for greater understanding of the decision-making process of why some 'offenders' with ASD enter the criminal justice system and others do not.

In terms of prevalence within forensic settings, current evidence suggests that although individuals with ASD represent a relatively small proportion of the total number of individuals in such settings, they are likely to be over-represented relative to the general 1% prevalence of ASD within the general population [9, 10]. For example, within UK prisons, one study of a London prison identified high levels of ASD traits among male prisoners [11]. Of the 186 prisoners approached, 10% were said to be screened positive or displaying significant autistic traits and within this group 2% were said to fulfil the diagnostic criteria for ASD following a detailed diagnostic assessment. Although likely to be an underestimate, based on this 2% estimate, it was suggested that it was likely that approximately 1,600 men and 120 women may have ASD within prisons. It was also suggested that the prevalence of ASD was likely to vary between different types of prisons, such as whether they are for remand or sentenced prisoners, high secure, mainstream or open prisons [12]. Internationally, a similar over-representation estimate was found in a screen of a US prison [13]. Outside of prison settings, such as in community probation services, it has been found that while individuals with ASD represented a small proportion of the total case load, they were also disproportionately represented relative to general population prevalence of ASD [14].

Perhaps because of the relative stability of the patient population, high secure psychiatric care (HSPC) within the UK has been the focus of early prevalence estimates. For example, in a frequently cited study of one HSPC hospital it was found, after an initial patient file screen to identify possible cases followed by interviews with primary nurses and obtaining patients consent, that from 17 individuals identified (from a total 392 male patients), 6 met the diagnostic criteria for Asperger syndrome (representing a prevalence rate of 1.5%). An additional three possible cases were identified raising the prevalence rate to 2.3%. The conclusion from this study was that Asperger syndrome was over-represented compared to the general population prevalence rate [15]. A significant limitation of this study, however, was that the diagnostic process was not based on contemporary best practice. It is also important to highlight that not only the admission criteria to HSPC have changed since this study was completed but also that the current total patient population in such settings is approximately two-thirds of that examined by Scragg and Shah [15]. Similar points can also be put against another study including all three of England's HSPC hospitals, where a total of 31 individuals with ASD were identified (1.6% of total patient population) [16]. Although the prevalence of ASD was not the focus of another study, an examination of incompatibilities and seclusions of patients with ASD in one HSPC hospital found approximately 4% of patients (out of a total of 198) with this diagnosis [17]. In contrast, a survey of a number of forensic and specialist settings in Scotland found the prevalence of ASD to be low (around 0.93% in prisons, 0.46% in secure units and 1.39% in mental health units). However, Myers also noted that many prison staff expressed the view that the number of individuals formally identified probably fell short of the actual number [18].

Another issue likely to skew the estimates of many studies and result in a significant number of undiagnosed individuals within different parts of the criminal justice system is the refusal to participate in any assessment. Indeed, it likely that a sizeable number of individuals with ASD in the system remain undiagnosed because they decline to engage with a formal assessment and where other co-occurring difficulties or psychiatric disorder mask a presentation. To date, there is also a significant absence of research examining the prevalence of offenders with ASD in terms of age, socio-economic factors and ethnicity. However, clinical experience of one author suggests that, while individuals admitted to one HSPC hospital come from a range of ethnic groups and socio-economic backgrounds, many individuals with ASD from lower socio-economic backgrounds receive a diagnosis in adulthood rather than childhood, and often not until their involvement with the criminal justice system. In terms of gaps in knowledge, while awareness is growing, there is also very little research to date examining the prevalence of women with ASD who enter the criminal justice system.

Risk and Protective Factors

There are a limited number of studies examining the application of conventional risk-assessment aids with offenders who have ASD. There is also a significant absence of research examining whether female offenders with ASD have additional needs to be considered when assessing risk for future offending, as well as the potential role of any cultural or ethnicity factors. However, some studies and the consensus opinion of most clinicians suggest that any formal risk assessment of an individual with ASD, regardless of offence type, needs to consider their strengths and difficulties associated with having ASD. The presence of any protective factors such as social inclusion, 'autism friendly' environments and pharmacological management of any comorbid psychiatric disorder also needs to be established [19]. A failure to assess and consider all these factors is likely to result in an inadequate formulation of an individual's difficulties and ultimately poor risk management plans. In terms of risk management, the most effective approach also needs to be collaborative with the individual, involve the family where possible, as well as be multidisciplinary and multi-agency. Other legal channels may also have to be established, such as those restricting an individual's access to some online material. Risk assessments for individuals who have ASD continue to develop, including exploring the application of existing risk measures with individuals who have ASD, as well as the evolution of some specific ASD risk tools. Within secure settings, the application of new technologies such as using virtual reality [20], with its potential to simulate many scenarios and ability to manipulate variables, will also play an increasingly important role in both assessing risk and delivering therapeutic interventions aimed at reducing risk. For a detailed discussion on risk assessment with individuals with ASD, see Chapter 14.

Influence of the Media

The influence of the media in shaping the public perception of ASD and offending should not be underestimated. However, while there is evidence to suggest that the media is important in influencing public attitudes about disability and mental health conditions [21] and can be more powerful in shaping beliefs than actual experience [22], there remains very little examination of how offenders (charged or convicted) with ASD are portrayed in the media. There is, though, a general view held by many that the portrayal in the media of individuals with ASD who offend is often distorted and can lead to public stigma, stereotyping and misunderstanding. For example, in an examination of the UK newspapers between 1999 and 2008, three categories of stories were identified, including the 'burden' of autism, 'sensationalising' and 'misconceptions and misuse of a label'. It was suggested that ASD tended to be portrayed in a rather standardised and homogenised way, which failed to recognise the diversity of the spectrum [23]. In another study examining Finnish newspapers from 1990 to 2016, it was found that while the majority of newspapers (around two-thirds) framed autism in a clinical and educational way, the portrayal of offenders with autism was less positive and tended to reinforce some form of association between ASD and violent behaviour [24].

In terms of potentially influencing the criminal justice system, there is recognition that the media's portrayal of individuals with ASD who offend can also influence the attitudes, views and decision making of those working in the legal profession, as well as members of the jury. For example, in a study of telephone interviews with 21 California Superior Court judges, asking about their views on how individuals with ASD who offend are portrayed in the media, it was found that while the majority of judges expressed the view that the media portrayed ASD in both positive and negative ways, they felt that the coverage of ASD and criminality was often misleading and created a false association between ASD and violent behaviour [25]. The potential influence of the media in reinforcing the perception of a link between ASD and offending was also found in an experimental study with students, where an 'offending' vignette was more likely to reinforce the perception of guilt than those that had 'no diagnostic information' or was more 'educational' in content [26]. However, while offenders with ASD who commit unusual or violent offences attract considerable media attention, it is unclear whether this is always negative. For example, Gary McKinnon and Laurie Love [27, 28], both UK citizens and charged with computer hacking related offences within the USA, were portrayed by the UK media in a sympathetic way, which in both cases resulted in an extradition request to the USA being blocked. This contrasts markedly with that of Jonty Bravery, an 18-year-old man with ASD convicted of the attempted murder of a child by throwing him off the roof gallery of the Tate Modern in London and where he it could be argued that was portrayed in an unsympathetic and negative light [29]. Requiring more detailed examination, it seems likely that the portrayal of offenders with ASD by the media is determined by a number of factors, such as offence type, as well as intent and victim characteristics. Of significance is also the presence of some media guidelines as to how best describe individuals with ASD promoted by the autism charities Autistica [30] and the National Autistic Society [31].

Influence of Government Policy

Within the UK, some key government legislation has impacted and continues to influence how offenders with ASD enter and are managed within the criminal justice system. For example, the Autism Act 2009 [32], the Think Autism Strategy [33], the UK's Department of Health and Social Care adult autism strategy [34] and transforming care [35] have placed ASD on the agenda of many institutions and established a duty to provide appropriate diagnostic assessments and staff training. There has also been a proposal that training in autism should be mandatory for all care staff within the UK's National Health Service (NHS), including those within secure psychiatric settings [36]. Although not specifically directed at ASD, the Equality Act 2010 [37] has also had some influence on how individuals with ASD are treated by the criminal justice system. In terms of the sentencing and release of offenders with ASD, a House of Commons briefing paper, the smart sentencing white paper [38] and some sentencing guidelines produced by the Sentencing Council [39] are also beginning to address and support the specific needs of this group of offenders at all levels of the criminal justice system. In addition to encouraging ASD awareness among police services, there is the aim that judges and magistrates take an informed, fair and consistent approach to the sentencing of individuals with ASD. Beyond the courts, there are also recommendations for many probation services and prisons to achieve accreditation with the National Autistic Society. Of significance is the recent 'call for evidence' by the Ministry of Justice to obtain more information on the prevalence and current national provision for offenders with neurodivergent conditions, including individuals with ASD.

Conclusion

Although individuals with ASD comprise a relatively small proportion of the overall offender population, they are likely to be over-represented relative to the general prevalence of ASD in the population. Current prevalence studies are also likely to reflect an underestimate of the actual number of individuals with ASD in many secure settings. The understanding of women and other demographic and ethnic characteristics of offenders with ASD also remains poorly understood. As a group of individuals, offenders with ASD also present with diverse difficulties, risk management issues and needs that can challenge the mainstream criminal justice system and specific services, whether that be a custodial environment or a secure psychiatric setting. The media also plays a role in influencing the public perception of individuals with ASD who offend and how they are subsequently treated within the criminal justice system. The influence of UK government legislation in how individuals with ASD are assessed and managed within the criminal justice system has also been highlighted. While some progress has been made in how individuals with ASD are viewed and managed within the criminal justice system, as for all individuals falling within the neurodiversity spectrum there remains a need for a more informed and joined-up approach to how individual difficulties and needs are best addressed.

References

1. Wing L. Asperger's syndrome: management requires diagnosis. *Journal of Forensic Psychiatry* 1997: 2(8): 253–7.

2. American Psychiatric Association. *Diagnostic and Statistical Manual of Mental Disorders, 5th edition: DSM-5.* American Psychiatric Association, 2013.

3. Brugha TS, McManus S, Bankart J, Scott F, Purdon S, Smith J, Meltzer H. Epidemiology of autism spectrum disorders in adults in the community in England. *Archives of General Psychiatry* 2011; 68(5): 459–65.

4. Wachtel L, Shorter E. Autism plus psychosis: A 'one-two punch' risk for tragic violence? *Medical Hypotheses* 2013; 81(3): 404–9.

5. Rogers J, Viding E, Blair J, Frith U, Happé F. Autism spectrum disorder and psychopathy: shared cognitive underpinnings or double hit? *Psychological Medicine* 2006; 36: 1789–98.

6. King C, Murphy G. A systematic review of people with autism spectrum disorder and the criminal justice system. *Journal of Autism and Developmental Disorders* 2014); 44(11): 2717–33.

7. Allen D, Evans C, Hider A, Hawkins S, Peckett H, Morgan H. Offending behaviour in adults with Asperger syndrome. *Journal of Autism and Developmental Disorders* 2008; 38(4): 748–58.

8. Rava J, Shattuck P, Rast J, Roux A. The prevalence and correlates of involvement in the criminal justice system among youth on the autism spectrum. *Journal of Autism and Developmental Disorders* 2017; 47(2): 340–6.

9. Baird G, Simonoff S, Pickles A, Chandler S, Loucas T, Meldrum D, Charman T. Prevalence of disorders of the autism spectrum in a population cohort of children in South Thames: the special needs and autism project (SNAP). *Lancet* 2006; 368 (9531): 210–15.

10. Maenner M, Shaw K, Baio J, Washington A. Prevalence of autism spectrum disorder among children aged 8 years: ADDM network, 11 sites, United States. *Morbidly and Mortality Weekly Report* 2016; 69 (4): 1–12.

11. Underwood L, McCarthy J, Chaplin E, Forrester A, Mills R, Murphy D. Autism spectrum disorder among prisoners. *Advances in Autism* 2016; 2(3): 106–17.

12. Underwood L, Forrester A, Chaplin E, McCarthy J. Prisoners with neurodevelopmental disorders. *Journal of Intellectual Disabilities and Offending Behaviour* 2013; 4(1/2): 17–23.

13. Fazio RL, Pietz CA, Denney RL. An estimate of the prevalence of autism spectrum disorders in an incarcerated population. *Open Access Journal of Forensic Psychology* 2012; 4: 69–80.

14. Bates A. The prevalence of autistic spectrum conditions in a community offender sample. *Advances in Autism* 2016; 2(4): 191–200.

15. Scragg P, Shah A. Prevalence of Asperger's syndrome in a secure hospital. *British Journal of Psychiatry* 1994; 165: 679–82.

16. Hare D, Gould J, Mill, R, Wing L. A preliminary study of individuals with autistic spectrum disorders in three special hospitals in England. National Autistic Society. 1999. Available at: www.aspires-relationships.com/3hospitals.pdf.

17. Murphy D, Bush EL, Puzzo I. Incompatibilities and seclusions among

individuals with an autism spectrum disorder detained in high secure psychiatric care. *Journal of Intellectual Disabilities and Offending Behaviour* 2017; 8(4): 188–200.

18. Myers F. On the borderline? People with learning disabilities and or autistic spectrum disorders in secure, forensic and other specialist settings. 2004. Available at: http://docs.scie-socialcareonline.org.uk/fulltext/asdsecure.pdf.

19. Kelbrick M, Radley J. Forensic rehabilitation in Asperger syndrome: a case report. *Journal of Intellectual Disabilities and Offending Behaviour* 2013; 4(1–2): https://doi.org/10.1108/jidob.2013.55404aaa.001.

20. Benbouriche M, Nolet K, Trottier D, Renaud P. Virtual reality applications in forensic psychiatry. In Proceedings of the Virtual Reality International Conference, Laval Virtual (VRIC' 14). April 9–11, 2014, Laval, France.

21. Lyons A. Examining media representations: benefits for health psychology. *Journal of Health Psychology* 2000; 5: 349–58.

22. Philo G. Changing media representations of mental health. *Psychiatric Bulletin Royal College Psychiatry* 1997; 21: 171–2.

23. Huw J, Jones R. Missing voices: representations of autism in British newspapers, 1999–2008. *British Journal of Learning Disabilities* 2010; 39(2): 98–104.

24. Pesonen H, Itkonen T, Saha M, Nordahl-Hansen A. Framing autism in newspaper media: an example from Finland. *Advances in Autism* 2020; DOI 10.1108/AIA-01-2020-0003.

25. Berryessa C. Judicial perceptions of media portrayals of offenders with high functioning autistic spectrum disorders. *International Journal of Criminology and Sociology* 2014; 3: 45–60.

26. Brewer N, Zoanetti J, Young R. The influence of media suggestions about links between criminality and autism spectrum disorder. *Autism* 2017; 21(1): 117–21.

27. McKinnon G. Theresa May saved my life: now she's the only hope for the Human Rights Act. *The Guardian* 2019, 15 November.

28. BBC News. Lauri Love case: hacking suspect wins extradition appeal. Available at: www.bbc.co.uk/news/uk-england-42946540.

29. BBC News. Jonty Bravery: Tate Modern balcony teen 'smiled' after attack. Available at: www.bbc.co.uk/news/uk-england-london-53177998.

30. Autistica. Media Communications Guide. Available at: www.autistica.org.uk/about-us/media-communications-guide.

31. National Autistic Society. How to talk and write about autism. Available at: www.autism.org.uk/what-we-do/help-and-support/how-to-talk-about-autism

32. Autism Act 2009. Available at: www.legislation.gov.uk/ukpga/2009/15/contents.

33. Think Autism: fulfilling and rewarding lives. The strategy for adults with autism in England: an update. (2014). Available at: Assets.publishing.service.gov.uk/government/uploads/system/uploads/attachment_data/file/299866/Autism_Strategy.pdf.

34. Department of Health and Social Care. Adult autism strategy: supporting its use. 2015. Available at: www.gov.uk/government/publications/adult-autism-strategy-statutory-guidance.

35. Department of Health and Social Care. 'Right to be heard': the government's response to the consultation on learning disability and autism training for health and care staff. 2019. Available at: https://assets.publishing.service.gov.uk/government/uploads/system/uploads/attachment_data/file/844356/autism-and-learning-disability-training-for-staff-consultation-response.pdf.

36. NHS England. Transforming care. Model service specifications supporting implementation of the service model. 2017. Available at: www.england.hns.uk / wp-content/uploads/2017/model-service-spec-2017.

37. Equality Act 2010. Available at: www.legislation.gov.uk/ukpga/2010/15.

38. Ministry of Justice. A smarter approach to sentencing. 2020. Available at: https://assets.publishing.service.gov.uk/government/uploads/system/uploads/attachment_data/file/918187/a-smarter-approach-to-sentencing.pdf.

39. Sentencing Council. Sentencing offenders with mental disorders, developmental disorders or neurological impairments. 2020. Available at: www.sentencingcouncil.org.uk/overarching-guides/magistrates-court/item/sentencing-offenders-with-mental-disorders-developmental-disorders-or-neurological-impairments/.

Associations between Autism Spectrum Disorder and Types of Offences

Clare S. Allely and David Murphy

Introduction

This chapter examines the literature relating to several different offences and their associations with neurodevelopmental disorders. Specifically, it explores the following types of offences: cybercrime (viewing of indecent child images and computer hacking/cyberdeviancy), violent offending (physical assault, mass shootings, arson or fire setting and terroristic behaviours) and sexual offending (sexual 'hands-on' offending and stalking behaviour). We explore how certain features or symptomology of autism spectrum disorder (ASD) can provide the context of vulnerability to engagement in these offending behaviours in a small subgroup of individuals with ASD.

Cybercrime

Viewing of Indecent Child Images

Some individuals may use the Internet for sexual education or to satisfy sexual needs because of a lack of sexual outlets with peers/friends. Many individuals with ASD have an average or above average intelligence while their social maturity can be comparable to that of someone much younger, which often leads them to be more interested and comfortable in befriending people who are much younger than them (they are at the same level as them socially and emotionally) [1]. Some individuals with ASD may be completely unaware that the viewing of indecent child images is actually a criminal offence. One reason that may contribute to this lack of awareness may be their impaired ability to recognise the facial expressions of the children in the material they are viewing. This impaired inability to recognise such expressions (such as fear or distress) has been well established in the empirical literature [2, 3]. Additionally, some individuals with ASD may inadvertently view indecent images of children due to their impaired ability to guess correctly the age of the individuals in the images. Also, the boundaries/distinction between an adult and a child can very often be unclear or blurry. Given that the legality and severity of the offence is determined by the age of the victims in the images being viewed by the defendant, this impaired ability to correctly guess age and the blurred boundaries between adult and child is important to consider [4–7].

Exploring sexuality on the Internet through child pornography is one way for some individuals with ASD to try to understand relationships and sexuality rather than being a precursor to sexual offending towards a minor. For some individuals with ASD, the desire for this material, as with many preoccupations and interests that individuals with ASD have, can end up being markedly excessive and compulsive [8]. Indeed, there are a significant number of cases of individuals with ASD who have been found to have amassed substantially large collections of pornographic material (e.g., involving children) due to the ritualistic nature of ASD. Very often in these cases, the individual with ASD has hundreds and hundreds of files which have never even been opened. Some of the broader issues, such as where and how they got those files, who else might be able to access them and what the consequences (and impact on) are for the minors in the images they are viewing are issues which many individuals with ASD who engage in this behaviour may be completely unaware of or fail to appreciate. Because individuals with ASD typically have a literal view of the world, they may not consider that something that is freely accessible online could be illegal [8]. The media also is saturated with marketing materials which show risky images of teenage models or images where older models have been made to look childlike. For individuals with ASD, these types of images can be confusing and challenging to discern as being illegal pornography [8]. Additionally, the viewing of sexual material that is extreme is not always a reflection of the presence of deviant sexuality. Rather it may be 'counterfeit deviance' (in other words, naïve curiosity) in individuals with ASD who engage in offending behaviour [4, 9].

Computer Hacking/Cyberdeviancy

There have been numerous high-profile cases and published case studies which suggest there may be some relationship between Asperger syndrome and cybercrime, in particular, computer hacking. One particularly high-profile example is the British computer hacker Gary McKinnon, who was accused of hacking into 97 United States military and NASA computers in 2001 [10]. Surprisingly, only a few studies have investigated the relationship between cybercrime or cyberdeviancy and ASD. Although some association has been found linking cybercrime and ASD [11], there was no evidence to support the notion that there is an over-representation of individuals with ASD who had committed cybercrime offences.

In order to investigate the relationship between ASD traits or characteristics and cyber deviancy (hacking, cyberbullying, identity theft and virus writing), Seigfried-Spellar and colleagues recruited a sample of 296 university undergraduate students who completed an internet-based anonymous survey, which measured self-reported computer deviant behaviour and features that are associated with Asperger syndrome (based on the Autism Spectrum Quotient (AQ) screening tool) [12]. Findings showed that 179 (60%) of the 296 university students who took part in the survey reported that they had been involved in computer deviant behaviour. However, of the 179 students only two (0.01%) reached the clinical threshold on the AQ. Additionally, it was found that, when compared to non-computer hackers, hackers did not exhibit higher scores on the AQ. Interestingly, when subtypes of cyber deviancy were examined, higher scores on the AQ were found in the virus writers, identity thieves and cyberbullies when compared to their computer non-deviant counterparts. Another interesting finding was that higher scores on the AQ and more impaired social skills, more impaired communication and poorer imagination were found in the individuals who engaged in hacking, identity theft, cyberbullying and virus writing when compared to all other individuals engaging in computer deviant behaviours.

In another investigation of the potential relationships between cyber-dependent crime and ASD, autistic-like traits, explicit social cognition and perceived interpersonal support, 290 internet users of which 194 were male and 96 were female (ages ranged from 14 to 74; mean age 24.24 years, standard deviation (SD) 9.25) took part in an online survey [13]. Of the 290 internet users who took part in this online survey, 23 self-reported that they had a diagnosis of ASD. The 290 individuals in the sample did not have a conviction or caution for cybercriminal activity. Participants were recruited through the University of Bath's participant databases containing computer science students and alumni. Additionally, computer science students in local schools were contacted, as was the 'Cyber Security Challenge'. This is an organisation which aims to promote the development of cyber-skilled individuals. These channels were used to recruit participants who had advanced digital skills. Findings from Payne and colleagues' study showed that there was an association between an increased risk of committing cyber-dependent crime and higher autistic-like traits. Specifically, the findings from this study revealed that a large proportion of the association (approximately 40% of the total effect) between scores on the AQ and cyber-dependent criminal activity is mediated by advanced digital skills. Findings also indicated that there was mediation by basic digital skills (about 23%) but not by perceived interpersonal support or explicit social cognition. It was likely that some participants would self-report that they had actually engaged in such behaviour, despite not having received a conviction or caution for cybercriminal activity. Findings revealed that 122 individuals (42%) reported having perpetrated 333 cyber-dependent crimes. Lastly, an ASD diagnosis was found to be associated with a decreased risk of engaging in cyber-dependent criminal activity [13].

Violent Offending

There are numerous single case reports or small case-series in the literature which describe individuals with ASD who have committed violent offences [14–29] or studies examining relatively small samples of males and females who are detained in high secure psychiatric hospitals [30, 31].

Numerous empirical studies have found no evidence that individuals with ASD are more at risk of being violent when compared to the general population [32–35]. However, it is important to consider how the unique features of ASD may contribute to violence. In other words, how some of the features of ASD may provide the context of vulnerability for engaging in offending behaviour. There are an increasing number of case studies in the literature involving individuals with ASD, which have described the way in which some of the unique features of ASD (including impaired social understanding and restricted empathy, lack of perspective taking, social naïvety, pursuit of special circumscribed interests, even more so when these comprise a morbid fascination with violence) may subsequently lead to violent offending behaviour in certain provocative situations [15, 24, 36, 37].

In their study, Woodbury-Smith and colleagues [38] compared the circumscribed interests of a group of 21 intellectually able 'offenders' with a diagnosis of ASD (18 males and 3 females; mean age 35.4 years, SD 11.6) to those of 23 individuals with no 'offending' history (20 males and 3 females; mean age 29.7, SD 7.9). Interests rated as having a 'violent' content were significantly more likely to be reported in the 'offenders'. In 29% of the sample Woodbury-Smith and colleagues identified that the 'index offence' appeared to be related to his or her interest(s). These findings indicate that a circumscribed interest which has a violent content (e.g., consisting of threat or harm to others) may increase the risk or vulnerability to engaging in offending behaviour in individuals with ASD [38]. Mawson and colleagues [22] described the case of a man who reported having violent fantasies and also an extensive interest in poisons. Additionally, he would assault women for 'idiosyncratic reasons'. In one instance, he struck a woman using a saw blade because she was wearing shorts. In another instance, he stabbed a woman with a screw driver because he disliked women drivers.

Mass Shootings

It has previously been suggested that it is not uncommon for school shootings and mass shootings to be perpetrated by individuals with neurodevelopmental disorders, who frequently exhibit warning signs in the weeks, months or even years leading up to their attack [39]. Allely and colleagues [40] used the 73 mass shooting events which were identified by Mother Jones (motherjones.com) in their database for their study, in order to avoid author bias in sample selection. This database included two mass shooting events, which were perpetrated by two individuals, resulting in a total of 75 mass shooter cases that were investigated. Information was found for 6 of the 75 mass shooter cases (8%) that referred to a formal diagnosis of ASD or where there was evidence of a strong suggestion of possible ASD made by family and friends. A further 16 cases (21% of the total sample) were identified where some suggestions of ASD traits (according to the authors of the study based on reports or articles published on the individual) were identified. These findings need to be treated with caution as an indication of ASD traits does not equate to a diagnosis. The study by Allely and colleagues is not suggesting that individuals with diagnosis of ASD are more likely to be perpetrators of extreme acts of violence like mass shootings. However, the findings indicate that there may exist a very small subgroup of individuals with a diagnosis of ASD who are more vulnerable to engaging in serious offending behaviour.

Additionally, in his theoretical paper, Lino Faccini [41] applied two different models in an attempt to understand the path to intended mass violence in the case of school shooter, Adam Lanza. The three factors of autism-based deficits, psychopathology and deficient psychosocial development were included in the 'path to intended violence' model in order to try to develop an understanding of the path to mass shooting in the very small number of individuals with a diagnosis of ASD who perpetrate such extreme acts of violence. According to Calhoun and Weston [42], the path to intended violence model consists of six behavioural stages including: holding a grievance (e.g., due to a perceived sense of injustice, a threat or loss, a need for fame, or revenge); ideation (believing violence to be the only option, sharing one's thoughts with others or modelling oneself after other assailants – such as high-profile mass shooters); research and planning (obtaining information on one's target, or stalking the target); preparations (obtaining one's costume, weapon(s), equipment, transportation or engaging in 'final act' behaviours); breach (assessing security levels, devising 'sneaky or covert approach'); and, finally, attack [43]. In order to demonstrate how the combination of the two models can be applied in order to try to understand the process which leads to someone perpetrating a mass shooting attack, Faccini (2016) used the case of the mass shooter, Adam Lanza. This model has also been applied to other contemporary mass shooters including Elliot Rodger, Anders Behring Breivik, Dylann Roof and Dean Allen Mellberg [44–47].

Arson or Fire Setting

The terms 'arson' and 'fire setting' are typically used when referring to deliberate acts of fire setting. The two terms are often used interchangeably in the literature but it is important to note the distinction between them. Arson is a 'restrictive legal term' [48, 49]. The term arsonist is used to describe an individual who has been convicted of the crime of arson. Fire setting refers to the deliberate setting of fires but there has been no conviction. There may be no conviction due to, for instance, the identity of the fire setter being unknown, the fire not being detected as being a deliberate act or the fire resulting in minimal damage [50].

Siponmaa and colleagues [51] conducted an interesting study which examined 126 individuals, aged 15–22 years, who had originally undergone evaluation in relation to serious, predominantly violent, criminal offending. In the initial diagnostic evaluation, two individuals who qualified for a pervasive developmental disorder (PDD) diagnosis during childhood were identified. Additional evaluations (which also included assessment for neuropsychiatric developmental disorders) found that 12% of the 126 individuals fulfilled the diagnostic criteria for pervasive developmental disorder not otherwise specified and 3% fulfilled the diagnostic criteria for Asperger syndrome). In the whole sample, a total of 16 individuals had committed arson (as a main or index crime). Of those who had been diagnosed with a pervasive developmental disorder, 10 (63%) had committed arson [51]. Additionally, Mouridsen and colleagues [34] carried out a study which investigated the prevalence and types of criminal behaviour. In their study, they compared a group of individuals with Asperger syndrome (n = 114) with a group of control participants (n = 342). Findings revealed that, in the group of individuals with Asperger syndrome, there was a higher prevalence of arson. Specifically, five individuals (four males and one female) had engaged in arson out of the 114 individuals with Asperger syndrome – all cases were identified as being intentional. There were no cases of arson in the control group. No history of previous convictions was found in three of the five cases of arson. Therefore, only cases of arson were identified as being statistically separate AS cases from the control group [34]. A preliminary study of individuals with ASD in three special hospitals in England was carried out by Hare and colleagues [30]. A total of 31 definite cases of ASD were identified from the information in hospital records. This group were compared to 31 individuals who formed an uncertain group – where there was a lack of sufficient information available to make a clear diagnosis of an ASD and/or diagnostic criteria were only partially met [30]. There were a total of 215 index offences. Findings from this study revealed that there were higher numbers of individuals in the ASD group and the uncertain group who had arson as an index offence (16% in each case, both n = 5) compared to 5% (n = 8) who had arson as an index offence in the non-autistic group.

Lastly, there are some features of ASD that can provide the context of vulnerability to engaging in arson or fire-setting behaviour. Some of the key symptoms include: a lack of understanding and appreciation of the possible harmful consequences of fire setting (e.g., damage to property, injury or death); considering fire setting as being a means to resolve issues; impaired victim empathy; and a preoccupation and special interest in fire and fire setting. Freckelton and List [52] have argued that often, in the arsonist with ASD, there is an obsessive preoccupation and interest with 'flames, cinders, colours and heat' rather than being any malicious intention to damage property, kill or cause harm or danger to others [52]. It is the fire itself which serves a psychological function for the fire setter with ASD [53, 54].

Terroristic Behaviours

Research carried out to date has not found evidence for an association between ASD and terrorism in the general population [55, 56]. However, when terrorist acts are planned or executed by individuals with ASD, it is crucial that there is 'an understanding of the individual's autistic functioning and how it may contextualise factors that push them towards terrorism and aspects of terrorism that may pull them in, in order to manage and reduce risk' ([56], p. 926). There has been research which is attempting to highlight how ASD can 'contextualise vulnerability and risk' [55, 56]. It is important that any work carried out with individuals with ASD who are vulnerable to extremism or have perpetrated acts of terrorism (herein referred to as 'terrorism' risk or vulnerability) needs to be informed by a nuanced understanding of the various facets of ASD (as well as high functioning autism) in addition to the complex dynamics of radicalisation and pathways to extremist causes/ groups and terrorist offending [56–61]. In a recent paper, Al-Attar [56] outlined and examined seven facets of ASD that may have different functional links with push and pull factors to terrorism:

Facet 1: circumscribed interests

Facet 2: rich vivid fantasy and impaired social imagination

Facet 3: need for order, rules, rituals, routine and predictability

Facet 4: obsessionality, repetition and collecting

Facet 5: social interaction and communication difficulties

Facet 6: cognitive styles

Facet 7: sensory processing.

Al-Attar [56] points out that all of these facets 'do not map onto discrete diagnostic symptoms or profiles but are a mixture of diagnostic and research-evidenced correlates of ASD, which have been postulated to contextualise risk and protection in offenders with ASD' [56–62]. Each of the seven facets is very briefly reviewed below.

Facet 1: Circumscribed Interests

Restricted or circumscribed interests may develop in any topic, even 'shocking' topics such as terrorism [56, 61, 62]. Restricted or circumscribed interests may also develop in technical topics. Technical topics appeal to a brain that naturally processes details, facts and theories. Some of these technical topics may be explosives, hacking and conspiracy theories [62]. For instance, a restrictive interest in explosives involves the chemical properties, etc. of the explosives. Individuals with ASD may collect the different chemicals and make all different types of explosive devices but not necessarily with the intent to use in a malicious way.

Facet 2: Rich Vivid Fantasy and Impaired Social Imagination

Al-Attar highlights that restricted interests and preoccupations may be expressed through vivid, typically visual, fantasy. Strong visual and rote memory coupled with an impaired social imagination and context blindness can be exhibited in some individuals with ASD [63]. Given this, the contents of their fantasy life tends to be derived from what they have seen and heard both offline and online in a direct and literal way. They tend to make minimal modifications to the fantasies in order to make the content realistic or related to their own life [57–62]. In the fantasies, the themes that occur may hold certain functions or general functions for the individual. An example of a certain function may be revenge or violent fantasies, which release anger or provide the individual with a sense of empower-ment against those who have perpetrated injustices towards them. An example of a general function may be to provide the individual with intellectual stimulation and excitement [56].

Facet 3:   Need for Order, Rules, Rituals, Routine and Predictability

Many individuals with ASD have a strong need for predictability and routine. They have a tendency to seek these features in their lives and rigidly adhere to rules. Unpredictability or loss of routine and order can lead to confusion, anxiety and distress. In some individuals with ASD, research indicates that aggression and offending behaviour may be related to unpredictability or loss of order [60]. For individuals with ASD, the social world can be unpredictable and extremist groups/causes that offer order and predictability may be intuitively appealing. Indeed, it is common for terrorist groups to brand themselves as 'organised, systematic and orderly' [56, p. 935].

Facet 4:   Obsessionality, Repetition and Collecting

Interests and preoccupations, in some individuals with ASD, may become obsessional in nature, with the individual pursuing the interest or preoccupation in a repetitive manner and in a pedantic detail [64]. Relating to terroristic behaviour, the individual may collate significant quantities of information/data relating to terrorism (it could be the terrorist group/cause or target). Additionally, they may also watch propaganda videos repeatedly, make terroristic items (such as improvised explosive devices) or engage in the pursuit of individuals who are related to terrorism. Under terrorism legislation, such activities/behaviours may constitute unlawful behaviour. The preoccupational interest in the terrorism-related material would also be considered evidence of an intense commitment to terrorism. However, the engagement in each act (e.g., watching a propaganda video) does not always indicate that there is a 'broader or longer-term moral or operational objective' [56, p. 937]. Al-Attar stresses that this does not in any way suggest that their behaviour is in some way less dangerous or harmful, rather that it is more accurate to see this behaviour as 'being driven or at least accentuated by obsessionality, repetition, pedantry for detail and compulsive collecting/pursuit, as opposed to evidence of broader or greater ideological objectives or greater operational involvement' [57]. For instance, an individual with ASD may have a preoccupation with improvised explosive devices and possess a number of them, which they made and are collecting. However, this behaviour may not be driven by any malicious intent or with the intention to use to harm or kill others. Rather, this particular terroristic behaviour may be driven by the individual's ASD-related preoccupation with chemicals, etc.

Facet 5:   Social Interaction and Communication Difficulties

Individuals with ASD exhibit a number of social communication impairments [65, 66]. Their ability to navigate the complex social world can be extremely challenging and exhausting. As a result, they may become withdrawn and be socially isolated and anxious. For many of these individuals, the online world provides them a safe place to spend their time. This environment feels predictable, they can choose when to start and end the online interactions, there is the absence of the social and sensory overload associated with physical social environments and, also, communication is devoid of subtle social cues; it is scripted, rote learnt and visual. Others online may validate them by positive comments regarding their strong online communication skills (e.g., in writing, detailed information recall and rote learning of scripts). The online space is also a place where the individual can communicate with like-minded individuals – individuals who share their interests, views, etc. – providing them with a social companionship and sense of belonging. Throughout their life, their social and communication impairments may have contributed to their experience of social adversities (e.g., bullying, lack of friendships and intimacy, social humiliation) which may subsequently lead to distress, resentment and anger. This can accumulate and fester for some time and, subsequently, leads to push factors towards revengeful ideologies and groups, including terrorism, political/celebrity assassinations, mass shootings, etc. [56].

Facet 6: Cognitive Styles

Research has indicated that ASD has been associated with numerous neurocognitive profiles. However, regarding their neuropsychological profiles, individuals with a diagnosis of ASD are extremely heterogeneous and an individual with ASD may even perform differently at various times and on different tasks [67]. Individuals with ASD have a profile of both strengths and weaknesses, and professionals are recommended to identify the profile for each individual with ASD on a case-by-case basis. Al-Attar [56] outlined four elements or features of neurocognitive functioning which may contribute to the push and pull factors. These four elements are briefly outlined in turn below.

- Theory of mind: The ability to understand how others think/feel when this differs from our own perspective is reliant on the theory of mind. This includes the ability to understand the desires, intentions and beliefs of others.
- Central coherence: Individuals with ASD often 'overfocus' on fine detail or strong 'local coherence', which is coupled with the tendency to miss the bigger picture or weak 'central coherence' [68, 69]. Weak central coherence can impair the ability for an individual to recognise the links between events and between one's own behaviour and the consequences [70].
- Systemising: A strong tendency towards systemising can be found in individuals with ASD. Individuals who are high in systemising tend to process and recognise the world around them (including the social world) and information as systems, facts and categories. This is coupled with an impaired ability to empathise and to understand the social and emotional nuances of events or the world more generally [71] (see Milton [72] for discussions around the double-empathy problem in autism). This may increase the need that the individual has 'for a logical world whereby people and events can be ordered into systems, categories, hierarchies, theories and facts and make the social and emotional aspects of the world and behaviour confusing and unpredictable' [56, p. 942].
- Attention switching: An impaired attention-switching ability can be displayed in individuals with ASD. This impairment can have a negative impact on their mental flexibility and ability to shift their attention from one topic/idea to another [70], which may impact to some degree on the individual's hyperfocus and fixation, particularly when they develop an interest or preoccupation [56].

Facet 7: Sensory Processing

Many individuals with a diagnosis of ASD experience differences in processing sensory information across the range of modalities including sound, sight, touch and smell [73]. Al-Attar highlights that sensory hypersensitivity may contribute to negative experiences and the loss of positive opportunities that may lead to success. This may indirectly serve as a push into terrorist involvement or behaviour if it were to aggravate or exacerbate grievance, anger and feelings of injustice (real or imagined). Terrorist propaganda and materials may have sensory appeal and hence a strong sensory pull (e.g., colours, lights, smells and noises of explosives). The colourful and detailed visual imagery/stimuli (terrorist imagery, magazines, diagrams, flags, murals, uniforms, weapons and paraphernalia that can be visually appealing) may also have a marked sensory appeal to the individual with ASD [56].

Al-Attar [74] also provided 20 recommendations to guide forensic interviewers working with terrorism suspects and offenders who have ASD. She also outlines some of the potential implications of each of the seven facets of ASD for the terrorism interview. Furthermore, she refers to some of the key medico-legal and ethical ramifications of making terrorism interviews responsive to the interviewee's autistic functioning [74].

In their recent study, Walter and colleagues [75] carried out 34 qualitative interviews with experts in the field including NHS staff, academics, educational staff and counter-terrorism officers, as well as young people with autism from the UK. In their paper, Walter and colleagues discuss their findings in relation to a number of areas, for instance, the key traits of ASD and environmental contexts that may contribute towards a susceptibility to radicalisation. The findings and discussion in this paper will help support clinicians and criminal justice professionals when working with individuals with ASD who present with radical ideology [75].

Sexual Offending

Sexual 'Hands-On' Offences

Case studies are described in the literature of individuals with ASD who have engaged in sexual offending behaviour [20, 24, 76–79]. However, Allen and colleagues [80] used a survey methodology which studied offending behaviour in those with Asperger syndrome in the UK. Only 3 of the 126 individuals in their sample had engaged in sexual offending behaviour. This indicates that there is insufficient support for the notion that individuals with ASD are more likely to engage in sexual offending behaviour or sexually harmful behaviour. Some research has highlighted the importance of recognising that there are innate vulnerabilities or features in individuals with ASD which may provide the context of vulnerability for engaging in sexual offending behaviour. Some of these innate vulnerabilities include: impaired theory of mind repetitive and stereotyped behavioural patterns, and persistent preoccupation [20, 81–83]. For instance, an impaired theory of mind can negatively impact on the individual's ability to understand social cues and it can also have a negative impact on impulse control and the ability to empathise. These features can make some individuals with ASD present as totally unaware of the harm their actions had on their victims [20].

Stalking

Some research indicates the possible association between features of ASD and stalking behaviour [84]. For instance, it has been suggested in the literature that the obsessive tendencies found in ASD may be problematic when they are directed into behaviours which include a sexual component [15, 36, 80, 85] including a sexual attraction to a person, a fixation on certain body parts or an obsession with pornography [86]. Such behaviours may increase the context of vulnerability to engaging in stalking behaviour or sexual advances which are unreciprocated [85, 86]. In their empirical study, Stokes and colleagues [87] found that individuals with ASD were more likely to engage in inappropriate courting behaviours and were also more likely to focus their attention upon celebrities, strangers, colleagues and ex-partners. Interestingly, the study also found that individuals with ASD were more likely to pursue their target for longer durations compared to controls. They struggled to understand why the pursued person was not responding to them in the way they wanted and also held the belief that they had done no wrong. Lastly, individuals with ASD were not reported as having had any learning about romantic skills from either parents, siblings, observation, the media, sex-education teachers or peers.

Conclusion

In this chapter we explored how certain features or symptomology of ASD can provide the context of vulnerability to engagement in cybercrime (viewing of indecent child images and computer hacking/cyberdeviancy), violent offending (physical assault, mass shootings, arson or fire setting and terroristic behaviours) and sexual offending (sexual 'hands-on' offending and stalking behaviour). ASD can have significant legal relevance. As a result, as previously pointed out by Freckelton [88], courts are frequently tasked with assessing how and if ASD should be taken into consideration during case proceedings. For example, in criminal cases, courts are charged with identifying whether the symptoms of ASD might have played a causal or contributory role in the criminal action for which the accused is on trial [88]. However, 'research and recent court decisions have shown that judges and jurors themselves often do not have the knowledge or background to properly assess an individual diagnosed with ASD and whether his or her symptoms may be related to the committed crime' [89, p. 578]. This raises questions relating to the fairness of decisions on procedural issues [89, 90] and highlights the necessity for the expertise of mental health professionals who can educate and assist the courts in making decisions that are fully informed by expert opinions associated with the complexities of ASD [88, 89]. In sum, expert insights into the nature of ASD and its symptomology are important [52, 88, 90].

References

1. Cutler E. (2013), Autism and child pornography: a toxic combination. Available at: http://sexoffender-statistics.blogspot.com/2013/08/autism-and-child-pornography-toxic.html.

2. Woodbury-Smith MR, Clare IC, Holland AJ, Kearns A, Staufenberg E, Watson P. A case–control study of offenders with high functioning autistic spectrum disorders. *Journal of Forensic Psychiatry and Psychology* 2005; 16(4): 747–63.

3. Uljarevic M, Hamilton A. Recognition of emotions in autism: a formal meta-analysis. *Journal of Autism and Developmental Disorders* 2013; 43(7): 1517–26.

4. Mahoney M. Asperger's syndrome and the criminal law: the special case of child pornography. 2009. Available at: www.har ringtonmahoney.com/content/Publications/AspergersSyndromeandtheCriminalLaw v26.pdf.

5. Allely CS, Dubin L. The contributory role of autism symptomology in child pornography offending: why there is an urgent need for empirical research in this area. *Journal of Intellectual Disabilities and Offending Behaviour* 2018; 9(4), 129–52.

6. Allely CS, Kennedy S, Warren I. A legal analysis of Australian criminal cases involving defendants with autism spectrum disorder charged with online sexual offending. *International Journal of Law and Psychiatry* 2019; 66: 101456.

7. Allely CS. Case report: autism spectrum disorder symptomology and child pornography. *Journal of Intellectual*

Disabilities and Offending Behaviour 2020; 11(3): 171–89.

8. Mesibov G, Sreckovic M. Child and juvenile pornography and autism spectrum disorder. In Dubin LA, Horowitz E, eds., *Caught in the Web of the Criminal Justice System: Autism, Developmental Disabilities, and Sex Offenses*. Jessica Kingsley Publishers, 2017, chapter 2.

9. Hingsburger D, Griffiths D, Quinsey V. Detecting counterfeit deviance: differentiating sexual deviance from sexual inappropriateness. *The Habilitative Mental Healthcare Newsletter* 1991; 10(9): 51–4.

10. Sharp J. *Saving Gary McKinnon: A Mother's Story*. Biteback Publishing, 2013.

11. Ledingham R, Mills R. A preliminary study of autism and cybercrime in the context of international law enforcement. *Advances in Autism* 2015; 1(1): 2–11.

12. Seigfried-Spellar K, O'Quinn C, Treadway K. Assessing the relationship between autistic traits and cyderdeviancy in a sample of college students. *Behaviour & Information Technology* 2014; 34(5): 533–42.

13. Payne KL, Russell A, Mills R, Maras K, Rai D, Brosnan M. Is there a relationship between cyber-dependent crime, autistic-like traits and autism? *Journal of Autism and Developmental Disorders* 2019; 49(10): 4159–69.

14. Baron-Cohen S. An assessment of violence in a young man with Asperger's syndrome. *Journal of Child Psychology and Psychiatry* 1988; 29(3): 351–60.

15. Barry-Walsh JB, Mullen PE. Forensic aspects of Asperger's syndrome. *Journal of Forensic Psychiatry and Psychology* 2004; 15(1): 96–107.

16. Chen PS, Chen SJ, Yang YK, Yeh TL, Chen CC, Lo HY. Asperger's disorder: a case report of repeated stealing and the collecting behaviours of an adolescent patient. *Acta Psychiatrica Scandinavica* 2003; 107(1): 73–76.

17. Chesterman P, Rutter SC. Case report: Asperger's syndrome and sexual offending.

The Journal of Forensic Psychiatry 1993; 4(3): 555–62.

18. Cooper SA, Mohamed WN, Collacott RA. Possible Asperger's syndrome in a mentally handicapped transvestite offender. *Journal of Intellectual Disability Research* 1993; 37 (2): 189–94.

19. Hall I, Bernal J. Asperger's syndrome and violence. *The British Journal of Psychiatry* 1995; 166(2): 262.

20. Kohn Y, Fahum T, Ratzoni G, Apter A. Aggression and sexual offense in Asperger's syndrome. *The Israel Journal of Psychiatry and Related Sciences* 1998; 35(4): 293–9.

21. Kumar S, Devendran Y, Radhakrishna A, Karanth V, Hongally C. A case series of five individuals with Asperger syndrome and sexual criminality. *Journal of Mental Health and Human Behaviour* 2017; 22 (1): 63.

22. Mawson DC, Grounds A, Tantam D. Violence and Asperger's syndrome: a case study. *The British Journal of Psychiatry* 1985; 147: 566–9.

23. Milton J, Duggan C, Latham A. Egan V, Tantam D. Case history of co-morbid Asperger's syndrome and paraphilic behaviour. *Medicine, Science and the Law* 2002; 42(3): 237–44.

24. Murrie DC, Warren JI, Kristiansson M, Dietz PE. Asperger's syndrome in forensic settings. *International Journal of Forensic Mental Health* 2002; 1(1): 59–70.

25. Silva JA, Ferrari MM, Leong GB. What happened to Jeffrey? A neuropsychiatric developmental analysis of serial killing behaviour. Proceedings of the American Academy of Forensic Sciences, Volume VIII, American Academy of Forensic Sciences, Atlanta, GA and Colorado Springs, CO, 11–16 February 2002.

26. Silva JA, Ferrari MM, Leong GB. The neuropsychiatric developmental analysis of serial killer behaviour. Annual meeting program, American Academy of Psychiatry and the Law, Newport Beach, CA and Bloomfield, CT, 24–27 October 2002.

27. Silva J.A. Wu JC, Leon GB. Neuropsychiatric developmental analysis of sexual murder. Annual meeting program, American Academy of Psychiatry and the Law, San Antonio, TX and Bloomfield, CT, October 16–19, 2003.

28. Silva JA, Leong GB, Ferrari MM. A neuropsychiatric developmental model of serial homicidal behavior. *Behavioral Sciences and the Law* 2004; 22(6): 787–99.

29. Simblett GJ, Wilson DN. Asperger's syndrome: Three cases and a discussion. *Journal of Intellectual Disability Research* 1993; 37(1): 85–94.

30. Hare D, Gould J, Mills R, Wing L. A preliminary study of individuals with autistic spectrum disorders in three special hospitals in England. National Autistic Society. 1999. Available at www.aspires-relationships.com/3hospitals.pdf.

31. Scragg P, Shah A. Prevalence of Asperger's syndrome in a secure hospital. *The British Journal of Psychiatry* 1994; 165(5): 679–82.

32. Woodbury-Smith MR, Clare ICH, Holland AJ, Kearns A. High functioning autistic spectrum disorders, offending and other law-breaking: findings from a community sample. *The Journal of Forensic Psychiatry and Psychology* 2006; 17 (1): 108–20.

33. Cederlund M, Hagberg B, Billstedt E, Gillberg IC, Gillberg C. Asperger syndrome and autism: A comparative longitudinal follow-up study more than 5 years after original diagnosis. *Journal of Autism and Developmental Disorders* 2008; 38(1): 72–85.

34. Mouridsen SE, Rich B, Isage, T, Nedergaard NJ. Pervasive developmental disorders and criminal behavior: a case control study. *International Journal of Offender Therapy and Comparative Criminology* 2008; 52(2): 196–205.

35. Långström N, Grann M, Ruchkin V, Sjöstedt G, Fazel S. Risk factors for violent offending in autism spectrum disorder: a national study of hospitalized individuals. *Journal of Interpersonal Violence* 2009; 24 (8): 1358–70.

36. Haskins BG, Silva JA. Asperger's disorder and criminal behavior: forensic psychiatric considerations. *Journal of the American Academy of Psychiatry and the Law Online* 2006; 34(3): 374–84.

37. Lazaratou H, Giannopoulou I, Anomitri C, Douzenis A. Case report: matricide by a 17-year old boy with Asperger's syndrome. *Aggression and Violent Behavior* 2016; 31: 61–5.

38. Woodbury-Smith M, Clare I, Holland AJ, Watson PC, Bambrick M, Kearns A, Staufenberg E. Circumscribed interests and 'offenders' with autism spectrum disorders: a case–control study. *The Journal of Forensic Psychiatry and Psychology* 2010; 21(3): 366–77.

39. Fitzgerald M. Autism and school shootings: overlap of autism (Asperger's syndrome) and general psychopathy. In Fitzgerald M, ed., *Autism Spectrum Disorder: Recent Advances*. InTech, 2015, chapter 1.

40. Allely CS, Wilson P, Minnis H, Thompson L, Yaksic E, Gillberg C. Violence is rare in autism: when it does occur, is it sometimes extreme? *The Journal of Psychology* 2017; 151(1): 49–68.

41. Fccini L. The application of the models of autism, psychopathology and deficient Eriksonian development and the path of intended violence to understand the Newtown shooting. *Archives of Forensic Psychology* 2016; 1(3): 1–13.

42. Calhoun FS, Weston SW. *Contemporary Threat Management: A Practical Guide for Identifying, Assessing, and Managing Individuals of Violent Intent*. Specialized Training Services, 2003.

43. Faccini L. The man who howled wolf: diagnostic and treatment considerations for a person with ASD and impersonal repetitive fire, bomb and presidential threats. *American Journal of Forensic Psychiatry* 2010; 31(4): 47.

44. Faccini L, Allely CS. Mass violence in individuals with autism spectrum disorder and narcissistic personality disorder: a case analysis of Anders Breivik using the 'path to intended and terroristic violence' model.

Aggression and Violent Behavior 2016; 31: 229–36.

45. Faccini L. Allely CS. Mass violence in an individual with an autism spectrum disorder: a case analysis of Dean Allen Mellberg using the 'path to intended violence' model. *International Journal of Psychological Research* 2016b; 11(1): 1–18.

46. Allely CS, Faccini L. 'Path to intended violence' model to understand mass violence in the case of Elliot Rodger. *Aggression and Violent Behavior* 2017; 37: 201–9.

47. Allely CS, Faccini L. Clinical profile, risk, and critical factors and the application of the 'path toward intended violence' model in the case of mass shooter Dylann Roof. *Deviant Behavior* 2019; 40(6): 672–89.

48. Williams D. *Understanding the Arsonist: From Assessment to Confession.* Lawyers and Judges, 2005.

49. Gannon TA, Pina A. Firesetting: psychopathology, theory and treatment. *Aggression and Violent Behavior* 2010; 15: 224–38.

50. Alexander RT, Chester V, Green FN, Gunaratna I, Hoare S. Arson or fire setting in offenders with intellectual disability: clinical characteristics, forensic histories, and treatment outcomes. *Journal of Intellectual and Developmental Disability* 2015; 40(2): 189–97.

51. Siponmaa L, Kristiansson M, Jonson C, Nydén A, Gillberg C. Juvenile and young adult mentally disordered offenders: the role of child neuropsychiatric disorders. *Journal of the American Academy of Psychiatry and the Law* 2001; 29(4): 420–6.

52. Freckelton S I, List D. Asperger's disorder, criminal responsibility and criminal culpability. *Psychiatry, Psychology and Law* 2009; 16(1): 16–40.

53. McEwan T, Freckelton I. Assessment, treatment and sentencing of arson offenders: an overview. *Psychiatry, Psychology and Law(* 2011; 18(3): 319–328.

54. Allely CS. Firesetting and arson in individuals with autism spectrum disorder: a systematic PRISMA review. *Journal of Intellectual Disabilities and Offending Behaviour* 2019; 10(4): 89–101.

55. Faccini L, Allely CS. Rare instances of individuals with autism supporting or engaging in terrorism. *Journal of Intellectual Disabilities and Offending Behaviour* 2017; 8(20): 70–82.

56. Al-Attar Z. Autism spectrum disorders and terrorism: how different features of autism can contextualise vulnerability and resilience. *Journal of Forensic Psychiatry and Psychology* 2020; 31(6): 926–49.

57. Al-Attar Z. Autism & terrorism links: fact or fiction? 15th International Conference on the Care and Treatment of Offenders with an Intellectual and/or Developmental Disability, National Autistic Society, April 19–20, 2016, Manchester.

58. Al-Attar, Z. Autism and terrorism links: baseless headlines or clinical reality? XIth AutismEurope International Congress, Autism-Europe and National Autistic Society, September 16–18, 2016, Edinburgh,

59. Al-Attar, Z. Interviewing terrorism suspects and offenders with an autism spectrum disorder. *International Journal of Forensic Mental Health* 2018; 17(4), 321–37.

60. Al-Attar Z. Terrorism and autism: making sense of the links in formulations of risk and protective factors. The Autism Professionals Annual Conference, March 7–8, 2018, Harrogate.

61. Al-Attar Z. Extremism, radicalisation and mental health: handbook for practitioners. 2019. Available at: https://home-affairs.ec.europa.eu/system/files/2019-11/ran_h-sc_handbook-for-practitioners_extremism-radicalisation-mental-health_112019_en.pdf.

62. Al-Attar Z. Development and evaluation of guidance to aid risk assessments of offenders with autism. Unpublished MA dissertation, Sheffield Hallam University, 2018.

63. Craig J, Baron-Cohen S. Creativity and imagination in autism and Asperger syndrome. *Journal of Autism and Developmental Disorders* 1999; 29(4): 319–26.

64. Klin A, Danovitch JH, Merz AB, Volkmar FR. Circumscribed interests in higher functioning individuals with autism spectrum disorders: an exploratory study. *Research and Practice for Persons with Severe Disabilities* 2007; 32(2): 89–100.

65. Tager-Flusberg H. The origins of social impairments in autism spectrum disorder: studies of infants at risk. *Neural Networks* 2010; 23(8–9): 1072–6.

66. Tager-Flusberg H. A psychological approach to understanding the social and language impairments in autism. *International Review of Psychiatry* 1999; 11 (4): 325–34.

67. Tager-Flusberg H, Joseph RM. Identifying neurocognitive phenotypes in autism. *Philosophical Transactions of the Royal Society of London B: Biological Sciences* 2003; 358(1430): 303–14.

68. Happé F, Frith U. The weak coherence account: detail-focused cognitive style in autism spectrum disorders. *Journal of Autism and Developmental Disorders* 2006; 36(1): 5–25.

69. Walęcka M, Wojciechowska K, Wichniak A. Central coherence in adults with a high-functioning autism spectrum disorder. In a search for a non-self-reporting screening tool. *Applied Neuropsychology: Adult* 2020; 29(4): 677–83.

70. Hill EL. Evaluating the theory of executive dysfunction in autism. *Developmental Review* 2004; 24(2): 189–233.

71. Baron-Cohen S. The extreme male brain theory of autism. *Trends in Cognitive Sciences* 2002; 6(6): 248–54.

72. Milton DE. On the ontological status of autism: the 'double empathy problem'. *Disability and Society* 2012; 27(6): 883–7.

73. Crane L, Goddard L, Pring L. Sensory processing in adults with autism spectrum disorders. *Autism* 2009; 13(3): 215–28.

74. Al-Attar Z. Interviewing terrorism suspects and offenders with an autism spectrum disorder. *International Journal of Forensic Mental Health* 2018; 17(4): 321–37.

75. Walter F, Leonard S, Miah S, Shaw J. Characteristics of autism spectrum disorder and susceptibility to radicalisation among young people: a qualitative study. *The Journal of Forensic Psychiatry and Psychology* 2020; 32(3): 408–29.

76. Fujikawa Y, Umeshita S, Mutura H. Sexual crimes committed by adolescents with Asperger's disorder: problems of management by the viewpoint of probation officers at a family court. *Japanese Journal of Child and Adolescent Psychiatry* 2002; 43 (3): 280–9.

77. Kellaher DC. Sexual behavior and autism spectrum disorders: an update and discussion. *Current Psychiatry Reports* 2015; 17(4): 25.

78. Kumagami T, Matsuura N. Prevalence of pervasive developmental disorder in juvenile court cases in Japan. *Journal of Forensic Psychiatry and Psychology* 2009; 20 (6): 974–87.

79. Sutton LR, Hughes TL, Huang A, Lehman C, Paserba D, Talkington V, et al. Identifying individuals with autism in a state facility for adolescents adjudicated as sexual offenders: a pilot study. *Focus on Autism and Other Developmental Disabilities* 2013; 28(3): 175–83.

80. Allen D, Evans C, Hider A, Hawkins S, Peckett H, Morgan H. Offending behaviour in adults with Asperger syndrome. *Journal of Autism and Developmental Disorders* 2008; 38(4): 748–58.

81. Allely C, Creaby-Attwood A. Sexual offending and autism spectrum disorders. *Journal of Intellectual Disabilities and Offending Behaviour* 2016; 7(1): 35–51.

82. Creaby-Attwood A, Allely CS. A psycho-legal perspective on sexual offending in individuals with autism spectrum disorder. *International Journal of Law and Psychiatry* 2017; 55: 72–80.

83. Allely C. Sexual offending behaviour in young people with intellectual disabilities and autism spectrum disorder: autism and

the criminal justice system. Available at: https://pure.strath.ac.uk/ws/portalfiles/por tal/87493838/Allely_CYCJ_2019_sexual_o ffending_behaviour_in_young_people_wi th_intellectual_disabilities_and_autism_ spectrum_disorder.pdf.

84. Mercer JE, Allely CS. Autism spectrum disorders and stalking. *Journal of Criminal Psychology* 2020; 10(3): 201–18.

85. Freckelton I. Asperger's disorder and the criminal law. *Journal of Law and Medicine* 2011; 18: 677–91.

86. Higgs T, Carter AJ. Autism spectrum disorder and sexual offending: responsivity in forensic interventions. *Aggression and Violent Behavior* 2015; 22, 112–19.

87. Stokes M, Newton N, Kaur A. Stalking, and social and romantic functioning among adolescents and adults with autism spectrum disorder. *Journal of Autism and Developmental Disorders* 2007, 37(10): 1969–86.

88. Freckelton I. Autism spectrum disorder: forensic issues and challenges for mental health professionals and courts. *Journal of Applied Research in Intellectual Disabilities* 2013; 26(5): 420–34.

89. Berryessa CM. Educator of the court: the role of the expert witness in cases involving autism spectrum disorder. *Psychology, Crime and Law* 2017; 23(6): 575–600.

90. Berryessa C. Defendants with autism spectrum disorder in criminal court: a judges' toolkit. *Drexel Law Review* 2021; 13(4): 841–68.

Overview of Young People with Neurodevelopmental Impairments in Contact with the Youth Justice System

Prathiba Chitsabesan, Nathan Hughes and Huw Williams

Introduction

Over the last decade, it has been highlighted that young people with disproportionately high and multiple needs have clustered in the youth justice system. These young people experience higher levels of diagnosable mental health problems and neurodevelopmental impairment than the general population.

Childhood neurodevelopmental impairment occurs when there is a compromise of the central or peripheral nervous system due to factors such as genetic vulnerability, birth trauma or brain injury in childhood. It is often the result of a complex mix of influences, including biological factors, such as genetics, and environmental factors, such as trauma and nutritional and emotional deprivation. Such compromises can lead to a wide range of specific neurodevelopmental disorders, with common symptoms including cognitive delay, communication difficulties and problems with emotional and behavioural control and social functioning. Such symptoms can occur in combination, as evidenced in a wide range of clinically defined disorders or conditions, including (though not restricted to): attention deficit hyperactivity disorder (ADHD); autistic spectrum disorder (ASD); learning (or intellectual) disability; communication disorders; fetal alcohol syndrome disorders (FASD); and traumatic brain injury (TBI) [1].

A review of studies across a range of international contexts reveals a consistently high incidence rate of neurodevelopmental impairment among young offenders in comparison to young people in the general population [2]. The findings of this review are summarised in Table 7.1; these data require careful interpretation. There are methodological and analytical challenges in comparing studies using different definitions of specific neurodevelopmental disorders. This variability is also reflected in the different measures and tools used to assess prevalence rates and the variation in samples and populations on which individual studies are focused.

However, despite these limitations, the evidence available consistently suggests a disproportionately high rate of neurodevelopmental disorders amongst young people in contact with the criminal justice system. Indeed, it suggests that a significant proportion of young people in the custodial estate have one or more neurodevelopmental disorders, signifying high levels of need. Additionally, the prevalence of clinically defined disorders is likely to be an underestimate of the proportion of young people affected by subclinical levels of impairment (see Chapter 9).

This weight of evidence therefore suggests a widespread failure of current practices and interventions intended to prevent offending and reoffending to recognise and meet the

Table 7.1 Comparing the prevalence of neurodevelopmental conditions

Neurodevelopmental condition	Prevalence rates amongst young people in custody* (%)	Prevalence rates amongst young people in the general population* (%)
Communication disorders	60–90	5–7
Intellectual/learning disability	23–32	2–4
ADHD	12	1.7–9
ASD	15	0.6–1.2
FASD	10.9–11.7	0.1–5
TBI	65.1–72.1	24–31.6

*References are provided and summarised by Hughes et al. [2].

needs of these vulnerable young people. Consequently, this promotes a rethinking of the approaches of the youth justice system, and of policy and services more generally.

Development Pathways to Offending and the Impact of Neurodevelopmental Impairment

Epidemiological studies suggest that the development of antisocial behaviour involves a complex interaction of intrinsic and psychosocial risk and protective factors [3]. Links between early adverse events in the prenatal period and the impact of parenting, family and peer relationships on behaviour in early childhood have been found. Heritable influences contribute towards a gene–environment interaction, suggesting pathways are complex, and some vulnerabilities become increasingly evident in the context of other risk factors. Intrinsic risk factors include socio-cognitive deficits (hostile attribution bias), temperamental factors (callous–unemotional traits) and low autonomic nervous system arousal [3]. However, antisocial behaviour also shows strong associations with psychosocial adversity. Parental mental illness, family breakdown, parenting style and association with other antisocial peers influence outcomes. Detachment from school through truancy and exclusion may increase the risk of offending through reduced supervision, loss of any positive socialisation effects of school and by creating delinquent groups of young people [4].

Moffitt and colleagues proposed a developmental taxonomy whereby early-onset conduct problems were more likely to be associated with individually based risk factors that increase vulnerability to the development of behaviour problems in the context of adverse family and parenting conditions [5]. In adolescent-onset conduct problems, by contrast, individual vulnerabilities may be less marked and the impact of environmental risk factors, including the influence of antisocial peers, is more evident. There is evidence that early-onset, life-course-persistent antisocial behaviour is more likely to be associated with a greater risk of neurodevelopmental impairment [6].

Neurodevelopmental impairments are expressed through a wide range of symptoms, including deficits in cognitive functions (reasoning, thinking and perception) and social–affective functions (the expression of emotion and formation of relationships). Such deficits can affect a child's daily functioning in the social world, also increasing vulnerability to certain behaviours in particular contexts.

Impairment in Executive Functioning, Cognitive Empathy and Emotional Regulation

'Executive functioning' is an umbrella term describing the various cognitive processes used to enable complex goal-oriented thought and action, and the self-regulation of socially appropriate behaviour. Such processes include the initiation, planning and sequencing of complex tasks, the utilisation of long-term memory, concentration, inhibitory and attention control and responsivity to novel or changing circumstances [7].

There is evidence of a statistically significant association between executive functioning and measures of antisocial and aggressive behaviour including: decreasing behavioural inhibition; impairing the ability to anticipate behavioural consequences and assess punishment and reward; and damaging the capability to generate socially appropriate behaviour in challenging contexts [8].

Deficits in executive functions are associated with a range of neurodevelopmental disorders. For example, the above descriptions of deficits in executive functioning closely relate to descriptions of the difficulties faced by those with ADHD, which include: setting goals and planning activity; organising and prioritising information; moving attention from one activity to another; and maintaining information in the working memory (see Chapter 4). Young people with FASD can also demonstrate a range of cognitive functioning deficits, including with regard to reasoning, planning ahead, anticipating and learning from the consequences of actions [9] (see Chapter 8).

Deficits in executive functioning are similarly related to TBI, which is any injury to the brain caused by impact. Typically, this may occur from a direct blow to the head or a force that causes the brain to move around inside the skull, as in a road traffic accident, fall or assault. The frontal and temporal areas of the brain are common sites of injury due to their location at the front of the brain and their proximity to the skull. These areas include the dorsolateral prefrontal cortex, associated with working memory, sustained attention, memory retrieval, abstraction and problem solving, and the orbitofrontal cortex, associated with emotional and social responses [10]. Sesma et al. report that between 20% and 40% of children aged between 5 and 15 years demonstrate significant executive dysfunction within the first year of TBI [11]. While motor deficits improve over time, there is evidence that executive functioning deficits are more enduring [12].

Low cognitive empathy is theorised as related to offending, on the assumption that people who can appreciate another's feelings are less likely to victimise them [13]. While low cognitive empathy was identified as strongly related to offending in a systematic review of 35 studies [14], the relationship was found to be greatly reduced after controlling for intelligence or socio-economic status [15]. This suggests that low empathy is a mediating or moderating variable in the presence of these other factors.

While its specific influence as a risk factor is unclear, poor cognitive empathy is a characteristic of several neurodevelopmental disorders, including learning disabilities, ADHD and ASD. Cognitive empathy is also related to TBI; for example, there is an inhibited ability amongst those who have experienced severe TBI to recognise and appropriately respond to other people's emotions [12]. Poorer emotional perception can create social misunderstandings that lead to the generation of inappropriate responses, which in turn may heighten the likelihood of rejection by peers or elicit psychological distress reflected in a range of externalising behaviours [16].

Emotional regulation involves complex cognitive and physiological components, which modulate affective states. Emotional regulation strategies develop throughout an individual's lifetime, but most critically during childhood, and reflect an interaction between factors, such as temperament and prior experience. Regulatory systems develop during adolescence through functional and structural changes within the brain, including within the prefrontal cortex and amygdala. The prefrontal cortex is associated with the integration of emotional experiences and cognition, including emotion regulation, while the amygdala is an important region for recognition of fear as well as emotion regulation [17].

Difficulties with emotional regulation have been shown in children with conduct disorder [18] as well as those with neurodevelopmental disorders, including those with; ADHD [19] learning disability [20] and TBI [21]. Therefore, problems with emotional recognition and regulation may be contributing mechanisms to the development of behavioural difficulties for this particular group of children and young people.

These examples provide a brief insight into the complex ways in which cognitive and emotional difficulties that are symptomatic of neurodevelopmental impairment might, in particular social contexts, increase the risk of aggressive or antisocial behaviour. The next sections identify a range of social or environmental risk factors that can lead to a greater likelihood of both criminality and criminalisation, and they illustrate how young people can be vulnerable by their underlying emotional or cognitive deficits.

Increased Exposure to Social and Environmental Risk Factors for Offending

Educational Disengagement

The relationship between neurodevelopmental impairment and social and environmental risk is most apparent in relation to education disengagement. For example, young people with learning disability can experience deficits in memory and problem-solving skills, which inhibit academic performance [22] and those with FASD [23] or ADHD [24] have difficulties with attention and concentration or impulse control.

Difficulties in pre-school and early educational experiences can have a cumulative effect on educational experience, with difficulties prior to the age of eight leading to subsequent challenges in engaging with further stages of education. For example, Snow and Powell describe the challenges facing young people with communication disorders or learning difficulties in recognising the shift from 'learning to read' to 'reading to learn', which typically occurs in the fourth year of formal education [25]. For boys in particular, this is often a time (around 8 years of age) when externalising behaviour difficulties becomes apparent in the classroom [25]. Young people who experience TBI in childhood, in contrast, may be prone to sudden and unanticipated educational problems, which are only realised at a later date.

Additionally, the transition from the more nurturing environment of primary school to a secondary school, which places significant academic, organisational and social demands on students, can be particularly challenging for young people with impairment [26].

Problematic transitions into secondary school can escalate disengagement from education and therefore represent a key developmental phase with regard to the risk of future criminal behaviour [27].

Peer Group Influence

A heightened risk of detachment from school, whether through disaffection, truancy or exclusion, can further act to increase the risk of offending [5]. There is evidence that susceptibility to risk factors associated with delinquent peer groups and a loss of positive socialisation through schools is itself heightened by the existence of specific neurodevelopmental impairments. This is supported by research studies that indicate challenges in peer group formation, and associated susceptibility to bullying and negative peer pressure.

Adolescents with neurodevelopmental impairment including ADHD present an increased risk of experiencing peer rejection [28]. Peer rejection may also lead to low self-esteem and a gravitation to an antisocial peer group, strongly associated with delinquent behaviour [29].

Deficits in social communication can influence the formation and maintenance of peer relationships by reducing the capacity for peer negotiation and effective interaction [30]. Baldry et al. argue that such deficits can promote a desire in a young person to want to be accepted by their peer group, which may contribute to the initiation or escalation of antisocial behaviour through a greater association with other deviant peers [31].

Parenting Practices

Parenting a child with a neurodevelopmental disorder can clearly bring a range of challenges, particularly when that disorder is not identified or supported. In particular, approaches to parenting that are excessively permissive or authoritarian may be adopted in response to the difficulties of parenting a child with challenging behaviour with negative consequences.

Wade et al. suggest that children who have experienced TBI may be particularly vulnerable to negative effects associated with 'maladaptive parent–child interactions' [32]. A study tracking the 10-year developmental trajectories of young people who experienced TBI during their school years found that poor long-term behavioural outcomes were predicted by such parenting approaches [33]. Similarly, Kaiser et al. also found evidence to support parenting (particularly negative parenting) as a mediator of the relation between ADHD severity and child social skill and aggression [34].

Discrimination, Criminalisation and the Rights of Children

In this section we now focus on experiences of disability, defined as 'the loss or limitation of opportunities to take part in the normal life of the community on an equal level with others due to physical and social barriers' [35, p. 2]. Adopting the lens of disability therefore focuses attention on how an individual with impairment experiences their environment, including day-to-day functioning, social relations and services and support.

Diagnosis can contribute to how a young person's needs are understood and responded to by their family and professionals. It determines service eligibility and subsequent support. Lack of identification hampers opportunities for early intervention and promotion of healthy development and resilience in young people. For example, failure to identify and respond to the learning needs resulting from neurodevelopmental impairment may result in potential disengagement with education. Without an awareness of an underlying cognitive or emotional deficit, classroom misbehaviour may simply be interpreted as a behavioural problem. Chitsabesan et al. found that the majority of young offenders with learning disability identified in their study had an intelligence quotient (IQ) in the 'mild learning disability range', and were therefore less likely to have had their learning needs identified in mainstream schools [36].

Disabling processes are also apparent in experiences of the criminal justice system, with various practices serving to increase the risk of criminalisation of young people with neurodevelopmental impairments. Inadequate assessment [37] or insufficient knowledge or training of neurodevelopmental impairment [38] can lead to a failure of services to identify and appropriately support those with a neurodevelopmental impairment. It is not unusual for children to find it difficult to communicate with the adults involved, to mistrust justice authorities and to lack basic information and understanding about processes and procedures, which prevents their full participation.

All of these issues are far worse for children when problems associated with their impairments prevent their effective engagement with criminal justice processes, including in the understanding of their rights or participating in interviews or court hearings (see Chapter 18). For example, cognitive impairment can inhibit narrative language skills, or the ability to tell one's story. Such skills are imperative given the forensic interviewing techniques applied in court or by police [39]. Additionally, monosyllabic, poorly elaborated responses and poor eye contact may be mistaken for deliberate rudeness or non-compliance [39]. If interpreted as behavioural and attitudinal, difficulties in communication may therefore lead to a greater risk of criminalisation.

Specialist service provision within the youth justice system is often limited [40]. Instead, young people with neurodevelopmental impairment are typically subject to generic youth justice interventions to reduce reoffending, which assume typical levels of language and cognitive competence. Such approaches may therefore be inappropriate for some young people with neurodevelopmental impairment, leading to a higher risk of reoffending and harsher responses from justice systems, including when sentencing and using disciplinary sanctions in detention.

All children who come into conflict with the law have rights that are established in international law and standards. Most notably, the United Nations Convention on the Rights of the Child (UNCRC) [41] is an international human rights treaty that sets out civil, political, economic, social and cultural rights for children. These include the right to a fair trial, to legal assistance and support, to participate in legal proceedings and to have their best interests as a primary consideration in decision making by courts. The recent publication of General Comment Number 24 in 2019 [42] further supports the implementation of the rights outlined in the UNCRC within 'child justice systems', including with respect to children with 'neurodevelopmental disorders or disabilities' for whom the case is made for prevention and diversion, where possible, and adjustments, when not.

Paragraph 28 states that children with 'neurodevelopmental disorders or disabilities . . . should not be in the child justice system at all, even if they have reached the minimum age of criminal responsibility'. This implies support to prevent criminalisation by addressing the causes of offending discussed above, or diversion from criminal justice systems when disability is identified. Paragraph 28 concludes that 'If not automatically excluded, such children should be individually assessed'. The awareness of an individual child's experience of disability is needed to ensure the protection of their rights without discrimination. This notion is represented in paragraph 40, which states that '[s]afeguards against discrimination are needed from the earliest contact with the criminal justice system and throughout the trial, and discrimination against any group of children requires active redress' [42, p. 7]. Children with disabilities are noted as a specific example of those requiring such safeguards through accommodations, which may include 'support for children with psychosocial disabilities, assistance with communication and the reading of documents, and procedural adjustments for testimony' [42, p. 8].

Implications for Policy and Practice

In this concluding section we highlight a selection of policy and practice implications, emphasising the need for early, responsive and tailored intervention and reform to criminal justice processes, all of which must be underpinned by effective screening and assessment to improve awareness of impairment.

Screening and Assessment

Timely screening and assessment are essential to the successful identification and management of neurodevelopmental impairment, and to the recognition of the possible relationship between offending behaviour and underlying needs in young offenders. Identifying offenders with neurodevelopmental impairment is therefore essential, not only to tailor interventions appropriately, but also because such impairments may affect the young person's capacity to engage in the legal process, including the court process.

This should be supported by regular supervision and access to consultation with specialist health professionals to enable staff to practice within a robust clinical governance framework. Seeking additional information from key informants in the young person's life is also essential to develop a better understanding of the young person's strengths and needs, as many young people may minimise symptoms for fear of stigma. Assessments should emphasise function and need rather than diagnosis, and should maintain a holistic approach.

In recognition of these difficulties, a health assessment tool has been developed and validated for use with young offenders within the secure estate across England and Wales. The Comprehensive Health Assessment Tool (CHAT) consists of five parts: an initial reception screen, followed by a physical health, mental health, substance misuse and neurodevelopmental impairment screen for all offenders [43]. The update to the 'Healthcare standards for children and young people in secure settings' [44] has also provided an opportunity to standardise good practice guidelines and support the use of the CHAT.

While being aware of the possible relationship between offending behaviour and these underlying needs is key, recognition of need does not necessarily imply the diagnosis of a disorder.

Early Intervention through Educational and Family Support

An awareness of the developmental pathways of young people with neurodevelopmental impairments who offend necessitates earlier intervention through family and educational support, so as to prevent the development of secondary risks such as problematic family functioning, detachment from education or negative peer group influence.

Families are a valuable resource in supporting young people; however, families need to be supported if they are to maintain an effective level of care to a child with complex needs such as those associated with neurodevelopmental impairment [45]. This might include greater investment in parenting support programmes known to be effective for young people with specific disorders, as well as through the provision of information and advice.

Young people at risk of later antisocial behaviour can often be identified early within the education system by their challenging behaviour or problems with academic engagement or attainment. Indeed, young people exhibiting early signs of difficulty should be routinely assessed for underlying cognitive and emotional needs. Where neurodevelopmental impairment has been identified, early and sustained interventions to maintain attachment to school have been shown to have a greater chance of success compared with attempting to re-engage young people [46]. Access to specialist consultation with health and educational professionals, such as educational psychologists, child and adolescent mental health professionals and speech therapists, is also essential. Given their complex needs and potential for associated challenging behaviour, some young people with neurodevelopmental impairment may benefit from support provided within a specialist educational placement, which is able to provide a small, flexible environment, and an adapted timetable with trained staff, as well the acquisition of life skills that could contribute to better social adaptation in later life.

This suggests a significant set of training needs across a range of services in order to ensure appropriate assessment and response. Staff in education services, social services, voluntary sector and primary healthcare settings, as well as in community youth justice services, require support to recognise and understand issues relating to neurodevelopmental impairment.

Responsive Youth Justice Interventions

As we have highlighted, young people with neurodevelopmental impairments typically have cognitive needs and learning styles that can affect their ability to engage in interventions intended to support rehabilitation. For example, research has suggested that individuals with a history of TBI may find it more difficult to engage with offence-related rehabilitation due to information processing difficulties or disinhibited behaviour [47].

Recognition is therefore essential in order to develop individual care plans for the young person, allowing for services that are responsive to specific cognitive and emotional deficits. Awareness of a young person's needs can help practitioners in regular contact with them to offer appropriate support in the development of better life skills and more adaptive coping mechanisms, with appropriate supervision and training. For example, the education of prison staff around the impact of TBI and management strategies to support offenders can lead to a reduction in the number of negative interactions [48].

Guidelines on how to support young people with specific neurodevelopmental disorders are already established and can be readily utilised, including, for example, those published by the National Institute for Health and Clinical Excellence regarding ADHD [49] and ASD [50]. An example of a specialist pathway for young offenders with TBI has also been developed by the Disabilities Foundation [51]. The service pathway is based on a successful model of interventions for adult offenders with TBI in an adult custodial secure facility [52]. There are also guidelines with specific reference to offending behaviour including 'recognition, intervention and management' of antisocial behaviour and conduct disorders [53]. There is also growing evidence of the efficacy of individual therapeutic approaches to address and manage aspects of neurodevelopmental impairment, including skills development using social stories and comic strip cartoons, which address emotional recognition and help develop coping strategies to manage stress and conflict [54].

Identifying offenders with neurodevelopmental impairment is also essential in order to ensure a young person's capacity to engage in the legal process, and consequently to effectively defend themselves. Only by recognising and responding to the specific needs of young people with such impairment can we counter experiences of neurodevelopmental impairment and criminalisation.

To achieve this, law, policy and practice must be in place to guarantee the following:

- Children in conflict with the law are screened for the presence of neurodevelopmental impairment.
- Justice professionals are supported to identify prominent disorders and to understand how they might affect a child's behaviour and engagement with the justice system.
- The adaptations that children need are identified at different stages of justice proceedings, for example, one-to-one mentoring to prepare for court hearings and targeted support with behaviour management in detention.
- Justice professionals are trained so they can communicate appropriately – for example, by using simple, everyday language, avoiding technical terms or abstract concepts, giving sufficient time for processing a question and by using visual aids.
- Judicial officers responsible for sentencing take account of the relevance of neurodevelopmental impairment to offending behaviour, including the potential impact on the child of difficulties with reading, processing and memory, maturity of judgement, impulsivity and an understanding of the perspectives of others.
- Diversion and rehabilitation measures are used, which include therapeutic treatments being prioritised.
- All children with neurodevelopmental impairment are provided with legal assistance and support when they are in conflict with the law.
- Justice responses are multidisciplinary and multisectoral, and include law enforcement officials, prosecutors, judges, social workers, probation services, civil society organisations, child protection and health and education workers working in close collaboration.

Conclusion

The disproportionately high prevalence of neurodevelopmental disorders among young people in custody in numerous countries suggests a heightened vulnerability to serious and/or persistent offending coupled with a failure of various policy and practice systems to address complex needs in seeking to prevent offending and reoffending. In this chapter we have provided some insight into the varied ways in which cognitive and emotional impairments might give rise to antisocial or aggressive behaviour in particular contexts or situations and how neurodevelopmental impairment may increase exposure to social and environmental risk factors for offending. This includes potential challenges to effective educational engagement and attainment, family functioning and negative peer group influences. We have also argued that experiences of neurodevelopmental impairment and risk of criminal justice engagement appears to be amplified by experiences of social marginalisation and inequality. Systemic failures to recognise and address the needs of young people with neurodevelopmental impairment have been shown to add further disadvantage and vulnerability, and ultimately to increase the likelihood of criminalisation.

Dismantling these barriers requires recognition, understanding, resources and awareness. The right to non-discrimination is not synonymous with equal treatment for everyone. Age-appropriate accommodations are needed to ensure that children affected by impairments have their rights respected, protected and fulfilled in criminal proceedings, on an equal basis to children without such impairments.

References

1. American Psychiatric Association. *Diagnostic and Statistical Manual of Mental D^{is}orders*, 5th edition: DSM-5. American Psychiatric Association, 2013.

2. Hughes N, Williams H, Chitsabesan P, Davies R, Mounce L. *Nobody Made the Connection: The Prevalence of Neurodevelopmental impairment in Young People Who Offend*. Office of the Children's Commissioner for England, 2012.

3. Murray J, Farrington DP. Risk factors for conduct disorder and delinquency: key findings from longitudinal studies. *Canadian Journal of Psychiatry* 2010; 55: 633–42.

4. Stevenson M. *Young People and Offending: Education, Youth Justice and Social Care Inclusion*. Williams Publishing, 2006.

5. Moffitt T, Caspi A, Rutter M, Silva P. *Sex Differences in Antisocial Behaviour: Conduct Disorder and Delinquency and Violence in the Dunedin Longitudinal Study*. Cambridge University Press, 2001.

6. Hughes N. Understanding the influence of neurodevelopmental disorders on offending: utilizing developmental psychopathology in biosocial criminology. *Criminal Justice Studies* 2015; 28(1): 39–60.

7. Meltzer L, ed. *Executive Function in Education: From Theory to Practice*. Guilford Press, 2007.

8. Ogilvie JM, Stewart AL, Chan RCK, Shum DHK. Neuropsychological measures of executive function and antisocial behavior: a meta-analysis. *Criminology* 2011; 49: 1063–107.

9. Burd L, Fast DK, Conry J, Williams A. Fetal alcohol spectrum disorder as marker for increased risk of involvement with correction systems. *Journal of Psychiatry and Law* 2010; 38(4): 559–83.

10. Williams WH. *Repairing Shattered Lives: Brain Injury and Its Implications for Criminal Justice*. Transition to Adulthood Alliance, 2013.

11. Sesma HW, Slomine BS, Ding R, McCarthy ML. Children's Health After Trauma (CHAT) study group. Executive functioning in the first year after pediatric traumatic brain injury. *Pediatrics* 2008; 121: E1686–95.

12. Catroppa C, Anderson V. Neurodevelopmental outcomes of pediatric traumatic brain injury. *Future Neurology* 2009; 4(6): 811–21.

13. Farrington DP, Welsh BC. *Saving Children from a Life of Crime: Early Risk Factors and Effective Interventions*. Oxford University Press, 2007.

14. Joliffe D, Farrington DP. Empathy and offending: a systematic review and meta-analysis. *Aggression and Violent Behaviour* 2004; 9: 441–76.

15. Jolliffe D, Farrington DP. Individual differences and offending. In McLaughlin E, Newburn T, eds. *The SAGE Handbook of Criminological Theory*, SAGE Publications, 2010: 40–56.

16. Ryan NP, Anderson V, Godfrey C, Eren S, Rosema S, Taylor K, et al. Social communication mediates the relationship between emotion perception and externalizing behaviors in young adult survivors of pediatric traumatic brain injury.

International Journal of Developmental Neuroscience 2013; 31: 811–19.

17. Davidson RJ, Putnam KM, Larson CL. Dysfunction in the neural circuitry of emotion regulation: a possible prelude to violence. *Science* 2000; 289: 591–4.

18. Fairchild G, Passamonti L, Hurford G, Hagan CC, von dem Hagen EAH. , van Goozen S, et al. Brain structure abnormalities in early onset and adolescent onset conduct disorder. *American Journal of Psychiatry* 2011; 168: 624–33.

19. Barkley RA. Deficient emotional self regulation is a core component of ADHD. *Journal of ADHD and Related Disorders* 2009; 1(2): 5–37.

20. Wishart JG, Cebula KR, Willis DS, Pitcairn TK. Understanding of facial expressions of emotion by children with intellectual disabilities of differing etiology. *Journal of Intellectual Disability Research* 2007; 51: 551–63.

21. Ganesalingam K, Sanson A, Anderson V, Yeates KO. Self-regulation as a mediator of the effects of childhood traumatic brain injury on social and behavioural functioning. *Journal of the International Neuropsychological Society* 2007; 13(12): 298–311.

22. British Psychological Society. *Learning Disability: Definitions and Contexts*. British Psychological Society, 2001.

23. Green JH. Fetal alcohol spectrum disorders: understanding the effects of prenatal alcohol exposure and supporting students. *Journal of School Health* 2007; 77 (3): 103–8.

24. Biederman J. Functional impairments in adults with self-reports of diagnosed ADHD: a controlled study of 1001 adults in the community. *Journal of Clinical Psychiatry* 2006; 67(4): 524–40.

25. Snow P, Powell M. Youth (in)justice: oral language competence in early life and risk for engagement in antisocial behaviour in adolescence. *Australian Institute of Criminology, Trends and Issues in Crime and Criminal Justice* 2012; 435: 421–44.

26. Pfiffner L, Barkley RA, DuPaul GJ. Treatment of ADHD in school settings. In Barkley, RA, ed., *Attention Deficit Hyperactivity Disorder: A Handbook for Diagnosis and Treatment*, 3rd ed. Guildford Press, 2006.

27. Public Health England. (2019). Collaborative approaches to preventing offending and re-offending in children (CAPRICORN). Available at: www.gov.uk /government/publications/preventing- offending-and-re-offending-by-children/c ollaborative-approaches-to-preventing- offending-and-re-offending-by-children- capricorn-summary.

28. Grygiel P, Humenny G, Rębisz S, Bajcar E, Świtaj P. Peer rejection and perceived quality of relations with schoolmates among children with ADHD. *Journal of Attention Disorders* 2018; 22(8): 738–51.

29. Piquero NL, Gover AR, MacDonald JM, Piquero AR. The influence of delinquent peers on delinquency. Does gender matter? *Youth & Society* 2005; 36(3): 251–75.

30. Botting N, Conti-Ramsden G. Social and behavioural difficulties in children with language impairment. *Child Language Teaching and Therapy* 2000; 16(2): 105–20

31. Baldry E, Dowse L, Clarence M. People with mental and cognitive disabilities: pathways into prison. Background Paper for National Legal Aid Conference, 2011, Darwin, Australia.

32. Wade SL, Taylor HG, Drotar D, Stancin T, Yeates KO, Minich NM. Parent–adolescent interactions after traumatic brain injury: their relationship to family adaptation and adolescent adjustment. *Journal of Head Trauma Rehabilitation* 2003; 18: 164–76.

33. Anderson V, Godfrey C, Rosenfeld JV, Catroppa C. Predictors of cognitive function and recovery 10 years after traumatic brain injury in young children. *Pediatrics* 2012; 129(2): 254–61.

34. Kaiser NM, McBurnett K, Pfiffner LJ. Child ADHD severity and positive and negative parenting as predictors of child social functioning: evaluation of three theoretical models. *Journal of Attention Disorders* 2011; 15(3): 193–203.

35. Barnes C. *Disabled People in Britain and Discrimination: A Case for Anti-Discrimination Legislation.* Hurst Publishers, 1991.

36. Chitsabesan P, Bailey S, Williams R, Kroll L, Kenning C, Talbot L. Learning disabilities and educational needs of juvenile offenders. *Journal of Children's Services* 2007; 2(4): 4–14.

37. Harrington R, Bailey S. *Mental Health Needs and Effectiveness of Provision for Young People in the Youth Justice System.* Youth Justice Board, 2005.

38. McKenzie K, Matheson E, Patrick S, Paxton D, Murray GC. An evaluation of the impact of a one day training course on the knowledge of health, day care and social care staff working in learning disability services. *Journal of Learning Disabilities* 2000; 4(2): 153–6.

39. Snow PC, Powell MB. Oral language competence in incarcerated young offenders: links with offending severity. *International Journal of Speech–Language Pathology* 2011; 13(6): 480–9.

40. Talbot J. Prisoner' voices: experience of the criminal justice system by prisoners with learning disabilities. *Tizard Learning Disability Review* 2010; 15: 33–41.

41. United Nations Children's Fund UK. The United Nations convention on the rights of the child. 1989. Available at: https://down loads.unicef.org.uk/wp-content/uploads/2 010/05/UNCRC_PRESS200910web.pdf?_g a=2.78590034.795419542.1582474737-1972578648.1582474737.

42. United Nations. Conventions on the Rights of the Child. General comment No. 24 on children's rights in the child justice system (CRC/C/GC/24*). Available at: https://doc uments-dds-ny.un.org/doc/UNDOC/GE N/G19/275/57/PDF/G1927557.pdf? OpenElement.

43. Offender Health Research Network. The Comprehensive Health Assessment Tool (CHAT): young people in the secure estate – version 3. 2013. Available at: www.yumpu.com/en/document/view/3490 7062/chat-tool-offender-health-research-network.

44. Royal College of Paediatrics and Child Health. Healthcare standards for children and young people in secure settings. 2019. Available at: www.rcpch.ac.uk/sites/defaul t/files/2019-09/RCPCH_Healthcare%20Sta ndards%20for%20Children%20and%20Yo ung%20People%201.2%20updated%20201 9-09.pdf.

45. Hughes N. Models and approaches to family-focused policy and practice. *Social Policy and Society* 2010; 9(4): 527–32.

46. Youth Justice Board. *Barriers to Engagement in Education, Training and Employment.* Youth Justice Board, 2006.

47. Williams HW, Giray C, Mewse AJ, Tonks J, Burgess CNW. Self-reported traumatic brain injury in male young offenders: a risk factor for re-offending, poor mental health and violence? *Neuropsychological Rehabilitation* 2010; 20 (6): 801–12.

48. Ferguson PL, Pickelsimer EE, Corrigan JD, Bogner JA, Wald M. Prevalence of traumatic brain injury among prisoners in South Carolina. *Journal of Head Trauma Rehabilitation* 2012; 27: E11–20.

49. National Institute for Health and Clinical Excellence. *Attention Deficit Hyperactivity Disorder; diagnosis and management. NICE Guideline [NG87].* NICE 2018.

50. National Institute for Health and Clinical Excellence. *Autism: Recognition, Referral and Diagnosis in Children and Young People on the Autism Spectrum. NICE Clinical Guideline 128.* NICE, 2011.

51. Chitsabesan P, Lennox C, Williams H, Tariq O, Shaw J. Traumatic brain injury in juvenile offenders: findings from the comprehensive health assessment tool study and the development of a specialist linkworker service. *Journal of Head Trauma Rehabilitation* 2015; 30(2): 106–15.

52. The Disabilities Trust Foundation. Brain injury and offending. Available at: www .thedtgroup.org/foundation/offenders-with-brain-injury.aspx.

53. National Institute for Health and Clinical Excellence. *Antisocial behaviour and conduct disorders in children and young people: recognition and management. Clinical Guideline [CG158]*, NICE Last updated 19 April 2017.

54. Murphy D. Extreme violence in a man with an autistic spectrum disorder: assessment and treatment within high-security psychiatric care. *Journal of Forensic Psychiatry and Psychology* 2010; 21: 462–77.

Overview of Offenders with Fetal Alcohol Spectrum Disorders

Raja Mukherjee, Penny A. Cook, David Gilbert and Clare S. Allely

Background, Assessment and Diagnosis

Background to Fetal Alcohol Spectrum Disorders: History and Challenges

Fetal alcohol syndrome was first reported within the English language scientific press in 1973 [1]. The paper described a case series of First Nation children who had characteristic features, linked to exposure to alcohol in utero. Earlier reports, for example a French case series of 127 people published by Paul Lemoine and his colleagues [2] had not come to the attention of the English-speaking scientific community, even though it had been published earlier.

Both of these publications focused primarily on the physical presentation and the observable stigmata. Over the subsequent years, it was identified that a spectrum of presentation existed. By 1996, a consensus guideline group was formed at the behest of the National Institute for Health in the USA. This defined the syndrome into broad categories of fetal alcohol syndrome (FAS) with or without knowledge of alcohol exposure, partial fetal alcohol syndrome (pFAS), alcohol-related birth defects (ARBD) and alcohol-related neurodevelopmental disorder (ARND)[3].

Several diagnostic approaches were subsequently developed including the four-digit approach [4], the Canadian 2005 [5], then updated 2016 [6] guidance and the Australian Guidance [7]. More recently, the *Diagnostic and Statistical Manual of Mental Disorders*, fifth edition (DSM-5) has proposed an approach, with a new category: neurobehavioral disorder associated with prenatal alcohol exposure (NDPAE) [8]. In 2019, the Scottish government sponsored the Intercollegiate Guidance Network (SIGN) to produce a review. This concluded that the 2016 Canadian guidance best suited the Scottish approach (SIGN 156) [9]. This has been adopted by the National Institute for Health and Care Excellence [10].

With time, it became clear that the neurological deficits involved were the more important area of focus. It was increasingly clear that the physical stigmata alone of short palpebral fissures, flattened philtrum and thin upper lip, as well as associated physical features, could not define the syndrome. While physical stigmata remain important, it was recognised that this had little impact on the behavioural presentation other than as a marker of the severity of the neurological deficit. Instead, it became clear that it was important to understand the underlying cognitive and brain-related presentations. Unfortunately, many of these do not present as discriminating features. Although characteristic symptoms were identified, it is not easy to delineate which features are caused by prenatal alcohol alone and which are due to other reasons.

There were early limitations in understanding because available investigations and wider diagnostic tools did not exist as they do now, for example in areas such as neuroimaging or genetic testing. Therefore, establishing fetal alcohol spectrum disorders (FASD), a term that collectively describes the various fetal-alcohol-related conditions, as a diagnosis was challenging. Over the nearly 50 years of research, this has changed. Despite this, many professionals refuse to diagnose without stigmata being present [11]. Relying solely on the three classic physical stigmata to diagnose is, however, becoming an outdated concept.

Early descriptors of facial stigmata highlighted numerous characteristics as well as discriminating features. Over time, the three core features were found to be the most consistently measurable, partly because they were more easily quantified. Other features, such as flat midface or micrognathia, were noted as common associated features. Specialist dysmorphologists but not most non-specialist clinicians could accurately assess these additional signs. More recently, with the advent of three-dimensional photographic technology, linked to highly specialist computer analysis, tens of thousands of facial 'landmarks' can be assessed. This can be used to differentiate normal from abnormal. Therefore, these wider features can now be used in addition to the core original features. This is allowing cases which were previously missed to be included. However, these techniques remain generally the behest of specialist clinics [12].

Another key development over the last 50 years has been the delineation of cognitive and neurodevelopmental profiles of FASD. These are considered aetiological syndromes, in that they are the cause of the underlying damage to brain and body and are more akin to genetic syndromes such as fragile X or Down syndrome. FASD have very specific profiles and characteristic symptoms but, when the physical stigmata of FASD are removed, the neurocognitive presentations in terms of intelligence quotient (IQ), executive function or language skills overlap with these other disorders. There are some discriminating differences but many overlapping presentations.

Recent evidence suggests that only around 5% to 10% of those affected cognitively by prenatal alcohol have classic facial stigmata. A recent study conducted on the ALSPAC (Avon Longitudinal Study of Parents and Children) database, looking at a screening prevalence in the UK, identified that between 6% and 17% of the population studied in a cohort of over 13,000 mothers and children could have met criteria for an FASD diagnosis [13]. It also highlighted that only around 2% had classic facial characteristics but all of those screening positive had the core cognitive features alongside alcohol exposure. This suggests that it is therefore difficult to identify people on the basis of physical stigmata alone; the majority would have been missed.

When considering the neurodevelopmental profiles in FASD, classic presentations can be seen. There are impairments exhibited across multiple domains such as with higher-level planning, memory, processing speed, receptive language skills and sensory integration. Much of this is not obvious, unless looked for.

Many of those with an FASD have only these cognitive impairments; however, in the worst cases, the severity of the presentation may mean that other neurodevelopmental conditions such as autism spectrum disorder (ASD) and attention deficit hyperactivity disorder (ADHD) can be diagnosed as comorbid outcomes. This means that, if present, ASD or ADHD are outcomes of the underlying neurological impairment caused by an FASD [14, 15]. The majority of cases with FASD, however, do not meet the clinical threshold for a diagnosis of ASD or ADHD and have the neurodevelopmental and neuro-cognitive profile typically expected with an FASD alone.

Diagnostic assessment is complicated further because often it is the more integrative neurocognitive processes that are most affected. In testing situations, where wider arousal or other environmental stressors are mitigated, individuals can present better than they function in real-world scenarios. There is evidence to suggest that it is only when multiple demands are experienced at the same time that these impact on the individual, which in turn leads to their function deteriorating. For example, in testing scenarios, people with FASD can sequence, or they can shift sets, but cannot do both together [16]. Real-world tasks, such as capacity and decision making, rely on multiple-level processing and are also, in the real world, influenced by emotion. This is not always the case in the testing scenario, and therefore real-world function is worse than performance assessed in a clinic environment [16].

Diagnostic Process

The process of diagnosis is challenging, both in terms of accessing services and the complexity of the diagnostic process in the face of limited resources. Individuals often present to services because of these other conditions, rather than for an assessment of an FASD alone, although requests for FASD assessment are increasing. A study completed in 2016 highlighted that there were 427 comorbid presentations linked to an FASD diagnosis [17]. The diagnostic process for FASD requires careful evaluation at every step. FASD diagnosis is one of exclusion as much as it is inclusion of characteristic symptoms. Much of the diagnostic time spent is to rule out, as far as possible, other common causes of a neurodevelopmental presentation. Box 8.1 highlights some of the core areas that are investigated and need to be considered before reaching an FASD diagnosis. The most common of these are genetic. Currently, the recommendation is that, as a minimum in those people who are non-dysmorphic, a microarray is arranged [18]. Where dysmorphic issues exist, it is always wise to include a clinical geneticist or dysmorphologist in the assessment, who can potentially direct the individual to more specific testing, including, potentially, a microarray or genome-wide assessment.

Where other possible reasons are found, this does not preclude alcohol also having a comorbid teratogenic effect. However, it does complicate the picture and obscure the

---

Box 8.1 Core areas to rule out when considering other aetiological causes of the neurodevelopmental presentation

(1) Genetic factors

(2) Other substances in pregnancy

(3) Prematurity (generally before 34 weeks)

(4) Perinatal hypoxia and significant physical trauma

(5) Extreme postnatal neglect

presentation of the unique phenotype. Due to the complexity and difficulty in delineating the different factors, in these cases, the diagnosis of an FASD cannot be confidently made. However, prenatal alcohol should be listed as an aetiological factor alongside the other factors.

Increasingly, through careful evaluation, it is becoming possible to delineate and rule out the influence of some of these other aetiological causes on the basis of the neurological deficits. Other drugs, rather than being considered as social constructs, must be looked at from the perspective of their differing biological mechanisms. For example, cocaine acts on dopaminergic reuptake and therefore can have some frontal lobe activation and effect; however, longer-term studies indicate that, where used alone, this has low potency for ongoing damage [19]. For heroin, while socially having significant impacts on the person and society, the biological impact is more limited. Studies that have monitored those using methadone, for example, show no long-term consequences [19]. However, the exact mix of substances used is often difficult to determine and, where there is chaotic multi-substance abuse, alcohol is often also consumed.

Box 8.1 also highlights postnatal neglect as a potential factor that can lead to behavioural presentations. However, as for drug use above, if alcohol exposure has also occurred in cases of postnatal neglect, alcohol is increasingly being seen as having a greater neurodevelopmental impact. Emerging research suggests that the neurological features are prenatal in origin and that postnatal neglect may not necessarily make this any worse [20]. Postnatal neglect does, however, impact on the wider vulnerabilities, and the subsequent psychological experience of life. This is increasingly understood as complex trauma, but must always be seen in the light of the underlying neurology.

There are multiple methods by which alcohol directs its effects on the developing fetus. This to some extent explains the different vulnerability of individuals. Exposure information is vital. Not everybody who was exposed to prenatal alcohol will develop an FASD. However, while prenatal alcohol in itself is insufficient to make the diagnosis, in most cases, the absence of information of exposure to the risk factors remains the most common reason to preclude diagnosis, rather than the lack of exposure itself.

When assessing individuals with FASD, a multidisciplinary approach is often needed [9]. Information can, however, be collated by a single clinician, where different assessments are brought together, allowing a diagnosis to be made. Reports by a psychologist, occupational therapist or speech and language therapist, are important to help identify the level of deficits and the identified needs. Box 8.2 highlights the cognitive domains that have been identified as being crucial to assess.

Given the difficulty and the lack of expertise on how to recognise and formulate conditions that may be caused by prenatal exposure to alcohol, cases of FASD are often missed or misdiagnosed. Therefore, those with undiagnosed FASD are likely to present later with secondary psychiatric mental health conditions. Table 8.1, taken from a long-term cohort study over 30 years, identifies that mental health problems are common, but also so is involvement with the criminal justice system and incarceration.

Box 8.2 Core cognitive domains where information needs to be gathered

(1) Hard or soft neurological signs

(2) Brain structure

(3) Cognition

(4) Communication

(5) Academic achievement

(6) Memory

(7) Executive function

(8) Attention/ hyperactivity

(9) Adaptive function

(10) Emotional dysregulation (not required in all criteria but a common comorbidity)

Table 8.1 Long term follow-up study into secondary outcomes in those with FASD by Streissguth and O'Malley [21]

Secondary disability	Percentage occurrence
Psychiatric problem	90
Disrupted school experience	60
Trouble with the law	60
Confinement	50
Inappropriate sexual behaviour	50
Alcohol/drug problems	30

Epidemiology of FASD in Young Offenders within the Criminal Justice System

Prevalence of FASD in General and in the Criminal Justice Setting

As outlined above, the complexity of diagnosis means that FASDs are rarely diagnosed, making healthcare records unreliable as a source of information for prevalence studies [22]. In a systematic review of active case ascertainment studies, the 'gold standard' method, prevalence in the general population of young people was estimated to be 7.7/1,000 globally, and 19.8/1,000 in Europe [23] (Table 8.2).

In the UK, there are no prevalence studies in young offender populations. In the USA, a survey of all states identified only one offender known to have FAS ([25]). Most studies originate from Canada (see Table 8.3), the USA and Australia. Interpreting data from these countries is challenging because specific sub-populations have a high FASD prevalence, for example 12% in indigenous populations in Australia and 19% in Canada [23]. The wider cycle of inequality experienced by these indigenous populations also increases their risk of incarceration, independently of FASD. In an Australian detention centre, the prevalence of FASD

Table 8.2 Prevalence of FASD in selected countries

Country	Source	FASD prevalence % (95% CI)	Method
South Africa	Lange et al. [23]	11.1 (7.1–15.8)	ACA
Croatia	Lange et al. [23]	5.3 (3.1–8.1)	ACA
Ireland	Lange et al. [23]	4.8 (2.8–7.4)	Est
US	Lange et al. [23]	1.5 (0.8–2.5)	ACA
	May et al. [24]	1.1 (7.8–1.6) to 5.0 (4.0–6.2)*	ACA
UK	Lange et al. [23]	3.2 (2.0–4.9)	Est

95%CI: 95% confidence interval. ACA: active case ascertainment; Est: estimated from pregnancy drinking prevalence for those countries without ACA estimates. *The variation in May et al.'s prevalence estimates was due to differences in sampling methods, sampling size and the locations of data collection.

Table 8.3 Summary of prevalence studies of FASD in offender populations in Canada from Popova et al. [27]

Location in Canada	Study population	Prevalence of FASD (%)
British Columbia	Youths	27
Manitoba	Adults	10
Yukon	Adults (18–40 years)	17.5
British Columbia	Youths	12

was 36%, and 47% of the young offenders with an FASD diagnosis were Aboriginals [26]. Studies in offender populations in Canada demonstrate prevalence of 10–27% (Table 8.3).

Another group at elevated risk of FASD are children in the adoption or social care system, with estimates of 17% prevalence of FASD in this subgroup globally [23] and prevalences of 30% [28] and 27% [29] found in two separate studies in the UK. Those young people who are currently or previously looked after, who have also had troubled and traumatic lives, may also be at an increased risk of incarceration [30]. However, worldwide, there are no data on the co-occurrence of FASD and incarceration in this group.

FASD Prevalence in Young Offenders: Comparison with Other Neurodevelopmental Disorders

Since there is a dearth of prevalence studies on young offenders with FASD within the criminal justice system, other related/co-occurring neurodevelopmental disorders such as ADHD and ASD are relevant to consider alongside FASD. Moreover, due to the paucity of diagnosis of FASD, a proportion of individuals with diagnosed ADHD and/or ASD in the criminal justice system will have an underlying undiagnosed FASD.

Table 8.4 Prevalence of ADHD in the criminal justice system

Country	Study population	Source	ADHD prevalence (%)
Germany	Female (all)	Rösler	10
	Female (young, <25 years)	et al. [34]	17.9
Germany	Male	Rösler et al. [35]	45
Finland	Violent offenders	Haapasalo and Hämäläinen [36]	48
UK	Incarcerated population	Young et al. [37]	25.5 (95% CI: 20.0–32.4)

Table 8.5 Prevalence of ASD in young offenders

Country	Study population	Source	Prevalence of ASD in the criminal justice system setting (per 10,000)	General population ASD prevalence for comparison (per 10,000)
UK	Children	Baird et al. [38]		−116·1 (95% CI: 90·4–141·8)
Japan	Juvenile justice setting	Kawamura et al. [39]; Kumagami and Matsuura [40];	180	130
Sweden	Criminal justice setting	Stahlberg et al. [41]; Gillberg et al. [42]	170	53.3 (95% CI: 48.8–57.8)

In a follow-up study, over 40% of children with ADHD received criminal convictions in adulthood and were five times more likely to sustain convictions compared to neurotypical peers [31], while ADHD populations were twelve times more likely to have violent convictions [32]. Adolescents with ADHD were over three times more likely to have trouble with the law and get arrested [33]. This leads to a high prevalence of ADHD in the criminal justice setting (Table 8.4). Evidence for the prevalence of ASD in the general population, and young people specifically, is mixed but suggests that the prevalence in the criminal justice system is significantly higher than in the general population (Table 8.5). In contrast, the FASD population is estimated to be 19 times more likely than the general population to encounter the criminal justice system [27].

The Relationship between FASD and the Criminal Justice System in Young Offenders

Patterns, Risk, and Protective Factors of Criminal Justice Encounters in Young Offenders with FASD

Individuals with neurodevelopmental disorders tend to encounter the criminal justice system earlier than their neurotypical counterparts [35]. Several risk factors contribute to the elevated risk of criminal justice system involvement in those with FASD, including low social economic status, placement instabilities, substance misuse, impairments in adaptive functioning domains, deficits in social functioning (which may worsen with age) and inability to comprehend the outcomes of actions [43]. Receptive language disorders identified in individuals with FASD may impact their ability to understand rules and the implication of contravening rules [44].

FASD disproportionately affect those who are disadvantaged, for example those who are part of the looked-after children system, or part of a community that already faces multiple deprivation (e.g., indigenous populations). Furthermore, lack of awareness within the justice system and poor identification of FASD exacerbate the risk [45]. Protective factors to reduce this risk include early diagnosis, placement stability and family and peer support [46]. Early diagnosis is essential for the implementation of early interventions and provision of other protective factors. However, as noted at the beginning of this chapter, obtaining an early diagnosis is difficult.

The Pathway to Criminal Justice Encounters in Young People with FASD

For young individuals with FASD, encounters with the criminal justice system could be as victims of crime, witnesses of crime or suspects in a crime [47]. Five major theoretical pathways leading to involvement with the criminal justice system have been identified [48] and are useful to consider in the context of young offenders with FASD: (1) prenatal-risk (resulting from fetal exposure to teratogenic substances); (2) childhood maltreatment (the impact of trauma); (3) adolescent-onset (young offenders with no history of exposure to offending risk factors); (4) extreme child temperament (extreme emotional reaction to events); and (5) personality-disorder pathways. Theoretically, four of these pathways (except for the adolescent-onset pathway) could influence the risk of criminal justice encounters for young people with FASD.

The most significant factor that contributes to the high criminal justice encounter rates of the FASD population is the spectrum of brain impairments, which may lead to behavioural problems such as lack of self-regulation, impulsivity and aggressive behaviour. These traits increase the risk of an initial encounter with the criminal justice system and, once encountered, lead to weaknesses in the ability to defend oneself in the system. The remaining sections of this chapter are chiefly concerned with the latter: the inability to defend oneself, starting with an explanation of the investigative interviewing process and why the process renders those with FASD potentially more vulnerable.

Investigative Interviewing Techniques in the Criminal Justice System

Investigative interviews are used in the criminal justice system in order to obtain evidence and confessions from suspects [49]. The PEACE model for interviewing, developed in the UK, comprises Preparation, Engagement, Account, Closure and Evaluation [50]. The Reid technique, used in the USA, involves a nine-step process that includes accusations levelled at the suspect and an analysis of the suspect's behaviour, known as a behaviour analysis interview [51].

Irrespective of the technique employed, different approaches may be used in interviews to obtain confessions from suspects. In an analysis of 182 custodial interrogations in the US, 85–90% of interrogators appealed to the self-interest of suspects and confronted the suspect with existing evidence of guilt; 40–43% asked specific 'behavioural analysis' interview questions, highlighted contradictions in the suspect's narrations, downplayed the confidence of the suspect in his/her denial and presented moral excuses for the committed crime; and 22–37% downplayed the seriousness of the offence, emphasised the importance of cooperation, confronted the suspect with false evidence of guilt or flattered the suspect [52]. Interviewers employed a median of 5 and a mean of 5.62 tactics per interrogation, with over 30% of interrogations lasting 31–60 minutes, and over 20% lasting 1–2 hours.

Vulnerabilities of Young Offenders with FASD during Investigative Interviewing

The vulnerabilities of young people with FASD during investigative interviewing are summarised in Box 8.3. Psychological vulnerabilities, the 'psychological characteristics or mental state which render a witness prone, in certain circumstances, to providing information, which is inaccurate, unreliable or misleading' [53] lead to a reduced capacity to prove innocence during an investigative interview. Investigative interviewers may employ sophisticated techniques, which may include deception and psychological coercion [54]. Those

---

Box 8.3 Summary of contemporary issues to consider with individuals impacted by FASD and their involvement with the criminal justice system

(1) Individuals with FASD may display verbal fluency, which may mask their vulnerabilities before the criminal justice system. This is termed 'frontal lobe paradox'.

(2) FASD-impacted individuals are susceptible to suggestions which may, in the first instance, render them vulnerable to accepting suggestions to break the law. Second, as suspects within the criminal justice system, individuals with FASD may easily accept interrogators' suggestions. This can lead to confessions of guilt that may not be true.

(3) During arrest, individuals with FASD may be more likely to waive their rights to remain silent (the 'Miranda rights') and then submit to questioning without the help of legal counsel.

(4) The IQ of FASD-impacted individuals may be above the threshold of 70. During mental capacity assessments, an IQ of 2 standard deviations below 100 (which equates to 70) is regarded as the basis of mental incapacity. This implies that individuals with FASD may be deemed as mentally capable when they may not be so in reality. This means that they would not qualify under the Mental Capacity Act 2005 for additional support during interrogation.

(5) Individuals with FASD have issues with poor memory and may confabulate during interviewing. Confabulation is the production of fabricated, distorted, or misinterpreted memories about an event. This can be misinterpreted as a deliberate attempt to conceal the truth.

with FASD, who are likely to be psychologically vulnerable, are predicted to perform poorly in these conditions and are less able to circumvent these interviewing techniques. These psychological vulnerabilities can lead to miscarriages of justice [55].

During investigative interviews, even when suspects are innocent, they must remain alert. Suspects require effective mental coordination to establish their innocence. Effective mental co-ordination is achieved through the executive function of the brain, impairments in which lead to weaknesses in handling complex neural processes. The predominance of expressive and receptive language disorders as comorbidities in individuals with FASD [43] may further increase vulnerabilities during encounters with the criminal justice system. Executive function impairments and damage to the frontal lobes in FASD leads to language and communication impairments, which may hinder individuals from effectively defending themselves verbally or from being competent witnesses during legal proceedings. However, individuals with frontal lobe damage may possess preserved verbal skills. Indeed, parents/carers of individuals with FASD often describe their children as 'chatty' [56], and this may mask their vulnerabilities. This phenomenon is termed the 'frontal lobe paradox' and was first described by Teuber in 1964 [57]. Investigative interviewers may not identify individuals as psychologically vulnerable, and this lack of recognition could lead to individuals with neurodevelopmental disabilities being interviewed without appropriate support.

Studies indicate that individuals with FASD may be more susceptible to suggestions [58], which could potentially act in two ways. First, individuals with a neurodevelopmental disorder and high suggestibility could readily accept suggestions from peers or associates to break the law. Second, even when innocent, individuals may be susceptible to accepting suggestions from investigative interviewers. The susceptibility to suggestions during an investigative interview is termed 'interrogative suggestibility' and is impacted by both interviewee- and interviewer-dependent factors [59]. Interviewer-dependent factors include factors that influence suggestibility due to the interviewer's behaviour, such as interviewer style during interviews [60]. Interviewee-dependent factors are dependent on the personality and characteristics of the interviewee and include self-esteem, age and the presence of psychological vulnerabilities [61]. The interaction of interviewee and interviewer-dependent factors impact suggestibility. In juvenile offenders, regardless of the presence of psychological vulnerabilities, it has been shown that younger individuals are more susceptible to suggestions during interrogation [62]. While the phenomenon of interrogative suggestibility is now fairly well understood in the general population, there is little research with neurodevelopmental disorders such as FASD.

Ability to Stand Trials in Young Offenders with Neurodevelopmental Disorders

It is crucial that the courts are informed of a diagnosis of a neurodevelopment disorder and the types of behaviours that someone with a particular neurodevelopmental disorder (such as ASD or FASD) may display. This will help the jury to understand and recognise the ways in which the diagnosis, in particular the different symptomologies of features of the neurodevelopmental disorder, may have contributed to the defendant's alleged offending behaviour [63]. Sorge conducted a review of 81 Canadian criminal cases and found that five impairments associated with an FASD diagnosis were considered at sentencing [64] (Box 8.4).

Box 8.4 Five impairments associated with an FASD diagnosis [64]

(1) The accused's difficulty linking punishment to crime

(2) Risk of being taken advantage of in prison

(3) Compromised ability to instruct counsel

(4) Difficulty with deciphering right from wrong

(5) Having been influenced by someone else to commit the crime

Sorge also found that on some occasions judges did consider lack of insight and impulsivity as being potential mitigating factors. However, significant variations were evident across provinces with regard to the frequency with which judges consider FASD-related mitigating factors in their dispositions [64]. The study also showed that the judges were more likely to consider an FASD when a previous diagnosis already exists compared to when an FASD is only suspected or not mentioned by counsel. This can perhaps be easily explained. The lack of a diagnosis and the subtle impairments that can be exhibited in individuals with FASD can make recognising this neurodevelopmental disorder challenging [65]. Individuals with such a disorder are likely to present with a negative demeanour, a lack of apparent remorse and atypical behaviours are likely to be displayed during judiciary proceedings. In the absence of expert testimony regarding the defendant's neurodevelopmental disorder, the jury is likely to form a negative perception of the defendant, which may have particularly negative consequences [63], such as longer sentences.

The complexity of judiciary proceedings is a challenge to individuals with intellectual abilities within the normal range but it is even more challenging and overwhelming to individuals with neurodevelopmental disorders [66]. Individuals with a neurodevelopmental disorder may say or do things which are not in their best interests during judiciary proceedings. It has been pointed out, for instance, that individuals with FASD often do not have the ability to fully appreciate and understand the judicial proceedings in which they participating [67]. Specifically, individuals with FASD may not be likely to comprehend the implications of consenting to a search, plea negotiations or sworn testimony [47].

Mela and colleagues carried out a study in a sample of 45 adults (average age 42) with serious mental illness in a Canadian outpatient forensic mental health program, including a subset with FASD [68]. The findings from this study revealed that, in both groups, there were similar high levels of lifetime adversity and varied offence histories. However, the study found that the rates of neurocognitive impairment such as verbal IQ, full-scale IQ, working memory, processing speed and expressive vocabulary were significantly greater in the group with FASD when compared to the adults with serial mental illness.

Finally, individuals with neurodevelopmental disorder may not be competent to participate in their own defence or serve as a witness. Due to their impulsive desire to please and to avoid uncomfortable/confrontational situations, exacerbated by their impaired reasoning abilities, they may testify falsely or confabulate during questioning in forensic contexts (e.g., court proceedings, investigative interviews) [47].

The Role That Providing Evidence of FASD Plays in Judicial Proceedings

In their study, Douds and colleagues [66] systematically reviewed all the relevant US federal case law in order to examine how federal courts receive FASD evidence and what role that evidence plays in the disposition of claims for mental incapacity, competency, sentence mitigation and ineffective assistance of counsel. In all federal court cases arising prior to 2011, the authors identified 1,713 cases, with 131 cases substantively relevant to mental capacity, criminal intent, sentencing and attorney malpractice. Most of the cases occurred following Atkins v. Virginia, the pivotal Supreme Court case that prohibits the death penalty for 'mentally disabled persons'. Douds and colleagues showed that FASD evidence usually defeats a death penalty sentence [66]. However, the study highlighted that the lower courts reflect inconsistencies in how courts receive and handle mental health evidence. All the courts in this study accepted FASD evidence as relevant. No court in this study was found to exclude evidence of FASD on the grounds that it was not probative of the matter raised. The courts were found to disagree on the persuasive value and effect of the FASD evidence but they did all consider the evidence to various degrees. The findings from this study also revealed that very few of the courts were found to analyse FASD evidence directly or independently of other evidence. Instead, this study showed that most of the courts took FASD evidence into consideration in conjunction with evidence of other mental health conditions – and subsequently finding that the aggregated mental health evidence was relevant to a defendant's mental state. This makes it difficult, if not impossible, to make any conclusions regarding the discrete significance of FASD diagnoses [66].

Fitness to Stand Trial

An individual is found unfit to stand trial if it can be demonstrated that the person does not understand the nature, object and potential consequences of the proceedings, and cannot effectively instruct counsel [65]. It is important to consider the ways in which the memory and language impairments that are associated with neurodevelopmental disorders such as FASD and ASD may impair a defendant's capacity to adequately communicate with counsel [69]. Additionally, individuals with neurodevelopmental disorders such as FASD and ASD are typically concrete thinkers and have a tendency to act impulsively. Such features may also make it a challenge for them to fully appreciate the possible outcomes of criminal proceedings [69]. To date, there have been relatively few cases in which a defendant with an FASD was found unfit to stand trial. This is in part due to the fact that the mental disorder defence was developed with the assumption that a disorder could be treated and mitigated, which is not the case with neurodevelopmental conditions such as FASD, which are lifelong conditions [69].

Recommendations for Questioning Individuals with Neurodevelopmental Disorders during Judicial Proceedings (and Other Forensic Contexts)

Several studies have shown poor knowledge and awareness of FASD among criminal justice professionals. For instance, in an Australian study, Mutch and colleagues [70] investigated knowledge of FASD among 427 justice professionals (e.g., judicial officers, lawyers, correctional staff, police) using an online survey. The findings highlighted that the majority of the justice professionals in this survey study (85%) reported having heard of FAS, but awareness of FASD was lower, and few were able to identify that an FASD is a lifelong impairment. These types of findings have been demonstrated in other similar studies internationally.

Some insights from research into other neurodevelopmental disorders are relevant for FASD [71]. These have been outlined in a number of sources, such as guidance provided by the advocacy services in the UK [72]. Briefly, the key recommendations are that: questions or statements which are potentially ambiguous in interpretation should not be used; questions should not include metaphors, sarcasm, non-literal language; questions should not require inference, insinuation, deduction or abstractive extrapolation; questions should be direct; and the use of 'tags' and double negatives should be avoided. An example of a 'tag' question is, 'You went to the park, didn't you?'. An example of a question with a double negative is, 'You would not disagree with that interpretation, Gilbert, would you?'. As highlighted earlier in this section, some individuals with FASD may also have an impaired autobiographical memory. Therefore, it is recommended that questions should be framed in the correct tense. Therefore, questions should avoid referring to a past event as if in the present, for instance. One example of such a question which should be avoided is, 'Now you are in the street and looking at the car' [71].

Conclusion

FASD is relatively common yet grossly underdiagnosed and under-recognised in part due to difficulties in diagnosis and overlaps with other disorders. While comprehensive data on the prevalence of FASD in the criminal justice setting is not available for most countries, including the UK, it is likely to be considerably higher than in the general population. The specific impairments experienced by those with FASD put them at significant risk of coming into contact with the criminal justice system. The spectrum of brain impairments may lead to behavioural problems, including lack of self-regulation, impulsivity and aggressive behaviour, all of which increase the risk of an initial encounter with the criminal justice system. Once encountered, these lead to weaknesses in the ability to defend oneself in the system including, for example, through false confessions. It is crucial that neurodevelopmental disorders are considered as being a potential mitigating factor and relevant to considerations surrounding the prospects of rehabilitation. It is important to highlight that it is highly possible that decision makers and legal professionals will overestimate a defendant's abilities and underestimate their needs if they have insufficient knowledge and understanding of the defendant's FASD diagnosis. The implications of this can be detrimental (e.g., harsher sentencing decisions and lack of appropriate treatment and support [73].

References

1. Jones KL, Smith DW. Recognition of the fetal alcohol syndrome. *Lancet* 1973; 302 (7836): 999–1001.

2. Lemoine P, Harousseau H, Borteryu JP, Menuet JC. les enfants des parents alcoholiques: anomolies observees a propos de 127 cas. *Quest Medical* 1968; 25(476): 482.

3. Institute of Medicine. *Fetal Alcohol Syndrome: Diagnosis, Epidemiology,* *Prevention, and Treatment.* National Academies Press, 1996.

4. Astley SJP, Stachowiak JR, Clarren SKM, Clausen CR. Application of the fetal alcohol syndrome facial photographic screening tool in a foster care population. *Journal of Pediatrics* 2002; 141(5): 712–17.

5. Chudley AE, Conry J, Cook JL, Loock C, Rosales T, LeBlanc N. Fetal alcohol spectrum disorder: Canadian guidelines for

diagnosis. *Canadian Medical Association Journal* 2005; 172(5 suppl): S1–S21.

6. Cook JL, Green CR, Lilley CM, Anderson SM, Baldwin ME, Chudley AE, et al. Fetal alcohol spectrum disorder: a guideline for diagnosis across the lifespan. *Canadian Medical Association Journal* 2016; 188(3): 191–7.

7. Bower C, Elliott EJ, Zimmet M, Doorey J, Wilkins A, Russell V, et al. Australian guide to the diagnosis of foetal alcohol spectrum disorder: a summary. *Journal of Paediatrics and Child Health* 2017; 53(10): 1021–3.

8. American Psychiatric Association. *Diagnostic and Statistical Manual of Mental Disorders*, 5th edition: DSM-5. American Psychiatric Association, 2013.

9. Healthcare Improvement Scotland. SIGN 156. Children and young people exposed to prenatal alcohol. 2019. Available at: www.sign.ac.uk/media/1092/sign156.pdf.

10. National Institute for Health and Care Excellence. FASD quality standards consultation. 2022. Available at: www.nice.org.uk/guidance/indevelop ment/gid-qs10139/documents.

11. Mukherjee RAS, Wray E, Curfs L, Hollins S. Knowledge and opinions of professional groups concerning FASD in the UK. *Journal of Adoption and Fostering* 2015; 39: 212–24.

12. Suttie M, Wetherill L, Jacobson SW, Jacobson JL, Hoyme HE, Sowell ER, et al. Facial curvature detects and explicates ethnic differences in effects of prenatal alcohol exposure. *Alcoholism: Clinical and Experimental Research* 2017; 41(8): 1471–83.

13. McQuire C, Mukherjee R, Hurt L, Higgins A, Greene G, Farewell D, et al. Screening prevalence of fetal alcohol spectrum disorders in a region of the United Kingdom: a population-based birth-cohort study. *Preventive Medicine* 2019; 118: 344–51.

14. Mukherjee RAS. The relationship between ADHD and FASD. *Thrombus* 2016; 8: 4–7.

15. Mukherjee RAS, Layton M, Yacoub E, Turk JT. Autism and autistic traits in people exposed to heavy prenatal alcohol: data from a clinical series of 21 individuals and a nested case control study. *Advances in Mental Health and Intellectual Disability* 2011; 5: 43–9.

16. Mohamed Z, Carlisle ACS, Livesey AC, Mukherjee RAS. Comparisons of the BRIEF parental report and neuropsychological clinical tests of executive function in fetal alcohol spectrum disorders: data from the UK national specialist clinic. *Child Neuropsychology* 2019; 25(5): 648–63.

17. Popova S, Lange S, Shield K, Mihic A, Chudley AE, Mukherjee RAS, et al. Comorbidity of fetal alcohol spectrum disorders: a systematic review and meta-analysis. *Lancet* 2016; 387: 978–87.

18. Douzgou S, Breen C, Crow YJ, Chandler K, Metcalfe K, Jones E, et al. Diagnosing fetal alcohol syndrome: new insights from newer genetic technologies. *Archives of Diseases in Children* 2012; 97(9): 812–17.

19. Preece PM, Riley EP. *Alcohol, Drugs and Medication in Pregnancy*. Mac Keith Press, 2011.

20. Mukherjee RAS, Cook PA, Norgate SH, Price AD. Neurodevelopmental outcomes in individuals with fetal alcohol spectrum disorder (FASD) with and without exposure to neglect: clinical cohort data from a national FASD diagnostic clinic. *Alcohol* 2019; 7: 23–8.

21. Streissguth AP, O'Malley K. Neuropsychiatric implications and long-term consequences of fetal alcohol spectrum disorders. *Seminars in Clinical Neuropsychiatry* 2000; 5(3): 177–90.

22. Morleo M, Woolfall K, Dedman D, Mukherjee RAS, Bellis MA, Cook PA. Under-reporting of fetal alcohol spectrum disorders: an analysis of hospital episode statistics. *BMC Paediatrics* 2011; 11: 14.

23. Lange, S., Probst, C., Gmel, G., Rehm, J., Burd, L., & Popova, S. (2017). Global prevalence of fetal alcohol spectrum disorder among children and youth: a

systematic review and meta-analysis. *JAMA pediatrics*, 171(10), 948–956.

24. May PA, Chambers CD, Kalberg Wo, Zellner J, Feldman H, Buckley D, et al., Prevalence of fetal alcohol spectrum disorders in 4 US communities. *JAMA* 2018; 319(5): 474–83.

25. Burd L, Selfridge R, Klug M, Bakko S. Fetal alcohol syndrome in the United States corrections system. *Addiction Biology* 2004; 9(2): 169–78.

26. Bower C, Watkins RE, Mutch RC, Marriott R, Freeman J, Kippin NR, et al. Fetal alcohol spectrum disorder and youth justice: a prevalence study among young people sentenced to detention in Western Australia. *BMJ Open* 2018; 8(2): e019605.

27. Popova S, Lange S, Bekmuradov D, Mihic A, Rehm J. Fetal alcohol spectrum disorder prevalence estimates in correctional systems: a systematic literature review. *Canadian Journal of Public Health* 2011; 102(5): 336–40.

28. Selwyn J, Wijedesa D. Pathways to adoption for minority ethnic children in England: reasons for entry to care. *Child and Family Social Work* 2011; 16(3): 276–86.

29. Gregory G, Reddy V, Young C. Identifying children who are at risk of FASD in Peterborough: working in a community clinic without access to gold standard dignosis. *Journal of Adoption and Fostering* 2015; 39(3): 225–34.

30. Fitzpatrick C. *Looked After Children and the Criminal Justice System*. John Wiley & Sons, 2009.

31. Young S, Moss D, Sedgwick O, Fridman M, Hodgkins P. A meta-analysis of the prevalence of attention deficit hyperactivity disorder in incarcerated populations. *Psychological Medicine* 2015; 45(2): 247–58.

32. Dalsgaard S, Mortensen PB, Frydenberg M, Thomsen PH. Long-term criminal outcome of children with attention deficit hyperactivity disorder. *Criminal Behaviour and Mental Health* 2013; 23(2): 86–98.

33. Satterfield J, Swanson J, Schell A, Lee F. Prediction of antisocial behavior in attention-deficit hyperactivity disorder boys from aggression/defiance scores. *Journal of the American Academy of Child and Adolescent Psychiatry* 1994; 33(2): 185–90.

34. Rösler M, Retz W, Yaqoobi K, Burg E, Retz-Junginger P. Attention deficit/ hyperactivity disorder in female offenders: prevalence, psychiatric comorbidity and psychosocial implications. *European Archives of Psychiatry and Clinical Neuroscience* 2009; 259(2): 98–105.

35. Rösler M, Retz W, Retz-Junginger P, Hengesch G, Schneider M, Supprian T, et al. Prevalence of attention deficit/ hyperactivity disorder (ADHD) and comorbid disorders in young male prison inmates. *European Archives of Psychiatry and Clinical Neuroscience* 2004; 254(6): 365–71.

36. Haapasalo J, Hämäläinen T. Childhood family problems and current psychiatric problems among young violent and property offenders. *Journal of the American Academy of Child and Adolescent Psychiatry* 1996; 35(10): 1394–401.

37. Young S, Moss D, Sedgwick O, Fridman M, Hodgkins P. A meta-analysis of the prevalence of attention deficit hyperactivity disorder in incarcerated populations. *Psychological Medicine* 2015; 45(2): 247–58.

38. Baird G, Simonoff E, Pickles A, Chandler S, Loucas T, Meldrum D, Charman T. (2006). Prevalence of disorders of the autism spectrum in a population cohort of children in South Thames: the special needs and autism project (SNAP). *Lancet* 368, 210–215.

39. Kawamura Y, Takahashi O, Ishii T. Reevaluating the incidence of pervasive developmental disorders: impact of elevated rates of detection through implementation of an integrated system of screening in Toyota, Japan. *Psychiatry and Clinical Neurosciences* 2008; 62(2): 152–9.

40. Kumagami T, Matsuura N. Prevalence of pervasive developmental disorder in juvenile court cases in Japan. *Journal of Forensic Psychiatry and Psychology* 2009; 20(6): 974–87.

41. Ståhlberg O, Anckarsäter H, Nilsson T. Mental health problems in youths committed to juvenile institutions: prevalences and treatment needs. *European Child and Adolescent Psychiatry* 2010; 19: 893–903.

42. Gillberg C, Cederlund M, Lamberg K, Zeijlon L. Brief report: 'the autism epidemic'. the registered prevalence of autism in a Swedish urban area. *Journal of Autism and Developmental Disorders* 2006; 36(3): 429–35.

43. Streissguth AP, Bookstein FL, Barr HM, Sampson PD, O'Malley K, Young JK. Risk factors for adverse life outcomes in fetal alcohol syndrome and fetal alcohol effects. *Journal of Developmental and Behavioral Pediatrics* 2004; 25(4): 228–38.

44. McLachlan K, Roesch R, Viljoen JL, Douglas KS. Evaluating the psycholegal abilities of young offenders with fetal alcohol spectrum disorder. *Law and Human Behavior* 2014; 38(1): 10–22.

45. Douglas H, Hammill J, Hall W, Russell E. Judicial views of foetal alcohol spectrum disorder in Queensland's criminal justice system. *Journal of Judicial Administration* 2012; 21(3): 178–88.

46. Reid N, Dawe S, Harnett P, Shelton D, Hutton L, O'Callaghan F. Feasibility study of a family-focused intervention to improve outcomes for children with FASD. *Research in Developmental Disabilities* 2017; 67: 34–46.

47. Fast DK, Conry J. Fetal alcohol spectrum disorders and the criminal justice system. *Developmental Disabilities Research Reviews* 2009; 15(3): 250–7.

48. Corrado R, Freedman L. Risk profiles, trajectories, and intervention points for serious and chronic young offenders. *International Journal of Child, Youth and Family Studies* 2011; 2(2.1): 197–232.

49. Gudjonsson GH. *The Psychology of Interrogations, Confessions and Testimony*. John Wiley & Sons, 1992.

50. Central Planning and Training Unit. *A Guide to Interviewing*. Central Planning and Training Unit, 1992.

51. Inbau F, Reid J, Buckley J, Jayne B. *Criminal Interrogation and Confessions*. Jones & Bartlett Publishers, 2011.

52. Leo RA. Inside the interrogation room. *Journal of Criminal Law and Criminology* 1996; 86: 266–303.

53. Gudjonsson GH. The psychological vulnerabilities of witnesses and the risk of false accusations and false confessions. In Heaton-Armstrong A, Shepherd E, Gudjonsson G, Wolchover D, eds., *Witness Testimony. Psychological, Investigative and Evidential Perspectives*. Oxford University Press, 2006: 61–75.

54. Kassin SM. The psychology of confession evidence. *American Psychologist* 1997; 52 (3): 221.

55. Gudjonsson GH. Psychological vulnerabilities during police interviews. Why are they important? *Legal and Criminological Psychology* 2010; 15(2): 161–75.

56. Streissguth AP, Bookstein FL, Barr HM, Press S, Sampson PD. A fetal alcohol behavior scale. *Alcoholism: Clinical and Experimental Research* 1998; 22(2): 325–33.

57. Stuss DT, Benson DF. Neuropsychological studies of the frontal lobes. *Psychological Bulletin* 1984; 95(1): 3–28.

58. Brown NN, Gudjonsson G, Connor P. Suggestibility and fetal alcohol spectrum disorders: I'll tell you anything you want to hear. *Journal of Psychiatry and Law* 2011; 39(1): 39–71.

59. Gudjonsson GH, Sigurdsson JF, Bragason OO, Newton AK, Einarsson E. Interrogative suggestibility, compliance and false confessions among prisoners and their relationship with attention deficit hyperactivity disorder (ADHD) symptoms. *Psychological Medicine* 2008; 38(7): 1037–44.

60. Baxter JS, Jackson M, Bain SA. Interrogative suggestibility: interactions between interviewees' self-esteem and interviewer style. *Personality and Individual Differences* 2003; 35(6): 1285–92.

61. Bain SA, McGroarty A, Runcie M. Coping strategies, self-esteem and levels of interrogative suggestibility. *Personality and Individual Differences* 2015; 75: 85–9.

62. Gudjonsson G, Vagni M, Maiorano T, Pajardi D. Age and memory related changes in children's immediate and delayed suggestibility using the Gudjonsson Suggestibility Scale. *Personality and Individual Differences* 2016; 102: 25–9.

63. Allely CS, Cooper P. Jurors' and judges' evaluation of defendants with autism and the impact on sentencing: a systematic Preferred Reporting Items for Systematic Reviews and Meta-Analyses (PRISMA) review of autism spectrum disorder in the courtroom. *Journal of Law and Medicine* 2017; 25(1): 105–23.

64. Sorge GB. Fetal alcohol spectrum disorder persons in Canadian criminal proceedings. York University, 2006.

65. Gagnier KR, Moore TE, Green JM. A need for closer examination of FASD by the criminal justice system: has the call been answered? *Journal of Population Therapeutics and Clinical Pharmacology* 2011; 18(3): e426–e39.

66. Douds AS, Stevens HR, Sumner WE. Sword or shield? A systematic review of the roles FASD evidence plays in judicial proceedings. *Criminal Justice Policy Review* 2013; 24(4): 492–509.

67. Clare ICH, Gudjonsson GH. Interrogative suggestibility, confabulation, and acquiescence in people with mild learning disabilities (mental handicap): implications for reliability during police interrogation. *British Journal of Clinical Psychology* 1993; 32: 295–301.

68. Mela M, Flannigan K, Anderson T, Nelson M, Krishnan S, Chizea C, et al. Neurocognitive function and fetal alcohol spectrum disorder in offenders with mental disorders. *Journal of the American Academy of Psychiatry and the Law* 2020; 48 (2): 195–208.

69. Roach K, Bailey A. The relevance of fetal alcohol spectrum disorder in Canadian criminal law from investigation to sentencing. *UBC Law Review* 2009; 42: 1–68.

70. Mutch RC, Jones HM, Bower C, Watkins RE. Fetal alcohol spectrum disorders: using knowledge, attitudes and practice of justice professionals to support their educational needs. *Journal of Population Therapeutics and Clinical Pharmacology* 2016; 23(1): e77–e89.

71. Murphy D. Interviewing individuals with an autism spectrum disorder in forensic settings. *International Journal of Forensic Mental Health* 2018; 17(4): 310–20.

72. Advocate's Gateway. Planning to question someone with autism spectrum disorder including Asperger syndrome. Advocate's Gateway Toolkit 3. 2013. Available at: http://files.campus.edublogs.org/blogs .city.ac.uk/dist/5/192/files/2012/06/Autism-spectrum-disorder-192pnxv.pdf.

73. Allely CS, Mukherjee RAS. Suggestibility, false confessions and competency to stand trial in individuals with fetal alcohol spectrum disorders: current concerns and recommendations. *Journal of Criminal Psychology* 2019; 9(4): 166–72.

The Role of Subthreshold Neurodevelopmental Disorder in Offending Behaviour

Eddie Chaplin and Jane M. McCarthy

Introduction

The theoretical debate of what constitutes a neurodevelopmental disorder and nosological classification are covered in Chapters 1 and 2. This chapter deals with those individuals who do not meet the diagnostic criteria threshold for a specific neurodevelopmental disorder and are considered as having a subthreshold disorder. This group is characterised as having multiple symptoms of one or more neurodevelopmental disorder, including intellectual disability (ID), attention deficit hyperactivity disorder (ADHD) or autism spectrum disorder (ASD), which have been identified by screening or clinical interview, but not sufficient symptoms to meet the criteria for a diagnosis as defined by the international classification systems of the ICD-11 or DSM-5 [1, 2]. The DSM-5 acknowledged for the first time that individuals with autism fall along a spectrum depending on the level of functioning and symptom severity. However, current clinical definitions of neurodevelopmental disorders may still not take into account a broader range of impairments [3]. Therefore, there has been an increasing recognition that there are a group of individuals with neurodevelopmental difficulties who do not meet the threshold for a disorder. This group may require specific support or are at risk of comorbid conditions, which without identification go unchecked, and may lead to a potential increased risk for offending type behaviours.

To begin to understand the role of subthreshold neurodevelopmental disorders (STNDs) in adults it is necessary to understand how neurodevelopmental impairments may impact on early life. Associated vulnerabilities and behaviours can continue into adulthood. This can be seen in research on male prisoners with STNDs who have been shown to have higher levels of disadvantage, such as poorer educational, housing and employment outcomes before imprisonment compared with other prisoners without STNDs [4]. Although neurodevelopmental disorders and impairments persist into adulthood the impact of impairments may lessen with age [5], and be subject to intervention to address factors that may decrease risk. These risk factors will differ and may diminish in adults through the attainment of social milestones and neurocognitive maturation [6]. Although an individual's risk profile may change, those who do offend will still have predictive traits consistent with current and future offending, which are rarely recognised or collated to determine future risk or interventions.

The study of similarities between clinical and non-clinical samples has shown the legitimacy of examining the role of traits and symptoms in subthreshold adult populations [7], which may help to develop targeted and effective treatment approaches. Although the correlation between neurodisability and higher offence rates in children has received attention, in adults this is not the case apart from a few dedicated studies on STNDs [4, 8] and other studies where STNDs are considered [9]. Studies into adults with neurodevelopmental disorders have tended to have been disorder-specific, without attention to prevalence and overlap of neurodevelopmental disorders, therefore missing the whole picture [5]. Research dedicated specifically to offenders with STNDs or neurodevelopmental impairments and those offenders with neurodevelopmental disorders is still in its infancy. There are several reasons for this including no agreed definition on what STNDs are, leading to a lack of recognition from funders and commissioners of services. When this population do come to the attention of services, they often do not meet the eligibility criteria for mental health and/or social service support. This is not unsurprising given those with a diagnosable neurodevelopmental disorder will also find it difficult to obtain support [10].

This chapter therefore examines offenders identified with STNDs, including definition, presentation, comorbidities, rates of offending, practice and research implications. As well as looking at studies that have purposefully included STNDs, we also examine studies that have reported on a single neurodevelopmental disorder where diagnostic criteria have not been met. Most of the studies to date include case studies or matched controlled studies.

Definitions and Identification of STNDs

Subthreshold disorders have been referred to as subclinical and subsyndromal disorders and are associated with negative consequences and increased disability [11]. The definition and scope are not always the same between disorders and research has suffered from lack of standardisation. In health settings, subthreshold disorder is a term that is often used to identify who is in the early stages of a disease or to identify those at high risk of the disease, in need of monitoring or treatments, either to prevent reaching diagnostic threshold or maintain well-being. However, with a neurodevelopmental disorder there is no prodrome or nascent stage given their developmental nature. Prevalence estimates vary depending on the definitions used, for example those falling short of accepted diagnostic classification and those with conditions widely recognised clinically but not accepted within diagnostic criteria, such as borderline intellectual functioning [4]. However, those diagnosed with a neurodevelopmental disorder are at increased risk for the presence of another neurodevelopmental disorder diagnosis and there may be a common genetic aetiology [12].

The current lack of definition or agreement of subthreshold disorders has historically divided methodological approaches in defining these populations. STNDs have been defined in a number of ways, including exceeding the threshold on one or more screening tools or a self-reporting of a diagnosis of ADHD, ASD or ID [13]. Tools such as the Adult Autism Subthreshold Spectrum (AdAS Spectrum) aim to highlight not only the core manifestations of ASD, but also the attenuated and atypical symptoms, the personality traits and the behavioural manifestations that may be associated with ASD but which may be present in subthreshold or partial forms. The AdAS Spectrum is a 160-item questionnaire so the size of the screen would therefore make it difficult to administer routinely in offender settings [14]. Screening tools used in practice need to be easy to administer, able to be used following basic training and brief in terms of the number of questions. Examples of screening tools that are used to support clinical decision making in criminal justice settings are given in Table 9.1. Often, subthreshold disorders are used to describe those with excessive levels of traits associated with a single neurodevelopmental disorder not meeting the diagnostic threshold. However, there is no agreement as to threshold and often the

Table 9.1 Examples of screening tools for neurodevelopmental disorders used in forensic settings

Screen	Threshold for identification	Reliability and validity
Learning Disability Screening Questionnaire (LDSQ) [15]	A score of < 46%	Sensitivity and specificity were found to be 82.3% and 87.5% in an offender population; a positive predictive power value of 92.9% and negative predictive power of 73.7% [15]
Rapid assessment of potential intellectual disabilities (RAPID) [16]	A score of 3 and above out of a possible 15	No published data found on reliability and validity
10-Item autism spectrum quotient (AQ-10) [17]	The cut-off value for the AQ-10 is ≥ 6	Sensitivity and specificity were found to be 0.88 and 0.91 and the positive predictive value was 0.85 [18]
Adult ADHD Self-Report Scale (ASRS) [19]	A score of 4 or more using the six screening items of the ASRS	Six-question ASRS screener vs the 18-question ASRS in sensitivity (68.7% vs 56.3%), specificity (99.5% vs 98.3%) [20]

decision is a reasoned judgement by clinicians or researchers. The reliability and validity of most screening tools for neurodevelopmental disorders among offender populations is not known. In studies to date, STNDs are often defined as those screening positive or just below for ADHD, ASD or ID as a single disorder or a combination of disorders. However, there is no current agreement on what tools should be used. This is made more difficult given different rates of neurodevelopmental disorder and mental health comorbidities between gender and different ethnic groups, which makes us question whether there is a gender bias and/or lack of cultural sensitivity within current measures [13].

Clinical Presentation

Those with STNDs may be less likely to present in the same way as those with a neurodevelopmental disorder, and therefore may only be detected by specialist screening or clinical interview. However, they may have similar needs and deficits experienced by individuals with a neurodevelopmental disorder diagnosis who require support. The complexity and overlap of presentation with other clinical presentations and offence-related behaviours may also be a factor in identification. The study of each specific neurodevelopmental disorder has occurred at different paces. This has led to different approaches to those not meeting diagnostic criteria, which are described below.

Borderline Intellectual Functioning

Borderline intellectual functioning (BIF) occurs in the developmental period and is defined by cognitive impairment (evidenced by an intelligence quotient (IQ) of between 70 and 85) and social impairment. It is estimated to affect between 12% and 14% of the population depending on diagnostic criteria [21]. BIF is characterised by significant impairments of social and adaptive functioning and as a result has been classified in individual cases as a mental disorder, as defined under the Mental Health Act for England and Wales. BIF may be used more particularly in those, with other comorbidities, such as genetic abnormalities, autism, cerebral palsy and brain injury [22]. Like other subthreshold groups, offenders with BIF have similar needs to those with mild ID but they are without access to forensic services in many cases, as they do not meet the eligibility criteria. Given scant attention for BIF, the true levels and type and need for support is unknown, unlike other levels of intellectual disability. In many cases, people with BIF are not seen or understood as vulnerable people and are therefore often excluded from support, despite similar difficulties in communication and adaptive problems to those persons with ID [23]. Despite similar clinical presentation to those with mild ID, there is evidence that the BIF group may be less likely to have a desire for help [24]. Some studies have chosen to look at those with both mild ID and BIF as one group which may reflect the wider eligibility for services of those with BIF in such countries as the Netherlands [25]. A Dutch study of young adults attending a diversion program aimed at the persistent violent offender reported on those identified with mild to borderline intellectual disability (MBID) and violent offending [26]. Of the 146 attendees, 30 (20.5%) were considered to have MBID. Growing up in unstable environments and psychosocial problems were evident for all offenders; however, the MBID offenders were more likely to display severe externalising and disruptive behaviour at a younger age, be more susceptible to peer pressure and neurological problems, while fewer had physically abusive parents [26]. Although the authors report these have implications for targeted interventions, they questioned, given the high criminogenic need in both groups, whether MBID group is a meaningful subpopulation. The inclusion of offenders across two levels of ID does highlight issues of defining populations with neurodevelopmental impairments. However, this often is not just a research issue as definitions may be dictated by policy, service and commissioning guidance, which can determine study populations.

Subthreshold Autism and Broader Autism Phenotype

Within autism, there exists a wide variation in presentation between individuals, both in nature and intensity, ranging from severe to subtle symptoms, which also present in non-autistic populations [27]. There are those not reaching the diagnostic threshold such as in the case of the broad autism phenotype (BAP), which is described as a continuum from almost no autistic traits to severe presentation of the condition. Research to date often concentrates on specific behaviours rather than the range of behaviours within a domain, for example social or communication [28]. Findings from this study showed how a continuous measure of autistic traits is related to a continuous measure of social functioning. The relationship between those with a diagnosis and those with traits not meeting the diagnostic threshold is central to using a dimensional approach, with current diagnostic criteria not always considering the dimensional nature of symptoms and other phenomena such as the BAP [29]. It is hypothesised that individuals with autistic traits have a higher vulnerability towards psychopathology and risk of comorbid mental health problems [30].

ADHD Traits into Adulthood

Although the link to ADHD and offending is well established [31–33], there may be problems recognising its occurrence in adulthood [33]. Often those diagnosed in childhood will lose their ADHD label, regardless of whether they are symptomatic. In the natural course, some adults with ADHD will grow out of their symptoms and may not meet diagnostic criteria [34], suggesting those who screen positive for symptoms of ADHD but not meeting the diagnostic threshold could be made up of those with a previous diagnosis of the condition. ADHD is a strong predictor for violent offending, with higher levels of general psychopathology and psychopathic traits found in ADHD prisoners [35]. A study examining the relationship between offending, ADHD and comorbid risk factors in 11,388 students in further education reported that the relationship between ADHD symptoms and offending could largely be explained indirectly by the presence of comorbid factors, such as substance use and relationships with delinquent peers [36]. A genetic link between ADHD and other neurodevelopmental disorders may be another explanation for those showing subthreshold symptoms of neurodevelopmental impairment [37].

Children with Impairments and Future Risk

Studies of children have shown high rates of behaviours that, if not addressed, will increase the risk of future offending but the evidence to date indicates those with neurodevelopmental disorders and other comorbidities are not having their needs identified. A National Institute Health Research funded study of young people with ASD and ADHD found this group to have significant unmet needs such as undiagnosed mental health symptoms throughout different transitioning stages, for example from child to adolescence to young adulthood, with the largest determinant of service provision being age rather than the severity of symptoms [38]. A twin study of subthreshold and threshold ADHD symptoms among Swedish children (n = 4,635), between the age of 9 and 12 years, who had a neuropsychiatric assessment, were followed up at age 15 years [39]. The children were divided into three symptom groups, screen-negative 91% (4,216), screen-intermediate 4% (183) and screen-positive for ADHD 4.9% (228). The higher screening scores were correlated with negative psychosocial outcomes. Girls in the intermediate group, that is, not meeting the diagnostic threshold, had the highest rates (48.5%) of internalising problems across all groups and higher rates of drug misuse. For those who screened as intermediate, only 24.8% of boys and 10.6% of girls were described as having no problem, 41.9% of boys and 33.3% of girls who were screened in the intermediate group had antisocial behaviours, of the boys, 29.1% alcohol misuse, 8.6% substance misuse, 27.4% peer problems and 16.2% truancy compared to 33.3% alcohol misuse, 18.8% substance misuse, 38.4% peer problems and 15.2% truancy for the girls. These vulnerabilities and behaviours often continue into adulthood as seen in research on male prisoners with STNDs who were found to have higher levels of disadvantage, such as poorer educational, housing and employment outcomes before imprisonment compared with other prisoners from the general population [4].

Mental Health and Offenders with STNDs

Studies to date on offenders with STNDs have highlighted the high levels of mental health needs and increased vulnerability for self-harm and suicide behaviour when compared to neurotypical offenders and in the general population [8, 13, 40–42]. See Table 9.2 for a summary of these studies. The findings through all these studies undertaken within the criminal justice system show a much higher risk for mental disorder, comorbidities of neurodevelopmental disorders and self-harm behaviour if looked at by specific difficulties, such as the presence of autistic traits, borderline functioning or symptoms of ADHD as well as when looked at as a broad group with STNDs.

Table 9.2 Studies in the criminal justice system on neurodevelopmental disorder and rates of comorbidity

Author	Chaplin et al., Characteristics of prisoners with intellectual disabilites [41]
Setting	UK prison
Sample size	240
ID	$N = 18$ (7.5%) with ID, i.e., a positive score on the LDSQ Only four known before study Of these, eight (44%) screened positive for either ASD or ADHD as well and five (28%) for both ADHD and ASD
Suicidality	ID 37.5% ($n = 6$) vs non-ID 7% ($n = 5$) ($X^2 = 10.552$, $p = 0.001$)
Psychiatric disorder	The following rates of psychiatric disorder were identified in those with ID: depression 2 (12.5%), psychosis 2 (12.5%) and antisocial personality disorder 10 (62.5%)
Screening and diagnostic measures	LDSQ, case notes for presence of ID Mini International Neuropsychiatric Interview (MINI) for psychiatric disorder and suicidality
Author	McCarthy et al., Prisoners with neurodevelopmental difficulties: vulnerabilities for mental illness and self-harm [8]
Setting	UK prison
Sample size	69 neurodevelopmental disorder vs 69 no neurodevelopmental disorder
Neurodevelopmental difficulties (ND)	69 with ND included: ADHD = 51, ASD = 37, ID = 28 Just over half (36, 52.2%) screened for more than one ND
Suicidality	In the ND group the following levels of suicide risk were recorded, High suicidality rating 15 (21.7%) ND vs 3 (4.3%) no-ND ($X^2 = 9.93$, $p < 0.002$)
Psychiatric disorder	In the ND group the following levels of psychiatric disorder were recorded: psychosis: 6 (8.7%) ND vs 1 (1.4%) no-ND ($X^2 = 4.15$, $p < 0.042$) depression: 15 (21.7%) ND vs 2 (2.9%) no-ND ($X^2 = 12.65$, $p = 0.000$) general anxiety disorder: 18 (26.1%) ND vs 3 (4.3%) no-ND ($X^2 = 13.82$, $p = 0.000$) antisocial personality disorder: 44 (63.8%) ND vs 16 (23.2%) no-ND ($X^2 = 23.87$, $p = 0.000$)
Screening and diagnostic measures	Screening tools used: AQ-10 and 20, ASRS, LDSQ plus self-report MINI for psychiatric disorder and suicidality
Author	Chaplin et al., 2021, Prisoners with attention deficit hyperactivity disorder: co-morbidities and service pathways [42]
Setting	UK prison
Sample size	240

Table 9.2 (cont.)

Symptoms of ADHD	Of the prisoners with ADHD, 65 (27.1%) screened positive for ADHD with 54 (22.5%) meeting the diagnostic criteria for ADHD, 28 of 54 had a previous diagnosis, 80% had combined type 20 (40.8%) screened positive for ID and 24 (49.0%) for autistic traits, 15 (30.6%) screened positive for both ID and autistic traits
Suicidality	4 (8.2%) of those with ADHD reported having tried to take their life in the last three months. Two-thirds had attempted suicide, 65.2%, in their lifetime (32) compared to 11.6% (8) of prisoners with no neurodevelopmental disorder
Psychiatric disorder	Prisoners with ADHD were significantly at risk of mental illness: ADHD 31 (63.2%) vs 12 (17.4%) no neurodevelopmental disorder ($X^2 = (n = 118)$ 28.03, $p > .001$) ADHD prisoners were significantly more likely to be diagnosed with a personality disorder 75.5% (37) to 23.2%, (16) of no neurodevelopmental disorder prisoners. The ADHD group also had significantly higher rates of mania/hypomania, general anxiety disorder, social phobia and obsessive–compulsive disorder
Screening and diagnostic measures	ASRS and Diagnostic Interview for ADHD in Adults (DIVA) MINI for psychiatric disorder and suicidality
Author	Chaplin et al., 2021, Self-harm and mental health characteristics of prisoners with elevated rates of autistic traits [40]
Setting	UK prison
Sample size	240
Autistic traits	46 (19.2%) were found to have high levels of autistic traits following screening, 12 (5%) met the diagnostic threshold using the Autism Diagnostic Observation Schedule (ADOS), of these 83.5% were previously unrecognised.
Suicidality	Prisoners with ASD traits significantly more likely to have attempted suicide, 64.9% over their lifetime compared to 11.6% for neurotypical prisoners
Psychiatric disorder	Those screening positive for autistic traits were most at risk of a comorbid mental disorder. They were more likely to be diagnosed with anxiety-related disorders. Generalised anxiety disorder 27% vs 4.3%, social phobia 40.5% vs 4.3%, psychotic disorders 8.1% vs 1.4% and depression 29.7% vs 15.4% when compared to neurotypical prisoners.
Screening measures used	ADOS, AQ-20 MINI for psychiatric disorder and suicidality

Offence History and Rates

There is a very limited literature on people with STNDs and types of offences committed. On the whole, the evidence indicates that the types of offences are comparable to other offenders but those with STNDs may be more likely to commit sexual offences. A Canadian prison study of ADHD [43] found 25.2% (n = 125) of prisoners were classified with subthreshold symptoms at the moderate level (using the ASRS [19]), and reported the following offence rates of homicide, 8.1%; sexual offence, 3.2%; robbery, 21.8%; other violent, 14.5%; drug-related, 15.3%; and other non-violent, 37.1%. In another study of 129 prisoners, prisoners with STNDs were significantly more likely to have been convicted of a sex offence than neurotypical prisoners and significantly less likely to have committed drug offences [8]. A study of sex offending among incarcerated male prisoners with low intellectual functioning, described as 'probable ID' and 'probable BIF' (equating to mild and borderline), reported many similarities apart from violent non-sexual offences, where those with mild ID were reported at rates of 93.5% compared to 61.5% for the BIF group [44].

Conclusion

The identification of similar social risk factors for offending has been used to support the call for similar support packages being available to help those with STNDs as a strategy to reduce further offending [44]. Vulnerability to offending needs to be addressed and the idea that symptoms cease to be a problem in adulthood needs to be challenged to ensure that support packages for those most at risk are available. There is a need for increased awareness and training on STNDs to assist identification and availability of reasonable adjustment within both the health and criminal justice services. Criminal justice staff often feel unequipped to deal with or recognise these groups and so these disorders often go unrecognised [45].

The study of STNDs and their implications for future health, social and criminal justice services is in its infancy. Current research points towards increased vulnerability that is likely to impact both the individual and future service demand. There are many similarities between offenders with STNDs and those formally diagnosed with a neurodevelopmental disorder in terms of increased vulnerability to mental health problems, self-harm and suicide and characteristics of poor support networks and lower socio-economic status. The future study of STNDs requires a coordinated strategy and an agreement to a common definition, taking a dimensional approach, if we are to improve the health outcomes of this group of offenders.

References

1. American Psychiatric Association. *Diagnostic and Statistical Manual of Mental Disorders*, 5th edition: DSM-5. American Psychiatric Association, 2013.

2. World Health Organization. International Classification of Diseases 11th revision. 2022. Available at: www.who.int/standards/classifications/classification-of-diseases.

3. Hughes N. Understanding the influence of neurodevelopmental disorders on offending: utilizing developmental psychopathology in biosocial criminology. *Criminal Justice Studies* 2015; 28(1): 39–60.

4. McCarthy J, Chaplin E, Underwood L, Forrester A, Hayward H, Sabet J, et al. Characteristics of prisoners with neurodevelopmental disorders and difficulties. *Journal of Intellectual Disability Research* 2016; 60(3): 201–6.

5. Billstedt E, Anckarsäter H, Wallinius M, Hofvander B. Neurodevelopmental disorders in young violent offenders: overlap and background characteristics. *Psychiatry Research* 2017; 252: 234–41.

6. Hilton NZ, Ham E, Green MM. The roles of antisociality and neurodevelopmental problems in criminal violence and clinical outcomes among male forensic inpatients. *Criminal Justice and Behavior* 2017; 45(3): 293–315.

7. McEwan TE, Strand S. The role of psychopathology in stalking by adult strangers and acquaintances. *Australian and New Zealand Journal of Psychiatry* 2013; 47(6): 546–55.

8. McCarthy J, Chaplin E, Forrester A, Underwood L, Hayward H, Sabet J, et al. Prisoners with neurodevelopmental difficulties: vulnerabilities for mental illness and self-harm. *Criminal Behaviour and Mental Health* 2019; 29(5–6): 308–20.

9. Underwood L, Forrester A, Chaplin E, McCarthy J. Prisoners with neurodevelopmental disorders. *Journal of Intellectual Disabilities and Offending Behaviour* 2013; 4(1–2): 17–23.

10. HM Inspectorate of Probation, HM Inspectorate of Constabulary, HM Crown Prosecution Service Inspectorate and the Care Quality Commission. A joint inspection of the treatment of offenders with learning disabilities within the criminal justice system – phase 1 from arrest to sentence. 2014. Available at: www.justiceinspectorates.gov.uk/hmicfrs/publications/joint-inspection-of-the-treatment-of-offenders-with-learning-disabilities-within-the-criminal-justice-system/.

11. Helmchen, H., & Linden, M. (2000). Subthreshold disorders in psychiatry: clinical reality, methodological artifact, and the double-threshold problem. *Comprehensive Psychiatry*, 41(2), 1–7.

12. Pettersson E, Anckarsater H, Gillberg C, Lichtenstein P. Different neurodevelopmental symptoms have a common genetic etiology. *Journal of Child Psychology and Psychiatry* 2013; 54 (12): 1356–65.

13. McCarthy J, Amanda K, Lisette Saunders P, Chaplin E, Underwood L, Forrester A, et al. Screening and diagnostic assessment of neurodevelopmental disorders in a male prison. *Journal of Intellectual Disabilities and Offending Behaviour* 2015; 6(2): 102–11.

14. Dell'Osso L, Gesi C, Massimetti E, Cremone I, Barbuti M, Maccariello G, et al. Adult Autism Subthreshold Spectrum (AdAS Spectrum): validation of a questionnaire investigating subthreshold autism spectrum. *Comprehensive Psychiatry* 2017; 73: 61–83.

15. McKenzie K, Michie A, Murray A, Hales C. Screening for offenders with an intellectual disability: the validity of the Learning Disability Screening Questionnaire. *Research in Developmental Disabilities* 2012; 33(3): 791–5.

16. Ali S, Galloway S. Developing a screening tool for offenders with intellectual disabilities: the RAPID. *Journal of Intellectual Disabilities and Offending Behaviour* 2016; 7(3): 161–70.

17. Booth T, Murray AL, McKenzie K, Kuenssberg R, O'Donnell M, Burnett H. Brief report: an evaluation of the AQ-10 as a brief screening instrument for ASD in adults. *Journal of Autism and Developmental Disorders* 2013; 43(12): 2997–3000.

18. Allison C, Auyeung B, Baron-Cohen S. Toward brief 'red flags' for autism screening: the short autism spectrum quotient and the short quantitative checklist in 1,000 cases and 3,000 controls. *Journal of the American Academy of Child and Adolescent Psychiatry* 2012; 51(2): 202–12.

19. Adler LA, Spencer T, Faraone SV, Kessler RC, Howes MJ, Biederman J, et al. Validity of pilot Adult ADHD Self-Report Scale (ASRS) to rate adult ADHD symptoms. *Annals of Clinical Psychiatry* 2006; 18(3): 145–8.

20. Kessler RC, Adler L, Ames M, Demler O, Faraone S, Hiripi E, et al. The World Health Organization Adult ADHD Self-Report Scale (ASRS): a short screening

scale for use in the general population. *Psychological Medicine* 2005; 35(2): 245–56.

21. Fernell E, Gillberg C. Borderline intellectual functioning. In Gallagher A, Bulteau C, Cohen D, Michaud JL, eds., *Handbook of Clinical Neurology*. Elsevier, 2020: 77–81.

22. Royal College of Psychiatrists. Forensic care pathways for adults with intellectual disability involved with the criminal justice system. 2014. Available at: www.rcpsych.ac.uk/docs/d efault-source/members/faculties/intellectual-disability/id-fr-id-04.pdf?sfvrsn=ba5ce38a_4.

23. Søndenaa E, Olsen T, Kermit PS, Dahl NC, Envik R. Intellectual disabilities and offending behaviour: the awareness and concerns of the police, district attorneys and judges. *Journal of Intellectual Disabilities and Offending Behaviour* 2019; 10(2): 34–42.

24. Luteijn I, Didden R, der Nagel JV. Individuals with mild intellectual disability or borderline intellectual functioning in a forensic addiction treatment center: prevalence and clinical characteristics. *Advances in Neurodevelopmental Disorders* 2017; 1(4): 240–51.

25. Woiez I, Eggink E, Putman L, Ras M. *An International Comparison of Care for People with Intellectual Disabilities: An Exploration*. The Netherlands Institute for Social Research, 2018.

26. Segeren MW, Fassaert TJL, Kea R, De Wit MAS, Popma A. Exploring differences in criminogenic risk factors and criminal behavior between young adult violent offenders with and without mild to borderline intellectual disability. *International Journal of Offender Therapy and Comparative Criminology* 2018; 62(4): 978–99.

27. Royal College of Psychiatrists. The psychiatric management of autism in adults College Report 228. 2020. Available at: www.rcpsych.ac.uk/improving-care/ca mpaigning-for-better-mental-health-policy/college-reports/2020-college-reports/cr228.

28. De Groot K, Van Strien JW. Evidence for a broad autism phenotype. *Advances in Neurodevelopmental Disorders* 2017; 1(3): 129–40.

29. Dell'Osso L, Luche RD, Gesi C, Moroni I, Carmassi C, Maj M. From Asperger's *Autistischen Psychopathen* to DSM-5 autism spectrum disorder and beyond: a subthreshold autism spectrum model. *Clinical Practice and Epidemiology in Mental Health* 2016; 12: 120–31.

30. Dell'Osso L, Lorenzi P, Carpita B. Autistic traits and illness trajectories. *Clinical Practice and Epidemiology in Mental Health* 2019; 15: 94.

31. Young S, Gudjonsson G, Chitsabesan P, Colley B, Farrag E, Forrester A, et al. Identification and treatment of offenders with attention-deficit/hyperactivity disorder in the prison population: a practical approach based upon expert consensus. *BMC Psychiatry* 2018; 18 (1): 281.

32. Young S, Gudjonsson GH, Wells J, Asherson P, Theobald D, Oliver B, et al. Attention deficit hyperactivity disorder and critical incidents in a Scottish prison population. *Personality and Individual Differences* 2009; 46(3): 265–9.

33. Kooij JJS, Bijlenga D, Salerno L, Jaeschke R, Bitter I, Balazs J, et al. Updated European Consensus Statement on diagnosis and treatment of adult ADHD. *European Psychiatry* 2019; 56: 14–34.

34. Young S, Gudjonsson GH. Growing out of ADHD. *Journal of Attention Disorders* 2008; 12(2): 162–9.

35. Machado A, Rafaela D, Silva T, Veigas T, Cerejeira J. ADHD among offenders: prevalence and relationship with psychopathic traits. *Journal of Attention Disorders* 2020; 24(14): 2021–9.

36. Gudjonsson GH, Sigurdsson JF, Sigfusdottir ID, Young S. A national epidemiological study of offending and its relationship with ADHD symptoms and associated risk factors. *Journal of Attention Disorders* 2014; 18(1): 3–13.

37. Du Rietz E, Pettersson E, Brikell I, Ghirardi L, Chen Q, Hartman C, et al. Overlap between attention-deficit hyperactivity disorder and

neurodevelopmental, externalising and internalising disorders: separating unique from general psychopathology effects. *British Journal of Psychiatry* 2021; 218(1): 35–42.

38. Murphy D, Glaser K, Hayward H, Eklund H, Cadman T, Findon J, et al. Crossing the divide: a longitudinal study of effective treatments for people with autism and attention deficit hyperactivity disorder across the lifespan. *Programme Grants for Applied Research* 2018; 6(2): 1–240.

39. Norén Selinus E, Molero Y, Lichtenstein P, Anckarsäter H, Lundström S, Bottai M, et al. Subthreshold and threshold attention deficit hyperactivity disorder symptoms in childhood: psychosocial outcomes in adolescence in boys and girls. *Acta Psychiatrica Scandinavica* 2016; 134(6): 533–45.

40. Chaplin E, McCarthy J, Allely CS, Forrester A, Underwood L et al. Self-harm and mental health characteristics of prisoners with elevated rates of autistic traits. *Research in Developmental Disabilities* 2021; 114: 103987.

41. Chaplin E, McCarthy J, Underwood L, Forrester A, Hayward H, Sabet J, et al. Characteristics of prisoners with intellectual disabilities. *Journal of Intellectual Disability Research* 2017; 61 (12): 1185–95.

42. Chaplin E, Rawat A, Perera B, McCarthy J, Courtenay K, Forrester, A, et al. Prisoners with attention deficit hyperactivity disorder: co-morbidities and service pathways. *International Journal of Prisoner Health* 2021; 18(3): 245–58.

43. Usher AM, Stewart LA, Wilton G. Attention deficit hyperactivity disorder in a Canadian prison population. *International Journal of Law and Psychiatry* 2013; 36(3–4): 311–15.

44. Athanassiou U, Cale J, Dowse L. A descriptive study of sex offending among incarcerated men with low intellectual functioning: offending parameters and sex offence characteristics in adulthood. *Current Issues in Criminal Justice* 2020; 32 (1): 76–90.

45. Chaplin E, McCarthy J, Underwood L. Autism spectrum conditions and offending: an introduction to the special edition. *Journal of Intellectual Disabilities and Offending Behaviour* 2013; 4(1/2): 5–8.

Chapter 10

Comorbid Mental Disorders and Neurodevelopmental Conditions

Kiriakos Xenitidis, Caryl Marshall and Jane M. McCarthy

Introduction

Comorbidity between neurodevelopmental disorders is common: one neurodevelopmental disorder diagnosis makes further diagnoses more likely [1–4]. Combined neurodevelopmental disorder diagnoses seem to carry a higher risk of behavioural disturbance. A UK study found that 32% of prison inmates had at least one neurodevelopmental disorder while there was significant comorbidity between neurodevelopmental disorders, as 63% of those with autism spectrum disorder (ASD) and 40% of those with intellectual disability (ID) also met the criteria for attention deficit hyperactivity disorder (ADHD) [1]. A combined ADHD/ASD and ADHD/ID diagnosis carried a raised risk for higher severity of psychiatric symptoms and behavioural disturbance, respectively [1].

The presence of a neurodevelopmental disorder is a risk factor for the development of additional mental health problems, commonly referred to as psychiatric comorbidity [3, 5, 6]. The link between neurodevelopmental disorders and psychiatric comorbidity is an important one, not least because of the association between mental health problems and criminality and also because of the range of specific treatments available for psychiatric disorders. In addition, mental health problems are likely to contribute further to the vulnerability of people with neurodevelopmental disorders who find themselves in the criminal justice system [7]. A UK prison study found that prisoners with neurodevelopmental difficulties were significantly more likely to have thoughts about self-harm and suicide in the last month and concurrent mental disorders, including psychosis, anxiety, depression, personality disorders and substance use disorders [2].

Comorbid Mental Disorders in Offenders with ID

Background

Individuals with comorbid ID and mental health problems are at increased risk of offending [7]. People with ID are often unidentified in the criminal justice system, thus creating barriers to support. Individuals with ID in the prison system are more likely to experience mental health problems, and inequality, in treatment and services, compared to their non-ID peers. Significant improvement in terms of identifying people with ID and mental health problems in the criminal justice system is required.

ID and Psychiatric Comorbidity

It is well established that adults with ID experience an increased risk of developing mental health problems compared to their non-disabled adult peers. Studies indicate that 10% of individuals with ID would meet the criteria for a clinical diagnosis of a psychotic or affective disorder. When all conditions including personality disorders, anxiety disorders, substance use disorder, other neurodevelopmental disorders and challenging behaviours are considered, this figure rises to 54% [3].

ID Comorbidity and Offending

In the UK, prevalence rates of 0.5–9% have been reported for people with ID in police custody [8]. This corresponds to a similar over-representation internationally in prisons with a prevalence of 7–10% identified [9]. The comorbidity of mental health problems and ID has been demonstrated to carry an increased risk of offending; a study showed this group were more than three times more likely to have been charged with an offence compared to ID-only peers [7]. Considering sexual and violent offending, ID alone has been shown to increase this risk, but the presence of a comorbid mental health disorder significantly exacerbates this, the rate being almost double [10]. The identification of mental health disorders in people with ID is a well-established challenge with atypical presentations being common. Limitations in communication can prevent conveyance of internal experiences, and behavioural changes can be falsely attributed to pre-existing difficulties. Adapted diagnostic criteria can support clinicians in the psychiatric assessment of individuals with ID [11].

Challenging behaviour occurs at significantly increased rates in individuals with ID. A UK population study found 36% of adults had a primary care record of challenging behaviour, including aggression, destructive acts, arson and sexual misconduct [12]. The underlying causes of challenging behaviour in this population are heterogeneous but, importantly, include comorbid mental disorders.

ID in Prison Settings

Prisoners with ID have been found to be twice as likely as non-ID peers to have probable psychosis (11.3% vs 5.7%), to attempt suicide and to engage in self-harm [13]. Further studies have replicated these findings with psychosis, anxiety, personality disorders, suicidality and self-harm all occurring at significantly higher rates in prisoners with ID [14]. A significant majority of offenders with ID have a mild disability and consequently are not easily identified [15].

Despite increased vulnerability to mental health problems, individuals with ID in forensic settings can experience inequality in accessing appropriate healthcare. Issues such as atypical presentations of mental health disorders, communication difficulties and diagnostic overshadowing may cause delays in support [16]. People with ID are less likely to self-report mental health symptoms, relying instead on family or carers. Furthermore, clinicians may lack confidence in diagnosing psychiatric disorders in this population [17]. These barriers are exacerbated in settings without specialist ID expertise.

ID Pathways in the Criminal Justice System

The need to identify individuals with ID and mental health problems, to support them and, if appropriate, divert them from the criminal justice system, is imperative to allow for provision of effective interventions. The benefits of screening for mental health problems and ID at the point of contact are well established [8]. In the UK, it is recommended that liaison and diversion services are available to police custody suites to facilitate screening of people with suspected ID; however, a concerning proportion have been shown to remain undetected. Studies indicate that identification can be improved with specific adaptations to current screening practice to detect ID in detained individuals [18].

Inspections relating to the identification of individuals with ID in UK prison settings have found that the screening for neurodevelopmental disorders is underdeveloped, leaving some individuals unidentified [19]. People with ID in the prison environment have been found to be subject to increased rates of segregation and restraint, to be at higher risk of bullying and be less likely to know how to seek support than their non-ID peers [20].

While it is recognised that some individuals with ID who offend are most appropriately managed in the criminal justice system, one of the key aims of screening for ID and mental health disorders is to consider diversion to a more appropriate setting. A UK retrospective case-notes study of adults with ID referred to services following offending or antisocial behaviour found that 20% were diverted to specialist ID community forensic services or non-forensic ID inpatient facilities and 30% to specialist ID secure inpatient services [21]. That a significant proportion required specialist forensic ID services, either community or inpatient, suggests the need for more appropriate provision for this complex patient group.

In the UK, there are currently 2,075 individuals with an ID admitted to a psychiatric hospital, 970 of them in secure units [22]. Patients admitted to secure specialist impatient provision have been identified as having complex needs, including comorbid mental health problems. A study of patients in a medium secure setting indicates approximately half have a mental illness, with a significant proportion of this heterogeneous group having additional needs, including past abuse, personality disorders and substance use disorders [23]. A study of patients with ID in medium and low secure settings found a readmission and reoffending rate of 20% and 22%, respectively [24]. The study noted that discharges were most often under the care of community ID services, with only a small proportion being supported by community forensic teams.

ID and Recidivism

Evidence also shows that those with comorbid difficulties are more likely to reoffend than those with ID alone [25]. Studies in the UK demonstrate that probation services struggle to meet the complex needs of people with ID. Less than half of assessments took account of the impact ID has on the ability to engage in rehabilitation and not all individuals received adapted interventions; complex social and health issues were cited as a factor that negatively impacts prevention of reoffending interventions for this group, with the recidivism rate being 38% [19]. It has been suggested that a remedy would be to coordinate probation services with ID services to provide a formalised, multi-agency, approach to support the management of complex individuals [26].

People with comorbid ID and mental health problems who offend are a heterogeneous group with complex needs for whom the criminal justice system can be difficult, and traumatic, to navigate. Failure to identify developmental and mental health needs at any stage of the criminal justice system can enhance the health and social inequality already experienced by these vulnerable individuals, including preventing access to healthcare and rehabilitation programmes. Addressing these inequalities starts with effective screening at each stage of the process and training of professionals to act on the findings. Without a commitment to the development of skills within existing health and criminal justice

---

Case Study 10.1 Person with ID, post-traumatic stress disorder and depression

John is a 21-year-old man with a history of educational and behavioural difficulties, who presented to secondary psychiatric services as a teenager with symptoms of significantly disturbed sleep and agitated and bizarre behaviour. John came to the UK, aged 11, with his family as asylum seekers. He had been exposed to war atrocities and suffered significant social and educational disruption through early childhood. Schooling in the UK proved difficult; he was unable to engage in learning and exhibited frequent behavioural outbursts. These difficulties were attributed to his migrant status, and having English as a second language. Aged 15, John was convicted of aggravated burglary after having been prompted by classmates. He was detained in a young offenders' institution, where he became more depressed and aggressive. On release he was referred to general adult mental health services due to his probation officer having concerns regarding vulnerability, mental health and possible ID. At that stage he was formally diagnosed with a mild ID, and a mental state examination revealed a poor sleep pattern with nightmares, low mood and hypervigilance and associated deterioration of his level of functioning. Diagnoses of post-traumatic stress disorder and depression were made in addition to ID, and medical and psychological treatment was offered by the community ID team.

---

teams, and the further development of specialist forensic ID psychiatric services, this population group will continue to suffer inequality in terms of rehabilitation and recovery and to be treated in overly restrictive and inappropriate environments (see Case Study 10.1).

Comorbid Mental Disorders in Offenders with ASD

ASD and Psychiatric Comorbidity

A systematic review of people with ASD and the criminal justice system concluded that people with ASD were not disproportionally over-represented in the criminal justice system [5]. Chapter 5 provides a detailed overview of the prevalence rates across different settings such as prison and forensic mental health services. The presence of psychiatric disorder can not only exacerbate the core autistic symptoms but also have a significant impact on functioning for a person with ASD [27]. This increased prevalence of psychiatric disorders has onset before adult life. A study of adolescents with ASD, compared to those without ASD, found a ratio of five episodes of psychiatric disorder to one episode [28]. It is increasingly recognised that adults with ASD are at risk for a number of comorbid psychiatric conditions, with rates of 16–35% being reported [29]. The main psychiatric disorders reported in people with ASD include mood and anxiety disorders, which encompass general anxiety disorders, agoraphobia, social phobias and obsessive compulsive disorders [29]. Both schizophrenia and bipolar affective disorder are frequently seen in adults with ASD [30]. ADHD is common with a recent systematic review finding ADHD to be the most prevalent condition in adults with ASD [31]. The relationship between psychopathology and challenging behaviour in adults with ASD and other neurodevelopmental disorders such as ID is complex, with those having ASD and challenging behaviour less likely to be diagnosed with a psychiatric disorder than those without ASD. This indicates that challenging behaviour and mental health problems are independent of each other in those with ASD and ID [32]. Trying to distinguish co-occurring psychiatric disorders from the core symptoms of ASD is often a challenge during the diagnostic evaluation of a person with ASD. Severe anxiety may present as a catastrophic meltdown. It may be very difficult to unravel the core symptoms of ASD, such as the routines and rituals, to make a diagnosis of obsessive–compulsive disorder. For those suffering from depression in the context of ASD, for example, an unravelling of whether increasing social isolation and not interacting is an established pattern or evidence of a developing mood disorder.

There are a number of risk factors linked to why people with ASD develop mental health problems. Communication difficulties and the existence of brain disorder are recognised risk factors for psychiatric disorders in general and they may partially explain this increased risk in people with ASD. People with ASD are also more likely to suffer poor self-esteem, bullying and loneliness, with rejection by their peers, so increasing their risk for mental illness [33]. Substance misuse and alcohol misuse are also reported for people with ASD, who may use alcohol or substances just to cope with everyday situations and experiences, such as bullying and loneliness [34].

Comorbidity with ASD and Offending

Psychiatric disorders and substance misuse increase the risk for violent criminal behaviour in the general population [35]. These conditions, when comorbid with ASD, may also play a significant role in violent offending, by diminishing an individual's ability to deal with everyday stressors [36]. A number of studies have found a history of psychiatric disorders, including schizophrenia and ADHD, to be common in individuals with ASD who have engaged in offending behaviour [37–39]. One study found depression, schizophrenia and anxiety disorders to be the most common diagnoses [37]. In a review of 37 cases of people with ASD who had committed violent offences, 31 (83.7%) were reported as having mental health problems, and 11 (29.7%) had an identifiable mental disorder at the time of the offence [38]. This study found a variety of psychiatric conditions, including conduct disorder, depression and psychotic disorder, to be present in those committing a violent offence. Although autistic individuals are no more prone to violence than neurotypical individuals, the presence of comorbid psychosis is associated with an increased risk for violent crime in those with ASD [39]. A study comparing 51 patients with ASD in a specialist autistic secure service, with 43 controls at a similar level of security, found almost three-quarters had psychiatric comorbidity, mainly schizophrenia, but personality disorders and substance use disorders were less commonly diagnosed in the autistic patients [40]. A retrospective study of all forensic examinations in Norway, over a 10-year period from 2001 to 2011, found 48 cases with ASD, which was 1.4% of all cases [41]. Of those, 33 had committed a sexual or violent offence of which 97% had previous mental health problems, with 27% having had a psychotic disorder, 24% an affective disorder, 21% a personality disorder, 36% an ID and 42% another neurodevelopmental disorder. The majority (64%) had no history of substance misuse, but those who did have a misuse problem it was typically linked to alcohol. At the time of the offence, of those who committed a violent offence ($n = 21$), 14% had a psychotic disorder identified during the forensic examination and 5% had an affective disorder, whereas those convicted of a sexual offence ($n = 12$) had neither a current psychotic nor an affective disorder.

Those with ASD who commit violent offences may not only present with mental illness but also may come from family environments in which adverse childhood experiences occur alongside additional stressors in the home situation at the time of the offence, as illustrated

> **Case Study 10.2** Person with ASD and psychotic disorder
>
> Peter was diagnosed in childhood with ASD and borderline ID. He had shown physical aggression since childhood and his biological father left in early childhood. At the age of 15 years, Peter developed a psychotic illness with auditory hallucinations including commands to harm his mother. He had witnessed domestic violence by mother's partner and it was not clear why his biological father left. Just prior to the index offence at the age of 19, he was reporting voices again and had not been taking his antipsychotic medication. One night, Peter took a kitchen knife, went upstairs and stabbed mother's partner, who was sleeping. He then attacked his mother. Peter was subsequently admitted to a secure hospital under Section 37/41. During the admission, he made threats to assault and kill staff. At one point he punched a female member of staff. Peter was prescribed olanzapine 10 mg daily and his mental state deteriorated on dose reductions. Peter was not able to talk about the time of the assault for a number of years but did say he was sorry for assaulting his mother.

by Case Study 10.2, which describes a young man with ASD who developed a psychotic disorder in adolescence, had witnessed domestic violence and was non-compliant with medication. The presentation is not atypical in that the person with ASD committed the violent offence against his parents. His underlying core difficulties of ASD may not have been the primary reason for his violent offending behaviour, with the untreated psychotic disorder being the significant risk factor that led to the index offence.

In summary, people with ASD experience a variety of mental health problems and they may suffer from more than one condition. It is important to recognise the presence of a co-occurring psychiatric disorder in offenders with ASD especially those who have committed violent offences.

Comorbid Mental Disorders in Offenders with ADHD

ADHD and Psychiatric Comorbidity

Both research evidence and clinical experience suggest that it is common for a person with a diagnosis of ADHD to attract additional psychiatric diagnoses. A multicentre study found that 66% of children and adolescents newly diagnosed with ADHD had at least one comorbid psychiatric disorder and those with the combined type of ADHD and with severe impairment were more likely to present with comorbidity [6]. Similar comorbidity has been shown in adults too [42]. Earlier studies in children and adolescents with ADHD showed that psychiatric comorbidity is not merely an artefact of overlapping symptoms between ADHD and comorbid disorders [43]. Moreover, an important reason for identifying both ADHD and its comorbidity amongst individuals with offending behaviour is that they then have the opportunity to receive appropriate treatment. There is some evidence that ADHD treatment has a protective effect on associated mental health problems [44] as well as reducing rates of criminality [45].

Specific Mental Disorders Comorbid with ADHD

Mood disorders, substance use disorders, anxiety disorders and personality disorders are amongst the commonest mental disorders that typically coexist with ADHD. In addition, other neurodevelopmental conditions such as ASD and ID are more likely to be diagnosed in people with ADHD.

Mood Disorders

In terms of comorbidity with mood disorders, it has been suggested that approximately 20% of adult patients with ADHD also have bipolar disorder and, conversely, 10–20% of those with bipolar disorder diagnosis also have ADHD [46]. Even higher rates of ADHD (37.8%) have been reported in children and young people with bipolar disorder; they are also more likely to have an earlier age of onset, a more chronic and disabling course of bipolar disorder and more psychiatric comorbidity [47].

Substance Use Disorders

ADHD rates between 15% and 25% were reported amongst adults with substance use disorders. The relationship between the two conditions has been described in detail elsewhere [48] but, briefly, substance misuse may arise in the context of impulsive behaviour or be used as 'self-medication' for the core symptoms of ADHD.

Anxiety Disorders

Data from the National Comorbidity Survey Replication in the USA suggest that adults with ADHD are at increased risk of anxiety [49]. Anxiety disorders are associated with ADHD, with rates of comorbidity approaching 25%, and it has been suggested that anxiety coexisting with ADHD may impair further working memory [50].

Personality Disorders

Personality disorders are common in people with ADHD. The two conditions are likely to be related in complex ways [51]. It has been suggested that at least one-third of children with ADHD of the combined or hyperactive type develop conduct disorder and one-fifth go on to develop antisocial personality disorder [52]. Another specific personality disorder, emotionally unstable personality disorder, has attracted a lot of clinical and research attention not least because of the symptom overlap with ADHD, namely symptoms arising from impulsivity, emotional dysregulation and mood instability. A study found that 60% of adults with borderline personality disorder probably met criteria for childhood ADHD [53].

ADHD Comorbidity and Offending

High levels of ADHD in incarcerated populations have consistently been reported. A meta-analysis found a prevalence rate of 26% amongst youth and adult prison populations [54]. Offending behaviour may be linked to the core ADHD symptoms of the offender and the link between the two is described in Chapter 4 of this book. Additional mental health problems co-occurring with ADHD are likely to contribute to the risk of offending.

Of all comorbid conditions, the role of substance use and personality disorders has been studied most extensively. A recent study found higher rates of alcohol dependence and stimulant misuse in association with ADHD in a sample of male prisoners [55]. Also, in a study of Scottish prisoners, the strongest predictors for violent offending was ADHD symptomatology, followed by alcohol dependence [56]. Thus, it was concluded that there is an urgent need to treat ADHD and substance misuse in order to reduce offending.

There is an overlap between substance use and personality disorders but a substance use disorder is a significant predictor of criminality amongst offenders with a history of childhood ADHD, even after allowing for the confounding effects of antisocial personality disorder [57]. Prisoners with ADHD, when compared to those without ADHD, have an increased risk for substance use disorder, and are more likely to have a second diagnosis and a higher number of comorbid disorders [58].

An Icelandic study found that ADHD contributed to the variance in non-violent and violent delinquency, but these effects were, to a large extent, mediated by comorbid factors such as substance use, conduct disorder and association with delinquent peers [59]. In a study using the Danish nationwide register, it was reported that ADHD was associated with conviction and incarceration [60]. Comorbidity with oppositional defiant/conduct disorder and substance use disorder significantly increased this risk. Thus, it is important to assess for substance use and additional comorbidity in those with ADHD in custodial settings.

Psychopathy has emerged as an important concept in the study of offending behaviour. ADHD has been linked with psychopathic traits, especially in incarcerated individuals, and this association seems to apply specifically to the behavioural but not the emotional aspects of psychopathy [61].

Although the majority of the studies in the field look at the effect of ADHD combined with substance use and/or personality disorders, there is some evidence that other psychiatric comorbidity also contributes to the risk of offending in people with ADHD [62].

Conclusion

It is clear from the evidence above that psychiatric disorders, including substance use disorders, are present in high rates in people with neurodevelopmental disorders who offend. Practitioners and clinicians working in healthcare and custodial settings must have the skills and expertise to evaluate the presence of comorbid psychiatric disorders in order to inform their diagnostic and risk formulation and consequent care and treatment plans. In addition, forensic, secure and custodial services must ensure that the resources are available for the full range of treatments for psychiatric disorders in this vulnerable group of offenders.

A key role of the clinician is, of course, the identification and treatment of neurodevelopmental disorders and any comorbidity in those who offend. It has increasingly been recognised that the role of mental health professionals also includes the assessment of whether symptoms of a neurodevelopmental disorder and associated comorbidity are likely to be made worse or to increase the offender's vulnerability in a prison environment. Finally, consideration has to be given to people with a neurodevelopmental disorder as witnesses or victims of violence, as there is some evidence that those who have been victims of violence have significantly increased odds for depression compared to those who have not experienced violence in the community [63].

References

1. Young S, González RA, Mullens H, Mutch L, Malet-Lambert I, Gudjonsson GH. Neurodevelopmental disorders in prison inmates: comorbidity and combined associations with psychiatric symptoms and behavioural disturbance. *Psychiatry Research* 2018; 1(261): 109–15.

2. McCarthy J, Chaplin E, Forrester A, Underwood L, Hayward H, Sabet J, et al. Prisoners with neurodevelopmental

difficulties: vulnerabilities for mental illness and self-harm. *Criminal Behaviour and Mental Health* 2019; 29(5–6): 308–20.

3. Cooper SA, Smiley E, Morrison J, Williamson A, Allan L. Mental ill-health in adults with intellectual disabilities: prevalence and associated factors. *British Journal of Psychiatry* 2007; 190(1): 27–35.

4. Public Health England. Learning Disabilities Observatory: people with learning disabilities in England 2015 – main report. Available at: https://assets .publishing.service.gov.uk/government/up loads/system/uploads/attachment_data/fil e/613182/PWLDIE_2015_main_report_N B090517.pdf#:~:text=People%20with%20l earning%20disabilities%20in%20England %202015%3A%20Main,is%2C%20within %20a%20single%20publication%2C%20to %20provide%20.

5. King C, Murphy G. A systematic review of people with autism spectrum disorder and the criminal justice system. *Journal of Autism and Developmental Disorders* 2014; 44(11): 2717–33.

6. Reale L, Bartoli B, Cartabia M, Zanetti M, Costantino MA, Canevini MP, et al. Comorbidity prevalence and treatment outcome in children and adolescents with ADHD. *European Child & Adolescent Psychiatry* 2017; 26(12): 1443–57.

7. Thomas SDM, Nixon M, Ogloff JRP, Daffern M. Crime and victimization among people with intellectual disability with and without comorbid mental illness. *Journal of Applied Research in Intellectual Disabilities* 2019; 32(5): 1088–95.

8. Department of Health. The Bradley Report: Lord Bradley's review of people with mental health problems or learning disabilities in the criminal justice system. Available at: https://lx.iriss.org.uk/sites/de fault/files/resources/The%20Bradley%20re port.pdf.

9. Hellenbach M, Karatzias T, Brown M. Intellectual disabilities among prisoners: prevalence and mental and physical health comorbidities. *Journal of Applied Research in Intellectual Disabilities* 2016; 30(2): 230–41.

10. Fogden B, Thomas S, Daffern M, Ogloff J, Crime and victimisation in people with intellectual disability: a case linkage study. *BMC Psychiatry* 2016; 16: 170.

11. Cooper SA, Melville CA, Einfeld SL. Psychiatric diagnosis, intellectual disabilities and diagnostic criteria for psychiatric disorders for use with adults with learning disabilities/mental retardation (DC-LD). *Journal of Intellectual Disability Research* 2003; 47 (1): 3–15.

12. Sheehan R, Hassiotis A, Walters K, Osborn D, Strydom A, Horsfall, L. Mental illness, challenging behaviour, and psychotropic drug prescribing in people with intellectual disability: UK population based cohort study. *BMJ* 2015; 351: h4326.

13. Hassiotis A, Gazizova D, Akinlonu L, Bebbington P, Meltzer H, Strydom A. Psychiatric morbidity in prisoners with intellectual disabilities: analysis of prison survey data for England and Wales. *British Journal of Psychiatry* 2011; 199 (2): 156–7.

14. Chaplin E, McCarthy J, Underwood L, Forrester A, Hayward H, Sabet J, et al. Characteristics of prisoners with intellectual disabilities. *Journal of Intellectual Disability Research* 2017; 61 (12): 1185–95.

15. Salekin KL, Olley JG, Hedge KA. Offenders with intellectual disability: characteristics, prevalence, and issues in forensic assessment. *Journal of Mental Health Research in Intellectual Disabilities* 2010; 3 (2): 97–116.

16. Marshall-Tate K, Chaplin E, Ali S, Hardy S. Learning disabilities: supporting people in the criminal justice system. 2019. Available at: www.nursingtimes.net/roles/learning-disability-nurses/learning-disabilities-supporting-people-in-the-criminal-justice -system-17-06-2019.

17. Scott H, Havercamp S. Comparison of self- and proxy report of mental health symptoms in people with intellectual disabilities. *Journal of Mental Health Research in Intellectual Disabilities* 2018; 11 (2): 143–56.

18. McKinnon I, Thorp J, Grubin D. Improving the detection of detainees with suspected intellectual disability in police custody. *Advances in Mental Health and Intellectual Disabilities* 2015; 9(4): 174–85.

19. HMI Probation and HMI Prisons A joint inspection of the treatment of offenders with learning disabilities in the criminal justice system – phase 2 in custody and the community. 2015. Available at: www.justiceinspectorates.g ov.uk>/cjji/wp-content/uploads/sites/2/2 015/03/Learning-Disabilities-phase-two-report.pdf.

20. Talbot J. Experiences of the criminal justice system by prisoners with learning disabilities. 2008. Available at: www.ojp.go v/ncjrs/virtual-library/abstracts/prisoners-voices-experiences-criminal-justice-system-prisoners-0

21. O'Brien G, Taylor J, Lindsay W, Holland A, Carson D, Steptoe L, et al. A multi-centre study of adults with learning disabilities referred to services for antisocial or offending behaviour: demographic, individual, offending and service characteristics. *Journal of Learning Disabilities and Offending Behaviour* 2010; 1(2): 5–15.

22. NHSDigital. Learning disability services monthly statistics. December 2020. Available at: https://digital.nhs.uk/data-and-information/publications/statistical/le arning-disability-services-statistics/learn ing-disability-services-monthly-statistics-at-november-2020-mhsds-september-2020 -final.

23. Alexander R, Hiremath A, Chester V, Green F, Gunaratna I, Hoare S. Evaluation of treatment outcomes from a medium secure unit for people with intellectual disability. *Advances in Mental Health and Intellectual Disabilities* 2011; 5(1): 22–32.

24. Wooster L, McCarthy J, Chaplin E. Outcomes of an inner city forensic intellectual disability service. *Journal of Intellectual Disabilities and Offending Behaviour* 2018; 9(1): 1–8.

25. Klimecki MR, Jenkinson J, Wilson L. A study of recidivism among offenders with an intellectual disability. *Australia and New Zealand Journal of Developmental Disabilities* 2009; 19: 209–19.

26. Royal College of Psychiatrists. Forensic care pathways for adults with intellectual disability involved with the criminal justice. Available at: www.rcpsych.ac.uk/d ocs/default-source/members/faculties/fore nsic-psychiatry/forensic-fr-id-04.pdf? sfvrsn=2fdf0def_2.

27. Levy SE, Mandell DS, Schultz RT. Autism. *Lancet* 2009; 374(9701): 1627–38.

28. Bradley E, Bolton P. Episodic psychiatric disorders in teenagers with learning disabilities with and without autism. *British Journal of Psychiatry* 2006; 189: 361–6.

29. Royal College of Psychiatrists. The psychiatric management of autism in adults College Report 228. 2020. Available at: www.rcpsych.ac.uk/improving-care/ca mpaigning-for-better-mental-health-policy/college-reports/2020-college-reports/cr228.

30. Selten JP, Lundberg M, Rai D, Magnusson C. Risks for nonaffective psychotic disorder and bipolar disorder in young people with autism spectrum disorder: a population-based study. *JAMA Psychiatry* 2015; 72(5): 483–9.

31. Lugo-Marin J, Rodríguez-Franco MA, Mahtani Chugani V, Magán Maganto M, Díez Villoria E, Canal Bedia R. Prevalence of psychiatric disorder in adults with ASD spectrum disorder: a systematic review and meta-analysis. *Research in ASD Spectrum Disorders* 2019; 59: 22–33.

32. McCarthy J, Hemmings C, Kravariti E, Dworzynski K, Holt G, Bouras N, Tsakanikos E. Challenging behaviour and co-morbid psychopathology in adults with intellectual disability and autism spectrum disorders. *Research in Developmental Disabilities* 2010; 31: 362–6.

33. Carey C, Clear D, Robertson D. Mental health morbidity across the lifespan. In Chaplin E, Spain D, McCarthy J, eds., *A Clinician's Guide to Mental Health Conditions in Adults with Autism Spectrum Disorders*, Jessica Kingsley Publishers, 2020: 24–39.

34. Chaplin E, McCarthy J. Substance use disorders. In Chaplin E, Spain D, McCarthy J, eds., *A Clinician's Guide to Mental Health Conditions in Adults with Autism Spectrum Disorders*, Jessica Kingsley Publishers, 2020: 373–86.

35. Arseneault L, Moffitt TE, Caspi A, Taylor PJ, Silva PA. Mental disorders and violence in a total birth cohort: results from the Dunedin Study. *Archives of General Psychiatry* 2000; 57(10): 979–86.

36. Langstrom N, Grann M, Ruchkin V, Sjostedt, G Fazel S. Risk factors for violent offending in autism spectrum disorder: a national study of hospitalised individuals. *Journal of Interpersonal Violence* 2009; 24 (8): 1358–70.

37. Allen D, Evans C, Hider A, Hawkins S, Pecket, H, Morgan H. Offending behaviour in adults with Asperger syndrome. *Journal of ASD and Developmental Disorders* 2008; 38(4): 748–58.

38. Newman SS, Ghaziuddin M. Violent crime in Asperger syndrome: the role of psychiatric comorbidity. *Journal of ASD and Developmental Disorders* 2008; 38(10): 1848.

39. Wachtel LE, Shorter E. ASD plus psychosis: a 'one–two punch' risk for tragic violence? *Medical Hypotheses* 2013; 81: 404–9.

40. Haw C, Radley J, Cooke L. Characteristics of male autistic spectrum patients in low security: are they different from non-autistic low secure patients? *Journal of Intellectual Disability & Offending Behaviour* 2013; 4(1/2): 24–32.

41. Søndenaa E, Helverschou SB, Steindal K, Rasmussen K, Nilsson B, Nøttestad JA. Violence and sexual offending behaviour in people with autism spectrum disorder who have undergone a forensic examination. *Psychological Reports: Disability & Trauma* 2014; 115(1): 32–43.

42. Wilens T, Biederman J, Faraone S, Martelon M, Westerberg D, Spencer T. Presenting ADHD symptoms, subtypes, and comorbid disorders in clinically referred adults with ADHD. *Journal of Clinical Psychiatry* 2009; 70(11): 1557–62.

43. Milberger S, Biederman J, Faraone SV, Murphy J, Tsuang ST. ADHD and comorbid disorders: issues of overlapping symptoms. *American Journal of Psychiatry* 1995; 152(12): 1793–9.

44. Boland H, DiSalvo M, Fried R, Woodworth KY, Wilens T, Faraone SV, et al. A literature review and meta-analysis on the effects of ADHD medications on functional outcomes. *Journal of Psychiatric Research* 2020; 123: 21–30.

45. Lichtenstein P, Halldner L, Zetterqvist J, Sjölander A, Serlachius E, Fazel S, et al. Medication for attention deficit-hyperactivity disorder and criminality. *New England Journal of Medicine* 2012; 367 (21): 2006–14.

46. Brus MJ, Solanto MV, Goldberg JF. Adult ADHD vs. bipolar disorder in the DSM-5 era: a challenging differentiation for clinicians. *Journal of Psychiatric Practice* 2014; 20(6): 428–37.

47. Masi G, Perugi G, Toni C, Millepiedi S, Mucci M, Bertini N, Pfanner C. ADHD-bipolar comorbidity in children and adolescents. *Bipolar Disorders* 2006; 8(4): 378–81.

48. Wilens TE. ADHD and the substance use disorders. In Buitelaar JK, Kan CC, Asherson P, eds., *ADHD in Adults: Characterisation, Diagnosis and Treatment*. Cambridge University Press, 2011: 174–90.

49. Kessler RC, Adler L, Barkley R, Biederman J, Conners CK, Demler O, et al. The prevalence and correlates of adult ADHD in the United States: results from the National Comorbidity Survey Replication. *American Journal of Psychiatry* 2006; 163(4): 716–23.

50. Schatz DB, Rostain AL. ADHD and comorbid anxiety: a review of the current literature. *Journal of Attention Disorders* 2006; 10(2): 141–9.

51. Van Dijk FE, Anckasaeter H. ADHD, personality and its disorders. In Buitelaar JK, Kan CC, Asherson P, eds., *ADHD in Adults: Characterisation, Diagnosis and Treatment*. Cambridge University Press, 2011: 174–90.

52. Hofvander B, Ossowski B, Lundstrom S, Anckarsaeter H. Continuity of aggressive antisocial behaviour from childhood to adulthood: the question of phenotype definition. *International Journal of Law and Psychiatry* 2009; 32(4): 224–34.

53. Fossati A, Novella I, Donati D, Donini M, Maffei C. History of childhood ADHD symptoms and borderline personality disorder: a controlled study. *Comprehensive Psychiatry* 2002; 43: 369–77.

54. Young S, Moss D, Sedgwick O, Fridman M, Hodgkins P. A meta-analysis of the prevalence of attention deficit hyperactivity disorder in incarcerated populations. *Psychological Medicine* 2015; 45(2): 247–58.

55. Young S, González RA, Wolff K, Xenitidis K, Mutch L, Malet-Lambert I, et al. Substance and alcohol misuse, drug pathways, and offending behaviors in association with ADHD in prison inmates. *Journal of Attention Disorders* 2020; 24(13): 1905–13.

56. Young S, Wells J, Gudjonsson GH. Predictors of offending among prisoners: the role of attention-deficit hyperactivity disorder and substance use. *Journal of Psychopharmacology* 2011; 25(11): 1524–32.

57. Mannuzza S, Klein RG, Moulton JL. Lifetime criminality among boys with attention deficit hyperactivity disorder: a prospective follow-up study into adulthood using official arrest records. *Psychiatry Research* 2008; 160(3): 237–46.

58. Vélez-Pastrana MC, González RA, Ramos-Fernández A, Padilla RR, Levin FR, García CA. Attention deficit hyperactivity disorder in prisoners: increased substance use disorder severity and psychiatric comorbidity. *European Addiction Research* 2020; 26(4–5): 179–90.

59. Gudjonsson GH, Sigurdsson JF, Sigfusdottir ID, Young S. A national epidemiological study of offending and its relationship with ADHD symptoms and associated risk factors. *Journal of Attention Disorders* 2014; 18(1): 3–13.

60. Mohr-Jensen C, Bisgaard CM, Boldsen SK, Steinhausen HC. Attention-deficit /hyperactivity disorder in childhood and adolescence and the risk of crime in young adulthood in a Danish nationwide study. *Journal of the American Academy of Child and Adolescent Psychiatry* 2019; 58(4): 443–52.

61. Eisenbarth H, Alpers GW, Conzelmann A, Jacob CP, Weyers P, Pauli P. Psychopathic traits in adult ADHD patients. *Personality and Individual Differences* 2008; 45(6): 468–72.

62. Karlén MH, Nilsson T, Wallinius M, Billstedt E, Hofvander B. A Bad Start: The combined effects of early onset substance use and ADHD and CD on criminality patterns, substance abuse and psychiatric comorbidity among young violent offenders. *Journal for Person-Oriented Research* 2020; 6(1): 39–55.

63. Stickley A, Koposov R, Koyanagi A, Inoue Y, Ruchkin V. ADHD and depressive symptoms in adolescents: the role of community violence exposure. *Social Psychiatry and Psychiatric Epidemiology* 2019; 54(6): 683–91.

Attention Deficit Hyperactivity Disorder: Assessment and Therapeutic Approaches within Forensic Settings

Bhathika Perera, Maheera Tyler and Zaid Al-Najjar

Introduction

Attention deficit hyperactivity disorder (ADHD) is a highly heritable neurodevelopmental disorder characterised by hyperactivity/impulsivity and inattention causing impairment in personal, social and occupational functioning. Significant research has been carried out on the symptoms, trajectory of the disorder and treatment. Certain groups of people are reported to have higher rates of ADHD. Among prisoners, the estimated prevalence rate for ADHD is around 20–25% [1]; worldwide, this equates to over 2.6 million prisoners. It is well established that identification, assessment and treatment of ADHD in prisoners leads to improved outcomes in social and personal domains, educational and occupational attainment, impulsivity, criminal behaviour and substance misuse, as well as better engagement with treatment for other comorbid psychiatric conditions. Therefore, it is important not to miss any opportunities to engage with people who are actively subject to the criminal justice system to detect, diagnose and treat ADHD if clinically indicated. In this chapter, we discuss assessment and treatment approaches, and also aim to address some of the challenges in identifying and managing ADHD in forensic settings.

Assessment of ADHD within Forensic Settings

Identification and Screening

The high prevalence of ADHD among offenders highlights the importance of screening for ADHD [2]. It can be argued that ADHD is a diagnosis that needs to be excluded among people in prison or forensic settings. Given the high number of individuals going through forensic and prison systems, screening for ADHD can be considered an effective way to identify individuals who need to undergo a full diagnostic assessment. Different countries have different systems in place to screen for mental health problems in prison settings. In the UK, it is recommended that all prisoners undergo a reception screen for mental health problems upon first arrival to prison. However, in practice, this often does not include specific questions aimed at screening for ADHD [1].

There are various ADHD screening instruments available for use in the general population. The World Health Organization (WHO) Adult ADHD Self-Report Scale (ASRS v1.1) symptom checklist has been widely used to screen for ADHD in community samples [3]. It has also been used to screen for ADHD among adults at an individual level. Various studies looking at the prevalence of ADHD in prison populations have used the ASRS v1.1 [2];

therefore, it could be argued that the ASRS can be utilised as a useful tool in prison and forensic settings. The ASRS v1.1 has 18 questions. The ASRS 5 has been developed as an update to ASRS v1.1 which fits in with modified *Diagnostic and Statistical Manual of Mental Disorders*, 5th edition (DSM-5) criteria [4, 5]. This is a short scale with six questions, which can be easily administered in different settings. ASRS screening tools have shown good sensitivity and specificity with a high positive predictive value. It is also available in several different languages. The Brief Barkley Adult ADHD Rating Scale (B-BAARS) is another assessment to screen for ADHD in adults in the criminal justice system. A study done in a prison population showed that the brief version of BAARS provided higher sensitivity and specificity in the prison population [6]. It is worth remembering that none of the screening tools are designed to be used as diagnostic instruments. They are purely used to identify individuals who need a full assessment for ADHD.

Incorporating ADHD screening methods into existing mental health assessments is a challenge. Lack of awareness of ADHD among health and prison care staff and well-established systems within prison settings can further compound these challenges. Staff training and increased awareness of ADHD presentation are of utmost importance. It can enable individuals with ADHD to be identified, screened, referred for further assessments and treatments and followed up by community services when released from prison/forensic settings. Developing and integrating screening and diagnostic pathways to existing systems in the criminal justice system can overcome barriers.

Diagnostic Assessment

Making the diagnosis itself can be therapeutic, as it can help the subject understand lifelong emotional and behavioural difficulties associated with a high risk of criminal behaviours. This can help the person with ADHD to gain an increased understanding and insight into what interventions may help to reduce symptoms and improve the functional impairment. Therefore, providing information about the reasons for the assessment as well as the process involved may help the person engage in the ADHD diagnostic process. The diagnostic assessment aims to establish whether a person meets the DSM-5 or the WHO's International Classification of Diseases 11th Revision (ICD-11) [7] criteria for adult ADHD. As in non-forensic settings, this includes a psychiatric history supported by a semi-structured interview focusing on ADHD symptoms. The psychiatric history should provide a detailed developmental perspective focusing on pregnancy, birth, early childhood, developmental milestones, educational achievements and emotional and behavioural development. A gold-standard ADHD assessment will include all of the above; however, this may not be practicable in a prison setting. In our experience, it is sometimes challenging to obtain a developmental history in early childhood. Therefore, a pragmatic view should be taken to decide on what is essential to make the diagnosis of ADHD in this patient group.

Although core symptoms of ADHD are clearly defined, they can be experienced and manifest differently in different individuals. This can often lead to underdiagnosis or misdiagnosis of ADHD and other mental disorders. The DSM-5 criteria (see Box 11.1) that are primarily based on ADHD symptoms in children and adolescents may not fully explain some of the symptoms experienced by adults. This can be even more marked amongst people going through forensic settings. Executive function deficits are another set of symptoms that have been shown to be present in adults with ADHD. Studies have proposed that executive function deficits are a reliable indicator of ADHD even though they

> **Box 11.1** DSM-5 criteria for adult ADHD [4]
>
> Five or more symptoms of inattention and/or five or more symptoms of hyperactivity/impulsivity persistent for six months, not consistent with the developmental level
>
> Several symptoms were present before the age of 12 years
>
> Several symptoms must have been present in two or more settings (e.g., home, school, social relationships, workplace)
>
> Clear evidence that symptoms have a negative effect on social, academic or occupational functioning
>
> Symptoms are not explained by any other psychiatric disorder

are not fully included in the DSM-5 [8]. Self-control, mood dysregulation, problem solving and difficulties in planning, enacting and organising activities that do not have immediate rewards are some of the executive function deficits seen among people with ADHD. This can be argued as one of the reasons for the functional impairment among people with ADHD who fall foul of the criminal justice system. Some authors argue ADHD as an executive function deficit disorder. Therefore, questions about executive function during an ADHD assessment can give a better understanding of the impairment due to ADHD.

There are several validated semi-structured interviews used in general adult ADHD clinics that can be used in the forensic population. The Diagnostic Interview for ADHD in adults (DIVA-5), Conners' Adult ADHD Diagnostic Interview for DSM-4 (CAADID) and ADHD evaluation for adults (ACE+) are some of the more commonly used semi-structured tools available. The Diagnostic Interview for ADHD in adults with intellectual disability (ID) (DIVA-5-ID) is advised if there is a diagnosis or suspicion of ID. While much of the information can be gathered from the clinical interview, utilising a semi-structured diagnostic tool as part of the assessment has the advantage of helping to complete the assessment in a systematic and structured way. It also provides reassurance that a diagnosis based on a validated semi-structured interview is clinically valid and reliable.

The diagnostic interview can be supplemented by completing questionnaires aimed at assessing the level of functional impairment such as the BAARS and the Weiss Functional Impairment Rating Scale. The time taken to complete a full assessment is variable and dependent on both the clinician, the individual being assessed and their clinical presentation. It is estimated that, in most cases, the full assessment can be completed in about two hours. This includes approximately an hour to complete the semi-structured interview with an additional hour to complete the psychiatric history. However, there can be practical difficulties such as not being able to have two hours of assessment time per prisoner or challenges in getting past information required for the assessment. Prisoners may also find it hard to engage in the interview process for two hours. Therefore, some assessments may require more than one appointment. The lack of availability of childhood symptoms in the clinical history should not exclude people from the diagnosis of ADHD. Overall symptom presentation as well as progression of symptoms can help make a balanced decision on the presence of ADHD in individuals despite missing childhood history. It is important to highlight that a pragmatic approach to the diagnostic process is needed to identify people with ADHD subject to the forensic and criminal justice system.

Differential Diagnosis

It is important to keep in mind when assessing patients for ADHD that there is increased comorbidity of mental disorders amongst people with ADHD [9]. As discussed earlier, common comorbid conditions include ID, autism spectrum disorder (ASD), obsessive–compulsive disorder, tic disorders, bipolar affective disorder (particularly hypomanic or manic presentations), personality disorders, anxiety disorders and substance use disorders [10]. Antisocial personality disorder, which is highly prevalent among prison and the forensic population, is also associated with ADHD [11]. Exploring childhood history can be helpful as a history of conduct disorder along with ADHD has shown to increase antisocial behaviours in adulthood compared to ADHD alone [12]. We have observed that there is a risk of not considering ADHD when people receive a diagnosis of severe mental illness or a personality disorder. Therefore, it is pertinent that diagnostic assessment for ADHD is carried out even though the person may have diagnosed mental illnesses.

It is also important to consider physical health conditions such as restless leg syndrome and hyperthyroidism as they may also cause hyperactivity and restlessness that may be mistaken for the hyperactivity of ADHD. Therefore, it is important to take an overview of physical health conditions in addition to psychiatric comorbidities. Additionally, people under the influence of or withdrawing from illicit substances may present as hyperactive and restless. However, it is still important to consider the possibility of existing ADHD as substance misuse is common among people with ADHD [13]. Even though ADHD is a condition starting in early childhood, a 'late-onset acquired ADHD' following traumatic head injury has been increasingly recognised. Given that the forensic population is at increased risk of head injury [14], it is worth considering the possibility of late-onset ADHD in this group of patients.

Simple vs Complex ADHD

It can be clinically helpful to divide ADHD in to two main categories: simple and complex. Simple ADHD is where an individual meets the criteria for ADHD without coexistent mental illnesses/disorders and/or neurodevelopmental disorders. Complex ADHD can be determined when a person with ADHD also has a mental illness/disorder and/or neurodevelopmental disorders. For an example, if a person has both ADHD and ASD, or ADHD and bipolar disorder or ADHD and ID, this can be defined as complex ADHD. It is important to make this distinction as the diagnostic process may be challenging in complex ADHD. More importantly, people with complex ADHD may need more support and interventions in addition to specific evidence-based pharmacological treatments. This is particularly relevant in the forensic and criminal justice system as a large number of people with ADHD are likely to have complex ADHD, given the significant psychiatric comorbidities in this population group [15]. This needs to be considered when developing treatment pathways, as complex ADHD patients may require more than pharmacological and psychological interventions for ADHD alone.

Challenges in Assessment and Diagnosis

There can be challenges in making an accurate diagnosis of ADHD in forensic settings, particularly in prisons. First, the diagnosis of ADHD is made from the patient's clinical history, as discussed above. The process of collecting information in prison settings, in particular, can be challenging for multiple reasons. Prisoners may not engage in a detailed ADHD assessment due to their emotional state. They may also be unreliable historians. Prisoners may look at engaging in a mental health assessment unfavourably; therefore, they may be reluctant to attend appointments with mental health staff in prison settings. There are also often difficulties in getting collateral information to support the diagnostic assessment. Some prisons, such as remand prisons, have a high turnover. This can present an additional challenge to the diagnostic assessment as prisoners may move out of the prison during the assessment process.

Substance misuse can be a significant complicating factor when assessing for ADHD. It can be challenging to differentiate between a primary substance misuse problem, resulting in high levels of activity and/or inattention, and a secondary substance misuse problem in which the individual attempts to 'self-medicate' in order to make their symptoms of ADHD manageable. Careful history taking and the involvement of a dual diagnosis specialist may be useful in such presentations.

It is well established that there is a high level of psychiatric comorbidity associated with ADHD; some estimates suggest that as many as 87% of people with ADHD have a comorbid psychiatric diagnosis [16], adding a further layer of complexity to the accurate diagnosis of ADHD, particularly in forensic settings where there may be a lack of other collateral information. There are commonalities between ADHD and the symptomatology of affective disorders, anxiety disorders and substance use disorders. Emotional dysregulation is considered as a common manifestation of ADHD. This can often lead to underdiagnosis of ADHD and interventions only focusing on a mood disorder even though it is also recognised that prevalence rates of affective disorders among people with ADHD is relatively high [9, 17]. Emotional dysregulation is also often seen in personality disorders and can therefore lead to diagnostic overshadowing. Some estimates suggest that up to 50% of people with ADHD have a comorbid personality disorder with the predominant symptoms being emotional dysregulation as opposed to inattentive symptoms [9].

Another significant challenge in assessing and diagnosing ADHD is the difference in symptoms reported by male and female patients. Historically, hyperactivity has been seen as a 'male' trait. It is well recognised that boys are more likely to be referred for assessment based on symptoms of hyperactivity in childhood. Girls and women are much more likely to report symptoms of internalised hyperactivity and mental restlessness. In forensic settings, these differences in presentation may mean that ADHD is significantly more likely to be missed in women, who do not present with hyperactivity and behavioural disturbance. Men and women with primarily inattentive ADHD are also likely to slip through the net as these symptoms are often missed.

While it is now widely recognised that ADHD remains underdiagnosed and undertreated, particularly in forensic settings, it is also important to address concerns that some patients may seek out a diagnosis for a secondary gain, such as access to stimulant medications and as an explanation for disturbed or violent and aggressive behaviour stemming from a different cause. It may also be viewed as a means to accessing time away from the general prison population or to avoid being placed in isolation for their safety or the safety of others. These risks should be assessed as a multidisciplinary team as part of the diagnostic process. A example is given in Case Study 11.1.

> **Case Study 11.1** Late diagnosis of ADHD in forensic patient group
>
> Adam is a 40-year-old man with mild ID, ADHD, antisocial personality disorder and bipolar affective disorder. He was a looked-after child from the age of 11, with multiple placement breakdowns. He attended mainstream school, but he was recognised as having special education needs and his behaviour has been challenging since an early age. This included aggression, disrupting the classroom, self-harming and sexually explicit language. His forensic history goes back to the age of 15 when he was charged for fire setting. He was convicted of several common assaults between the ages of 15 and 21 and admitted to a forensic hospital through the criminal justice system at the age of 20. He continued to present with behavioural challenges, needing regular seclusion and PRN ('when required') medications. Although he was treated for his bipolar affective disorder, his ADHD was not treated until he was about 40 years of age. Treatment with ADHD medications significantly improved his behaviour, including a reduction in the use of seclusion. The diagnosis of ADHD helped staff to understand some of his behaviours and make necessary adaptations when providing behavioural and psychological interventions.

Therapeutic Approaches

General Approaches to Management

ADHD is a highly treatable condition, with good results achieved from a multimodal approach combining psychoeducation (for both staff and patients), non-pharmacological interventions and pharmacological treatment. These interventions can be adapted for the prison and forensic population and achieve a significant reduction in the core symptoms and functional impairment. Studies have highlighted longer-term benefits such as a reduction in recidivism and reduced rates of criminal reconviction following commencement and optimisation of appropriate ADHD treatment [18].

As discussed earlier, it is well established that a diagnosis of ADHD is associated with an increased risk of serious mental illness. Treatment for severe affective or psychotic illnesses before commencing treatment for ADHD is recommended. There are anxieties amongst psychiatrists when treating patients with ADHD and psychotic or bipolar disorder using stimulant medications, due to a theoretical risk of relapse. Population-based observational data from the Swedish Prescribed Drug Register looking at the use of methylphenidate in patients with ADHD and psychosis found no evidence to support an increased risk of psychosis with methylphenidate [19].

It is important to commence multimodal treatment at the earliest opportunity for those with comorbid neurodevelopmental conditions such as ASD, mild affective disorders, substance use disorders and behavioural disturbance given that adequate treatment of the underlying ADHD may result in an improvement in overall psychological and behavioural distress.

Psychoeducation

As acknowledged in the ADHD Consensus Statement in 2018, all effective treatment for ADHD relies on a good understanding of the diagnosis of ADHD, how it may manifest and the specific challenges associated with a diagnosis [20].

Staff awareness of ADHD is linked closely with higher levels of engagement with treatment programmes, both pharmacological and non-pharmacological. Conversely, a lack of awareness from staff may be detrimental to the therapeutic rapport and result in poor adherence with medication regimes and engagement with psychological interventions. It is important for staff to understand the specific needs of prisoners and patients with ADHD, for example, noting that use of segregation and isolation for those with ADHD is likely to result in a worsening behavioural presentation, due to the exacerbation of ADHD symptoms from being additionally confined and restricted. These should therefore only be used as a last resort to manage acute risk and behavioural disturbance, for the shortest duration of time possible. It is also helpful for staff to understand the importance of administering the ADHD medication on schedule, and some flexibility may be required in allowing stimulant medication to be kept with non-restricted medications to allow for timely dispensing; this has been shown to improve adherence with longer-term pharmacological treatment.

For prisoners and patients, it is important that psychoeducation takes a holistic approach to foster an understanding of ADHD symptoms and their psychological and behavioural manifestations. It may be helpful to adopt a goals-based approach, with a focus on life skills to equip individuals to successfully manage the transition from highly restrictive to unrestrictive settings in due course; although not specific to ADHD, those with ADHD are likely to particularly struggle with planning and so benefit from this approach. It is also important to discuss both pharmacological and non-pharmacological treatments and to clearly explain the purpose, risks, benefits and response rates to different modalities of treatment. This is a necessary part of obtaining informed consent, but also has the benefit of improving engagement with the treatment plan.

Non-Pharmacological Treatment

Non-pharmacological treatment focused on psychosocial, neurocognitive and behavioural aspects is an important part of the multimodal approach to ADHD treatment. If the ADHD is assessed as being of mild to moderate severity, it may be that non-pharmacological treatment is sufficient and pharmacological intervention is not required (although this can be revisited at a later stage if needed). It is, however, important to acknowledge that there is often a dearth of trained practitioners who are able to deliver non-pharmacological interventions targeted at ADHD in forensic settings and, therefore, the following options may be under-utilised at present, due to a lack of resource. This may be mitigated by drawing from a wide pool of available staff from different training backgrounds, as well as (if appropriate) other prisoners to deliver interventions and form mentoring and coaching relationships with individuals.

Cognitive–behavioural therapy (CBT), and cognitive restructuring/reframing, can be delivered in groups or individually and allows the individual to develop a reflective, goal-oriented approach to different activities and social interactions. It takes into account the in-built resilience and protective factors of each individual and allows them to develop their own approach to problem solving and managing their thoughts and behaviours. There is good evidence that CBT alone or in combination with medication offers a reduction in functional impairment from ADHD.

R&R2ADHD is a cognitive skills programme based on CBT and aimed at young people and adults with ADHD [21]. The programme consists of group sessions supplemented by one-to-one sessions with a mentor, who is tasked with supporting the individual to transfer their learning from the group sessions to their daily life. Evidence shows that short- and long-term outcomes are improved as a result of engaging with this programme, with particular benefits in educational and occupational functioning as well as a reduction in symptoms of emotional dysregulation and anxiety.

Dialectical behavioural therapy can offer some benefits in coping with self-regulation, emotions and managing social situations. The treatment can be delivered in a group or individually. Although not originally developed for use in ADHD, it can offer benefits to patients whose main difficulties lie in emotional regulation and, in particular, those with comorbid diagnoses of a personality disorder.

Pharmacological Treatment

Pharmacological treatment for ADHD in forensic settings should be initiated and titrated by clinicians trained in the assessment, diagnosis and treatment of ADHD. It is important to conduct a risk assessment including the risks of potential abuse. However, we recommend positive risk taking when prescribing ADHD medications given potential significant benefits. ADHD medications (both stimulants and non-stimulants) (see Tables 11.1 and 11.2) are safe and well-tolerated medications and, broadly speaking, can be prescribed to people of all ages and genders. It is advisable to prescribe with caution in pregnancy, with a slow titration, lower dose and enhanced antenatal care in consultation, with a perinatal psychiatrist if required.

It is important to consider the full range of symptoms to be addressed and to balance these against the potential side effects. A baseline assessment of physical health is advised before commencing medication, to include a review of any pre-existing physical health conditions, blood pressure, heart rate and cardiovascular assessment. It may be necessary to consult a cardiologist in case of pre-existing cardiac conditions or strong family history of hereditary cardiac conditions.

Table 11.1 Medications available in the UK [22]

Stimulant medications*	Non-stimulant medications*
Methylphenidate	Atomoxetine
• methylphenidate immediate release	
• methylphenidate modified release	
Dexamfetamine	Guanfacine
• dexamfetamine immediate release	
• dexamfetamine sulfate	
• dexamfetamine slow release	
Lisdexamfetamine	
	Clonidine

* Note: the availability of ADHD medications varies from one country to another and they come under different tradenames.

Table 11.2 ADHD medication guidance

Medication	Starting dose	Titration	Maximum adult dose	Duration of action	Monitoring
Methylphenidate immediate release	5–10 mg, two–three times a day	Increments of 5–10 mg weekly	100 mg daily in divided doses	2–4 hours	Blood pressure, pulse, weight, insomnia, appetite, mood
Concerta XL (methylphenidate modified release)	18 mg once a day	Adjust weekly according to dose response	108 mg daily	8–10 hours	
Equasym XL (methylphenidate modified release)	10 mg once a day	Adjust weekly according to dose response	100 mg daily	6–8 hours	
Medikinet XL (methylphenidate modified release)	10 mg daily once a day	Adjust weekly according to dose response	100 mg daily	6–8 hours	
Dexamfetamine immediate release	10 mg daily in divided doses	Adjust weekly according to dose response	60 mg daily in divided doses	3–4 hours	
Elvanse (lisdexamfetamine)	20 mg daily in the morning	Increase by 10–20mg weekly according to dose response	70 mg daily	12–14 hours	
Strattera (atomoxetine)	40 mg daily	Increase according to dose response	120 mg per day; may be given in single or divided doses	24-hour symptom control	

Medication doses can be titrated as recommended by the UK's National Institute for Health and Care Excellence (NICE) guidelines, with regular reviews for stimulants. Those titrated or non-stimulants may be reviewed less frequently for dose adjustments.

Stimulant Treatment

As with the NICE guidelines relating to non-forensic population, stimulant medications are recommended as first-line agents [23]. They have a significant advantage in the speed of response and have a well-established large effect size. It is important to note that stimulant medications are classed as controlled substances in the UK, and are therefore subject to stringent rules about dispensing and storage. This has the potential to cause logistical difficulties with dispensing in a timely manner and may cause individuals to feel stigmatised if they are not able to receive medication in the same manner as their peers. This may then have a consequent reduction in adherence to the treatment.

Lisdexamfetamine is a long-acting stimulant medication with a duration of action of approximately 14 hours. Modified-release preparations of methylphenidate (Concerta XL, Medikinet XL and Equasym XL) and immediate-release preparations of methylphenidate can also be used as first-line treatment alternatives to lisdexamfetamine. A joint discussion on target symptoms and treatment outcomes help to decide on the choice of stimulant medication. Longer-acting stimulants may be preferred when functional impairment lasts most of the day. Shorter-acting stimulants can be used if symptom control is required for shorter periods with more flexible dosing. Stimulant treatment needs to be personalised to achieve better outcomes as well as good compliance.

Non-Stimulant Treatment

Non-stimulant medications are listed as second-line agents in the pharmacological management of ADHD as per NICE guidelines. We advise to make treatment decisions based on what is required for each patient, as non-stimulants may be more suitable for some individuals. They are particularly helpful in cases that require 24-hour symptom control; however, it is important to note that it may take several weeks to achieve a steady state. There is also the added advantage that non-stimulants are not controlled substances and therefore not subject to the strict dispensing restrictions as stimulants, which allows for greater ease of administration and can have a beneficial effect on treatment adherence.

Atomoxetine is the most commonly used non-stimulant agent and offers the benefits listed above. The side-effect profile is generally tolerable and is the medication of choice for patients with a history of drug-seeking behaviour, stimulant misuse or those who require long-acting control of their symptoms.

Guanfacine and clonidine can also be used for treatment of ADHD; however, they are not used as first or second line drugs. Our experience is that they are prescribed along with other ADHD medications to achieve fine control of symptoms.

Care Planning

People with ADHD in the criminal justice system can be easily lost to follow-up when released from prison. It is often hard to access mental health services for ADHD in the community. Very often, people with ADHD in forensic settings have complex needs and require input from multiple professional agencies and streams [24]. Therefore, it is important that aftercare is planned when a person is ready to be released from prison. Various different models of care exist when people are released from prison. We believe a named care coordinator to coordinate care when released from prison is helpful to maintain continuity of care. This allows the individual to form trusting therapeutic relationships with named responsible care coordinators, so individual needs can be identified and addressed. People with ADHD often need support and advice with regard to planning and structuring day-to-day activities at the beginning. This can be even more important for people released from prison settings. Such psychosocial interventions need to be cater to needs of the person, once again highlighting the importance of personalised interventions.

Conclusion

ADHD is a common neurodevelopmental disorder that affects the general population; however; its prevalence rate is higher in prison and forensic settings. The assessment of ADHD in prison and forensic populations is important given the high prevalence rate and availability of effective treatment. It includes establishing the presence of ADHD symptoms, a full psychiatric history and assessing for comorbidities and functional impairment. The assessment of ADHD in a prison setting can also be challenging, so a pragmatic approach is needed to decide what information is needed to make the diagnosis within the confines of this environment, the resources available and the limited information in the clinical history. It is important to separate simple ADHD from complex ADHD, as people with complex ADHD may need more support and therapeutic interventions. Prison and forensic settings are more likely to have patients with complex ADHD.

In terms of treatment, pharmacological interventions such as stimulants or non-stimulants are effective in treating the core symptoms of ADHD and reducing the functional impairment. There are also various psychosocial interventions that are equally important in addition to pharmacological treatment, especially in the complex ADHD patient group.

References

1. Young SJ, Adamou M, Bolea B, Gudjonsson G, Müller U, Pitts M, et al. The identification and management of ADHD offenders within the criminal justice system: a consensus statement from the UK Adult ADHD Network and criminal justice agencies. *BMC Psychiatry* 2011; 11: 32.

2. Ginsberg Y, Hirvikoski T, Lindefors N. Attention deficit hyperactivity disorder (ADHD) among longer-term prison inmates is a prevalent, persistent and disabling disorder. *BMC Psychiatry* 2010; 10(1): 112.

3. Kessler RC, Adler L, Ames M, Demler O, Faraone S, Hiripi E, et al. The World Health Organization Adult ADHD Self-Report Scale (ASRS): a short screening scale for use in the general population. *Psychological Medicine* 2005; 35(2): 245–56.

4. American Psychiatric Association. *Diagnostic and Statistical Manual of Mental Disorders*, 5th edition: DSM-5. American Psychiatric Association, 2013.

5. Ustun B, Adler LA, Rudin C, Faraone SV, Spencer TJ, Berglund P, et al. The World Health Organization Adult Attention-Deficit/Hyperactivity Disorder Self-Report Screening Scale for DSM-5. *JAMA Psychiatry* 2017; 74(5): 520–7.

6. Young S, González RA, Mutch L, Mallet-Lambert I, O'Rourke L, Hickey N, et al. Diagnostic accuracy of a brief screening tool for attention deficit hyperactivity disorder in UK prison inmates. *Psychological Medicine* 2021; 46(7): 1449–58.

7. World Health Organization. International Classification of Diseases 11th revision. 2022. Available at: www.who.int/standards/classifi cations/classification-of-diseases.

8. Kessler RC, Green JG, Adler LA, Barkley RA, Chatterji S, Faraone SV, et al. Structure and

diagnosis of adult attention-deficit/ hyperactivity disorder: analysis of expanded symptom criteria from the Adult ADHD Clinical Diagnostic Scale. *Archives of General Psychiatry* 2010; 67(11): 1168–78.

9. Katzman MA, Bilkey TS, Chokka PR, Fallu A, Klassen LJ. Adult ADHD and comorbid disorders: clinical implications of a dimensional approach. *BMC Psychiatry* 2017; 17(1): 302.

10. Das D, Cherbuin N, Butterworth P, Anstey KJ, Easteal S. A population-based study of attention deficit/hyperactivity disorder symptoms and associated impairment in middle-aged adults. *PLOS One* 2012 ;7(2): e31500.

11. Storebø OJ, Simonsen E. The association between ADHD and antisocial personality disorder (ASPD): a review. *Journal of Attention Disorders* 2016; 20(10): 815–24.

12. Mordre M, Groholt B, Kjelsberg E, Sandstad B, Myhre AM. The impact of ADHD and conduct disorder in childhood on adult delinquency: a 30 years follow-up study using official crime records. *BMC Psychiatry* 2011; 11: 57.

13. Young S, Thome J. ADHD and offenders. *World Journal of Biological Psychiatry* 2011; 12(sup1): 124–8.

14. Shiroma EJ, Ferguson PL, Pickelsimer EE. Prevalence of traumatic brain injury in an offender population: a meta-analysis. *Journal of Correctional Health Care* 2010; 16(2): 147–59.

15. Baranyi G, Scholl C, Fazel S, Patel V, Priebe S, Mundt AP. Severe mental illness and substance use disorders in prisoners in low-income and middle-income countries: a systematic review and meta-analysis of prevalence studies. *Lancet Global Health* 2019; 7(4): e461–71.

16. McGough JJ, Smalley SL, McCracken JT, Yang M, Del'Homme M, Lynn DE, et al. Psychiatric comorbidity in adult attention deficit hyperactivity disorder: findings from multiplex families. *American Journal of Psychiatry* 2005; 162(9): 1621–7. DOI: https://doi.org/10.1176/appi .ajp.162.9.1621.

17. Sandstrom A, Perroud N, Alda M, Uher R, Pavlova B. Prevalence of attention-deficit/ hyperactivity disorder in people with mood disorders: A systematic review and meta-analysis. *Acta Psychiatrica Scandinavica*; 2021; 143(5): 380–91.

18. Lichtenstein P, Halldner L, Zetterqvist J, Sjölander A, Serlachius E, Fazel S, et al. Medication for attention deficit– hyperactivity disorder and criminality. *New England Journal of Medicine* 2012; 367 (21): 2006–14.

19. Hollis C, Chen Q, Chang Z, Quinn PD, Viktorin A, Lichtenstein P, et al. Methylphenidate and the risk of psychosis in adolescents and young adults: a population-based cohort study. *Lancet Psychiatry*; 20196(8): 651–8.

20. Kooij JJS, Bijlenga D, Salerno L, Jaeschke R, Bitter I, Balázs J, et al. Updated European Consensus Statement on diagnosis and treatment of adult ADHD. *European Psychiatry* 2019; 56: 14–34.

21. Young S, Khondoker M, Emilsson B, Sigurdsson JF, Philipp-Wiegmann F, Baldursson G, et al. Cognitive–behavioural therapy in medication-treated adults with attention-deficit/hyperactivity disorder and co-morbid psychopathology: a randomized controlled trial using multi-level analysis. *Psychological Medicine* 2015; 45(13): 2793–804.

22. National Institute for Health and Care Excellence. British National Formulary 2021. Available at: hhtps://bnf.nice. org.uk.

23. National Institute for Health and Care Excellence. Attention deficit hyperactivity disorder: diagnosis and management. NICE guideline [NG87]. 2018. Available at: www.nice.org.uk/gui dance/ng87.

24. Chaplin E, Rawat A, Perera B, McCarthy J, Courtenay K, Forrester, A, et al. Prisoners with attention deficit hyperactivity disorder: co-morbidities and service pathways. *International Journal of Prisoner Health* 2021; 18(3): 245–58.

Chapter 12

Autism Spectrum Disorder: Assessment and Therapeutic Approaches within Forensic Settings

David Murphy and Jane Radley

Introduction

As highlighted previously in this book, while there is no evidence to suggest individuals with autism spectrum disorder (ASD) are more likely to offend than those without ASD and may actually more likely be victims of crime [1], it is generally accepted that vulnerability towards offending behaviours and subsequent involvement with the criminal justice system can be linked to a combination of an individual's specific difficulties directly related to their ASD (such as a tendency towards literal thinking, focusing on specific details at the expense of appreciating the wider context, perspective-taking difficulties and pursuing preoccupations, as well sensory sensitivities and emotional regulation difficulties) within a particular set of environmental circumstances. Such circumstances typically involve high stress situations perhaps involving a lack of structure to life, social isolation and alienation, transition periods and significant change in life demands, as well as being exploited by others. While methodological differences between studies prevent a clear view on the prevalence of ASD in forensic settings they are likely to be disproportionately represented relative to the 1% general UK population rate [2]. Within forensic settings, it has also been suggested that due to the high prevalence of social, communication and behavioural difficulties present among individuals in the criminal justice system, it is likely that increasing numbers of them will receive an ASD diagnosis, perhaps further inflating the number of cases [3]. Regardless of the forensic setting, offenders with ASD present with difficulties and needs that challenge mainstream services, which require special consideration. Within the UK, the assessment and management of offenders with ASD has also been influenced by various pieces of legislation.

Assessment within Forensic Settings

Obtaining a Diagnosis

While many offenders with ASD enter forensic settings with an established diagnosis, many do not. Attempting to obtain a diagnosis for these individuals can present many challenges. For example, individuals may decline to engage with an assessment, refuse for relatives or past care providers to be involved and there may be a lack of reliable background information to confirm an individual's developmental history. The presence of co-occurring disorders such as psychosis can also complicate the diagnostic process. Other issues with using diagnostic aids such as the Autism Diagnostic Observation Schedule (ADOS) [4] may also be present when used in some secure forensic settings. Many high secure forensic settings place limitations as to what materials can be taken into such environments, and there may be a need to make context-specific adaptations for eliciting features of autism. For example, within forensic settings there are typically 'unwritten' rules about individuals not asking for personal information or views of staff, therefore making this item of the ADOS difficult to rate. There may also be a general reluctance by individuals to share personal information. If an individual has been detained in secure environments for some time, institutional behaviour can also be difficult to disentangle from any pre-institutional need for predictability and routines, as well as limited opportunities being confused with having a restricted range of interests. In terms of a request for an ASD diagnosis in forensic settings, the question of symptom validity may also arise. In some cases, obtaining an ASD diagnosis may be potentially advantageous for an individual, where it could be viewed as a mitigating factor and have implications for sentencing. Although clinical experience suggests that attempts to 'fake' autism are unusual, there remains to be any exploration of whether it is possible to feign ASD and, if so, in what contexts. Any influence of ethnicity in the diagnosis of ASD also remains to be explored [5].

Assessing ASD Factors Relevant to Offence Formulations

As highlighted elsewhere in this book, a crucial aspect of managing individuals with neurodevelopmental disorders who offend is the assessment of their risk for future offending. While there exists a number of formal risk-assessment aids targeting specific offending behaviours (e.g., interpersonal violence, sexual offending and extremism, etc.), the application of most of these with offenders who have ASD remains to be adequately explored. However, clinical experience, and the consensus opinion held by most professionals working with offenders who have ASD, suggests that if these formal risk-assessment aids are used in isolation, without adequately assessing an individual's specific strengths and difficulties associated with having ASD (such as literal thinking style, problems with central cohesion and perspective taking, as well as preoccupations, sensory sensitivities and emotional regulation issues), the likely result will be an inadequate risk assessment, a poor formulation of offending behaviours and subsequently limited risk management plans, including inadequate interventions [6, 7]. As with many offenders, the role of past traumas in understanding difficulties, as well as treatment needs of offenders with ASD, also remain to be examined, where a possible association between past traumas and increased risk of violence has been suggested [8]. See Case Study 12.1.

Role of Psychopathy

An area of assessment relevant to understanding the difficulties and needs of a subgroup of offenders with ASD is the potential presence of psychopathy – another neurodevelopmental condition characterised by a lack of remorse and empathy deficits, as well as a number of other features. While similarities have been drawn between some features of ASD and psychopathy [9], evidence is limited. For example, within high secure psychiatric care, Murphy [10] examined the Hare Psychopathy Checklist Revised (PCL R) [11] profiles of 'high risk' male patients with ASD. Findings from this study suggested that although these individuals had lower overall PCL-R profiles compared to other patient groups, they also tended to have profiles characterised by elevated facet-two scores (notably affective features such as lack of remorse or guilt, shallow affect, lack of empathy and a failure to accept

Case Study 12.1 Trauma-informed care following an ASD diagnosis

RC, aged 30 years with a history of early neglect, was admitted to high secure psychiatric care due to concerns within medium secure care that he was at risk of attempting to abscond and immediate threats of violence to nursing staff, who he perceived as abusing his rights. RC's original index offence (the offence leading to his conviction and detainment in forensic services) was for sending explosive devices to a probation officer, who he believed had wrongly portrayed him as a paedophile (where the reality was that there was no evidence to support this view). Prior to admission, RC had never been assessed for ASD and had received a diagnosis of an antisocial personality disorder and possible psychosis (based on assumed paranoid ideas about probation services).

Following a detailed and extended assessment of RC's presenting difficulties and history, which included a comprehensive psychiatric assessment, a neuropsychological assessment (focusing on identifying thinking style), an ASD diagnostic assessment (following the observation of intolerance to noise and a need for routines, predictability and preoccupations) and a detailed risk assessment, a formulation of difficulties and multidisciplinary 'treatment' plan was devised. The formulation was based on the findings that RC's early experience of neglect in combination with his thinking style associated with having ASD – notably literal thinking, perspective taking difficulties and focus on details, as well as social isolation and low self-esteem – led to his mistrust of authority together with a vulnerability towards making negative interpretations of others, grudge bearing and defensive/aggressive reaction. RC's management plan included individual psychoeducation, exploring his experience and acceptance of the ASD diagnosis, and individual ASD-adapted CBT to address his tendency to form negative interpretations of others' actions and comments and to react in a defensive way. A collaborative risk management plan was also devised, including encouraging prosocial interests and opportunities to promote self-esteem through further education and work activities. A psychiatric assessment and management plan also led to the exclusion of a psychosis and the introduction of a short-term low-dose mood-stabiliser medication. Autism awareness training was provided to staff and the SPELL guidelines were encouraged to be followed by all staff involved in RC's management.

In terms of outcome, RC was initially reluctant to accept the diagnosis of ASD and externalised responsibility for all perceived wrongdoings onto others. However, with some initial motivational work, over several sessions it was possible to encourage RC to acknowledge the diagnosis, to challenge his negative bias in thinking and consider alternative perspectives, as well as view his thinking style (literal, with a tendency to focus on details) as an advantage in many situations. More adaptive ways of challenging perceived negative comments of others were also developed, including a shared collaborative formulation of understanding the risks for interpreting and acting on perceived wrongdoing (linked with his early experiences of neglect and abuse), along with the development of protective factors (such as improved self-esteem through education, positive relationships, social inclusion and valued work activities). Working in combination to address dysfunctional thinking patterns, reframe negative early experiences, grudge bearing and work towards positive goals, all these interventions led RC to move back to medium secure care and eventual transfer back into community care. Of particular significance was the shift in the formulation of RC's difficulties by those involved in his management from a purely personality-disorder-driven view to an ASD/trauma-informed one.

responsibility). When psychopathy might be present, other researchers have also suggested the idea of a so called 'double hit' [12], where both features of ASD and psychopathy co-occur independently. However, within this study of adolescent boys, 'psychopathic tendencies' were assessed using the antisocial process screening device [13], raising questions about whether the same features of psychopathy were assessed and where there was a focus on callousness rather than other features of psychopathy. Other researchers have also suggested that individuals with ASD are more likely to display 'naïvety' and 'reactive violence', as well as being more likely to confess to violence compared to individuals with psychopathy, who may be more manipulative, proactive with violence and more likely to deny or minimise violence [14]. If using a formal measure to assess psychopathy such as the PCL-R, Hare highlights to *exercise clinical judgement with the interpretation of psychopathic traits among individuals with unusual presentations*. Clinical experience also suggests these individuals are often a difficult group to engage with therapeutic work, as well as interview. In addition to displaying a lack of remorse for offending or acts of aggression, these individuals often present as deliberately inconsistent with the information provided during interviews despite relatively good verbal communication skills [15].

Assessment of Co-occurring Conditions

Offenders with ASD can present with a range of other neurodevelopmental conditions and psychiatric disorders, all of which can help to inform the formulation of an individual's offending behaviour and future risk of offending [16, 17]. Among the other neurodevelopmental conditions potentially present, attention deficit hyperactivity disorder (ADHD) [18, 19] and intellectual disability [20] are frequently observed. Other developmental disorders including tic disorders may also be present. Where co-occurring neurodevelopmental conditions are suspected, it is important that these are assessed and the contribution to the presenting difficulties evaluated. For some individuals, comorbid psychiatric disorders, such as anxiety, mood disorders, obsessive–compulsive disorder, psychosis or a personality disorder, may be present [21, 22]. Although alcohol and illicit substance misuse can be present among offenders with ASD, this appears to be less common compared to offenders without ASD [16]. While clinical assessment of these conditions is crucial, there are often unusual features to presenting symptoms, which can be difficult to disentangle from an individual's core symptoms of ASD. Conventional measures and assessment tools can be helpful, but most lack validation research applied to offenders who have ASD, and there is a need to consider how an individual's specific features of ASD may influence apparent presenting problems.

Therapeutic Approaches

Psychological Interventions

In terms of psychological interventions with offenders who have ASD, a distinction may be made between those targeting behaviours and issues relevant to offending and those that may improve the everyday functioning of an individual but may not be directly relevant to offending. In reality, however, such a distinction may be difficult to make, where improving or enhancing apparently unrelated issues (e.g., promoting pro-social interests, social inclusion and mood) may serve as protective factors against the risk for future reoffending. While there is evidence that individuals with ASD without forensic histories can benefit from a range of psychological interventions such as adapted cognitive–behavioural therapy (CBT) (see Case Study 12.1), dialectical behavioural therapy and mindfulness [23], there remains some uncertainty with regard to how much offenders with ASD might benefit from offence-focused interventions and, to date, there are no accredited ASD offending programmes.

In terms of prison settings, some studies suggest that many offenders with ASD who participate in mainstream groups may experience both sensory overload and exclusion [24, 25]. Other studies of specific offence behaviour groups suggest that individuals with ASD who take part in adapted sex offender treatment programmes designed for individuals with intellectual difficulties [26] tend to function at a much higher level compared to other group members and present with different needs [27]. Other research has also suggested that men with ASD with non-contact sexual offending histories who participate in such groups may also have higher recidivism rates [28]. Within forensic psychiatric settings, it remains debatable as to whether it is harmful to include individuals with ASD in conventional groups and there is some argument that some individuals with ASD report benefitting from participating in mixed groups by hearing different points of views and listening to other individual experiences [29]. Although requiring more empirical examination, key factors that seem to be associated with more positive experiences and outcomes appear to be facilitator ASD awareness and sensitivity to making appropriate adjustments, as well as other group members being sensitive to such difficulties.

Evidence for the effectiveness of individual psychological work addressing the offending behaviours of offenders with ASD also remains mixed. For example, Melvin and colleagues [30] carried out review of four quantitative studies and nine case studies describing interventions and outcomes for offenders with ASD. Differences were reported both in the study population and how outcomes were measured. Many of the studies included individuals with co-occurring intellectual and psychiatric difficulties, with no single therapeutic approach followed between the studies. However, while there may not be any published consensus regarding the effectiveness of psychological interventions with offenders who have ASD, this should not be interpreted as evidence of absence. Indeed, many individuals with ASD who offend can engage with, and benefit from, a range of psychological interventions addressing offence-specific and non-offence-specific behaviours. Clinical experience suggests that if a cognitive–behavioural approach is used to address risk and criminological issues (such as improving victim awareness and empathy and an appreciation of consequences), there is a need to identify clear realistic goals and potentially make specific adaptations allowing for the presence of any cognitive, communication and sensory and emotional regulation difficulties, as well as any co-occurring psychiatric disorder [31]. For many individuals, a personalised education plan about their ASD may also be useful in identifying past and current difficulties. However, regardless of setting, it may be the case that while many individuals do respond to individual psychological interventions (addressing general problem-solving skills, working on basic social-inference skills, encouraging appropriate assertiveness, reducing individual social anxieties, shifting preoccupations and obsessive thoughts and negative ruminations, and developing perspective-taking skills), it may be unrealistic to expect significant changes in cognitive style compared to 'neurotypical' offenders. Indeed, individuals who present with significant egocentricity, take limited personal responsibility and reject their diagnosis can be particularly difficult to engage in therapy. In general, Hare [32] suggests that a primary goal in CBT with individuals who have ASD should be to focus on behavioural changes that increase an individual's ability to function in everyday life rather than focus on cognitive changes. However, whatever therapeutic model is used, other specific adaptions may also be required, such as working on so-called 'Asperger time' [33], where individuals with ASD may require additional time to process information. Other adaptations may also be required when interviewing and working with offenders who have ASD, whether that be with considering the sensory sensitivities of individuals, using appropriate language or being mindful of thinking styles [15].

Beyond detention, there is a lack of research examining the difficulties offenders with ASD may experience during the transition back from secure environments into the community. Indeed, returning to the community can be difficult for many offenders, but may be particularly problematic for someone with ASD who might experience difficulties dealing with a change in routine and reduced structure [34]. Within the UK, where some prison to community services are present, it has been found that accessing these for many individuals with ASD can be confusing and that success depends on a coordinated multi-agency approach, including health, social care and the criminal justice system [35].

Pharmacological Interventions

While there are no specific pharmacological interventions targeting the core difficulties associated with having ASD, there is some evidence suggesting pharmacological treatments can improve outcomes associated with psychological interventions aimed at the core ASD features [36]. However, the National Institute of Clinical Excellence review [37] highlights that psychosocial interventions should always be considered before pharmacological interventions with individuals who have ASD. Within the UK, the policy Stop Over-Medication in People with a learning disability and autism (STOMP) (www.england.nhs.uk/stomp) also aims to reduce the reliance on psychotropic medication in the management of behavioural problems in these conditions.

Beyond the conventional treatment of any co-occurring conditions, there remains a lack of robust evidence to demonstrate the efficacy of psychotropic medications with offenders who have ASD to address some associated difficulties. Among the studies that have been published, some show that antipsychotics such as risperidone can be effective in reducing levels of irritability, arousal and aggression among adults with ASD in the absence of any overt psychosis [38]. Psychotic disorders may be overlooked and vigorous treatment of these can lead to considerable improvement and allow the patient to successfully engage in psychological therapies. Mood disorders should be treated with mood-stabilising drugs and antidepressants as required. Co-occurring ADHD can be treated with stimulant medication, although care should be taken as stimulant medication can lead to worsening of psychotic symptoms or even development of a first episode of psychosis [39]. Depression and anxiety responds well to the use of selective serotonin reuptake inhibitors or serotonin–norepinephrine reuptake inhibitors, but bipolar disorder should be suspected if the administration of these drugs leads to increased irritability and aggression. In such cases, a mood-stabilising drug such as semi-sodium valproate or lithium may be more effective.

In terms of future research, much remains to be established regarding the use of 'off licence' medications with adults who have ASD, including whether different dose requirements and side-effect profiles are present.

Role of ASD Awareness and Organisational Training

While psychological and pharmacological therapies can make a significant difference in addressing the needs of offenders with ASD, they do not operate in isolation. Indeed, within forensic settings, a wide range of factors can influence outcomes; for example, access to occupational and educational activities, environmental factors such as noise, structure to everyday lives and how all staff interact with individuals. Awareness of ASD within certain forensic settings such as prisons varies, with some surveys suggesting that many staff report lacking sufficient skills to work with such individuals [25]. However, awareness of ASD within some prisons does seem to be improving, including some such as the young offender institution at Feltham achieving 'accreditation' with the National Autistic Society [40], as well as other prisons such as HMP Wakefield developing a wing devoted to prisoners with ASD. Within secure forensic psychiatric services in the UK there are also a number of mainstream National Health Service (NHS) and private-sector units that are ASD sensitive, as well as specialist ASD units.

In terms of the importance of staff awareness of ASD, it is noteworthy that the UK government has proposed that all NHS clinical staff (including those working in secure forensic psychiatric settings) receive some form of compulsory autism awareness training [41]. Within high secure psychiatric care, ASD awareness training is valued by staff and appears to make a significant difference in how individuals with ASD are managed [42]. In addition to providing information on the current understanding of what ASD is, including the characteristic difficulties and features, the training introduces the so-called SPELL guidelines, which place an emphasis on a structured approach, a positive approach, empathy, low arousal and links with other professionals [43]. The aim of the SPELL approach is to encourage staff to work with an individual's strengths and minimise the likelihood of problem behaviours by making the immediate environment and interactions more autism friendly. With regard to recognising the importance of having the 'right' type of environment for offenders with ASD in secure settings, and the role of staff awareness of ASD, it is also worth considering the views of Wing [44], who highlighted that the crucial elements for appropriate care lie in carefully structuring the environment and daily programme, and in training staff in the psychological strategies to be used. Indeed, Wing noted that some, perhaps most of those who commit violent or other serious offences may require long-term care and supervision in a secure environment; the emphasis is that 'in the right kind of environment, the individual may behave in an exemplary way, but if he or she is moved to a setting that does not provide the right type of programme, the criminal behaviour may very well reoccur' ([44], p. 256).

Women Offenders with ASD

Although an under-researched group, some evidence suggests that women with ASD who offend present different assessment and therapeutic needs to males [45, 46]. Among the issues that might complicate the process of addressing the needs of women with ASD in the criminal justice system can be obtaining an accurate diagnosis. For example, so-called 'social camouflaging' might be present (where interpersonal difficulties are hidden by well-rehearsed social skills or where some stereotypes of social shyness might be more accepted), as well as diagnostic overshadowing, where another psychiatric diagnosis may be more likely. Like many offenders, women with ASD may also have histories of trauma and being victims of abuse [47]. As a group, women with ASD may be particularly vulnerable to experiencing post-traumatic stress disorder [48]. As such, in addition to an ASD-sensitive approach to offender management is the need for a trauma-informed approach [49].

Direction of Future Assessment and Therapeutic Research

While offenders with ASD represent a small proportion of the total offender population, they are a diverse group with specific assessment and therapeutic needs. Although there is a growing body of research examining the assessment and management of offenders with ASD, key areas of psychological and pharmacological practice remain poorly understood. While the variation in therapy outcomes is not surprising given the diversity of presentations, there is a need to have a much better understanding of why some individuals have better levels of engagement and outcome than others. Some authors have suggested specific typologies for offenders with ASD based on the presence of psychopathy, psychosis and behavioural problems, which in turn guide treatment needs [50]. However, a limitation of these typologies is the failure to appreciate the diversity of presentations found among individuals with ASD, notably within different aspects of social and non-social cognition, social naïvety, need for routine and predictability and emotional regulation and sensory sensitivities, as well as perhaps the presence of other neurodevelopmental disorders such as ADHD. Other authors [30] also highlight the potential role of 'severity' of ASD in determining an individual's capacity to benefit from interventions. However, this in turn raises questions around what aspects of ASD are relevant to define 'severity', where any cut-off of ability or dysfunction might be, as well as any co-occurring difficulties.

Of particular importance with regard to determining an individual's capacity to engage and benefit from therapeutic intervention appears to be their cognitive style. Clinical experience suggests that many offenders with ASD, who present with flexible thinking and relatively less egocentricity, engage well with interventions addressing a range of issues that are sensitive to their ASD. In contrast, individuals who present with significant social cognition difficulties and extreme literal thinking, as well as perhaps a greater degree of co-occurring intellectual difficulties, struggle to benefit from 'insight-orientated' psychological or occupational interventions [31], and require a more behavioural approach directed by staff. Regardless of what offence-focused interventions are followed, these do not operate in isolation and typically form part of a coordinated multi-agency/multi-professional approach to individual management. Indeed, the most economically and clinically effective method of addressing the needs of offenders with ASD remains in promoting an awareness of ASD among all those involved with their management. Although there is no specific research evidence devoted to examining how organisational awareness of ASD specifically improves the outcomes of offenders with ASD or the impact on reducing recidivism, staff surveys consistently find most staff feel underskilled with regard to how they work with offenders who have ASD and that training is valued. Clearly, any service or intervention that is sensitive to, and makes reasonable adjustments for an individual's ASD is more likely to result in positive outcomes than those that do not. It is also possible that having staff with ASD-sensitive qualities (including autism knowledge and 'empathy' towards an individual's difficulties) is particularly beneficial in encouraging positive outcomes [51].

In terms of promoting positive outcomes for offenders with ASD detained within forensic psychiatric settings, it also remains to be established whether specialist ASD services result in better 'outcomes' for individuals than more generic secure units, which aim to be ASD sensitive. There is clearly a role for both and, as suggested by one study examining patient experiences in high secure psychiatric care, some individuals with ASD report a preference to be around mixed patient groups rather than just those with ASD [29]. In terms of the future of offender-focused assessments and interventions within forensic settings, new technologies such as computer simulation and virtual reality are likely to play an increasingly important role [52]. With the low cost now associated with such technologies, as well as the ability to manipulate and replicate a wide range of variables, they offer significant assessment and therapeutic potential for this group of patients.

References

1. King C, Murphy G. A systematic review of people with autism spectrum disorder and the criminal justice system. *Journal of Autism and Developmental Disorders* 2014; 44(1): 2717–33.

2. Baird G, Simonoff E, Pickles A, Chandler S, Loucas T, Meldrum D, et al. Prevalence of disorders of the autism spectrum in a population cohort of children in South Thames: the Special Needs and Autism Project (SNAP). *Lancet* 2006; 368: 210–15.

3. Woodbury-Smith M. Conceptualising social and communication vulnerabilities among detainees in the criminal justice system. *Research in Developmental Disabilities* 2020; 100: 103611.

4. Lord C, Rutter M, DiLavore P, Risi S, Gotham K, Bishop S. Autism Diagnostic Observation Schedule – second edition (ADOS 2). Available at: https://pdfs .semanticscholar.org/1fbb/3f886a582ec19c0 db48721a6dc8241a8ce78.pdf.

5. Grochowska A. P02-62: autism spectrum disorder and ethnicity in a forensic psychiatric assessment. *European Psychiatry* 2010; 25(S1): DOI: https://doi.org/10.1016/ S0924-9338(10)70676-3.

6. Murphy D. Risk assessment of offenders with an autism spectrum disorder. *Journal of Intellectual Disabilities and Offending Behaviour* 2013; 4(2): 33–41.

7. Shine J, Cooper-Evans S. Developing an autism specific framework for forensic case formulation. *Journal of Intellectual Disabilities and Offending Behaviour* 2016; 7 (3): 127–39.

8. Im D. Trauma as a contributor to violence in autism spectrum disorder. *Journal of the Academy of Psychiatry* 2016; 44(2): 184–92.

9. Fitzgerald M. Callous/unemotional traits and Asperger's syndrome? *Journal of the American Academy of Child and Adolescent Psychiatry* 2003; 42(9): 1011.

10. Murphy D. Brief communication: Hare PCL-R profiles of male patients with Asperger's syndrome detained in high security psychiatric care. *Journal of Forensic Psychiatry and Psychology* 2007; 18 (1): 120–6.

11. Hare R. *The Psychopathy Checklist Revised.* Multi-Health Systems Inc., 2003.

12. Rogers J, Viding E, Blair J, Frith U, Happé F. Autism spectrum disorder and psychopathy: shared cognitive underpinnings or double hit? *Psychological Medicine* 2006; 36: 1789–98.

13. Frick P, Hare RD. *The Anti-Social Process Screening Device.* Multi-Health Systems Inc., 2001.

14. Bjørkly S. Risk and dynamics of violence in Asperger's syndrome: a systematic review of the literature. *Aggression and Violent Behaviour* 2009; 14: 306–12.

15. Murphy D. Interviewing individuals with an autism spectrum disorder in forensic settings. *International Journal of Forensic Mental Health* 2019; 17(4): 310–20.

16. Haw C, Radley J, Cooke L. Characteristics of male autistic spectrum patients in low security: are they different from non-autistic low secure patients? *Journal of Intellectual Disabilities and Offending Behaviour* 2013; 4: 24–32.

17. Esan F, Chester V, Gunaratna IJ, Hoare S, Alexander ST. The clinical, forensic and treatment outcome factors of patients with autistic spectrum disorder treated in a forensic intellectual disability service.

Journal of Applied Research in Intellectual Disabilities 2015; 28: 193–200.

18. Gillberg C, Billstedt E. Autism and Asperger syndrome: coexistence with other clinical disorders. *Acta Psychiatrica Scandinavica* 2000; 102(5): 321–30.

19. Matson J, Rieske R, Williams L. The relationship between autism spectrum disorders and attention deficit hyperactivity disorder: an overview. *Research in developmental Disabilities* 2013; 34(9): 2475–84.

20. Matson J, Shoemaker M. Intellectual disability and its relationship to autism spectrum disorders. *Research in Developmental Disabilities* 2009; 30(6): 1107–14.

21. Joshi G, Wozniak J, Petty C, Martelon M, Fried R, Bolfek A, et al. Psychiatric comorbidity and functioning in a clinically referred population of adults with autism spectrum disorders: a comparative study. *Journal of Autism and Developmental Disorders* 2013; 43(6): 1314–25.

22. Russell A, Murphy C, Wilson E, Gillan N, Brown C, Robertson D, et al. The mental health of individuals referred for assessment of autism spectrum disorder in adulthood: a clinic report. *Autism* 2016; 20(5): 623–7.

23. Spain D, O'Neil L, Harwood L, Chaplin E. Psychological interventions for adults with ASD: clinical approaches. *Advances in Autism* 2016; 2(1): 24–30.

24. Higgs T, Carter A. Autism spectrum disorder and sexual offending: responsivity in forensic interventions. *Aggression and Violent Behaviour* 2015; 22: 112–19.

25. Robertson C, McGillivray J. Autism behind bars: a review of the research literature and discussion of key issues. *Journal of Forensic Psychiatry and Psychology* 2015; 2(6), 719–36.

26. Sex Offender Treatment Services Collaborative – Intellectual Disabilities (SOTSEC-ID). Effectiveness of group cognitive behavioural treatment for men with intellectual disabilities at risk of sexual offending. *Journal of Applied Research in Intellectual Disabilities* 2010; 23: 537–51.

27. Haaven J. Suggested treatment outline using the old me/new me model. In Blasingame G, ed., *Practical Treatment Strategies for Forensic Clients with Severe and Sexual Behaviour Problems Among Persons with Developmental Disabilities.* Wood N Barnes/Safer Society Press, 2006: 85–114.

28. Heaton K, Murphy G. Men with intellectual disabilities who have attended sex offender treatment groups: a follow up. *Journal of Applied Research in Intellectual Disabilities* 2013; 26(5): 489–500.

29. Murphy D, Mullens H. Examining the experiences and quality of life of patients with an autism spectrum disorder detained in high secure psychiatric care. *Advances in Autism* 2017; 3(1): 3–14.

30. Melvin C, Langdon P, Murphy G. Treatment effectiveness for offenders with autism spectrum conditions: a systematic review. *Psychology, Crime and Law* 2017; 23(8): 748–76.

31. Murphy D. Extreme violence in a young man with an autistic spectrum disorder: assessment and intervention within high security psychiatric care. *Journal of Forensic Psychiatry and Psychology* 2010; 21(3): 462–77.

32. Hare DJ. Developing psychotherapeutic interventions with people with autism spectrum disorders. In Taylor JL, Lindsay WR, Hastings R, eds., *Psychological Therapies for Adults with Intellectual Disabilities.* John Wiley & Sons, 2013: 193–206.

33. Gaus V. *Cognitive Behaviour Therapy for Adults with Asperger Syndrome.* The Guildford Press, 2007.

34. Royal College of Psychiatrists. *Psychiatric Services for Adolescents and Adults with Asperger Syndrome and Other Autistic Spectrum Disorders.* Royal College of Psychiatrists, 2006.

35. Prison Reform Trust. Behaviour that challenges: planning services for people with learning disabilities and or autism who sexually offend. 2018. Available at: https://prisonreformtrust.org.uk/publica tion/behaviour-that-challenges-planning

-services-for-people-with-learning-disabilities-and-or-autism-who-sexually-offend/.

36. Findling RL. Pharmacological treatment of behavioural symptoms in autism and pervasive developmental disorders. *Journal of Clinical Psychiatry* 2005; 66: 26–31.

37. National Institute for Clinical Excellence. Autism, recognition, referral, diagnosis and management of adults on the autism spectrum. Clinical guideline [CG142]. Available at: www.nice.org.uk/guidance/cg142.

38. Fitzpatrick S, Srivorakiat L, Wink L, Pedapati E, Erickson C. Aggression in autism spectrum disorder: presentation and treatment options. *Neuropsychiatric Disorder and Treatment* 2016; 12: 1525–38.

39. Hollis C, Chen Q, Chang Z, Quinn P, Victorin A, Lichtenstein P, et al. Methylphenidate and the risk of psychosis in adolescents and young adults: a population based cohort study. *Lancet Psychiatry* 2019; 6(8): 651–8.

40. Lewis A, Pritchet R, Hughes C, Turner K. Development and implementation of autism standards for prisons. *Journal of Intellectual Disabilities and Offending Behaviour* 2013; 6(2): 68–80.

41. Department of Health. 'Right to be heard': the Government response to the consultation on learning disability and autism training for health and care staff. 2019. Available at: https://assets .publishing.service.gov.uk/government/up loads/system/uploads/attachment_data/fil e/844356/autism-and-learning-disability-training-for-staff-consultation-response.pdf.

42. Murphy D, Broyd J. Evaluation of autism awareness training for staff in high secure psychiatric care hospital. *Advances in Autism* 2019; 6(1): 35–47.

43. National Autistic Society. The SPELL framework. Available at: www.autism.org.uk/what-we-do/professional-development/the-spell-framework.

44. Wing L. Asperger's syndrome: management requires diagnosis. *Journal of Forensic Psychiatry* 1997; 2(8): 253–7.

45. Ashworth S, Bamford J, Tully R. The effectiveness of a CBT based intervention for depression symptoms with a female forensic inpatient with cognitive disability and autism. *The Journal of Forensic Psychiatry and Psychology* 2020; 31(3): 432–52.

46. Markham S. Diagnosis and treatment of ASD in women in secure and forensic hospitals. *Advances in Autism* 2019; 5(1): 64–76.

47. Roberts A, Koenen K, Lyall K, Robinson E, Weisskopf M. Association of autistic traits in adulthood with childhood abuse, interpersonal victimization and posttraumatic stress. *Child Abuse and Neglect* 2015; 45: 135–42.

48. Haruvi-Lamdan N, Horesh D, Zohar S. Autism spectrum disorder and post traumatic stress disorder: an unexplored occurrence of conditions. *Autism* 2020; 24 (4): 884–98.

49. Fuld, S Autism spectrum disorder: the impact of stressful and traumatic life events and implications for clinical practice. *Clinical Social Work Journal* 2018; 46: 210–19.

50. Alexander R, Langdon P, Chester V, Barnoux M, Gunaratna I, Hoare, S. Heterogeneity within autism spectrum disorder in forensic mental health: the introduction of typologies. *Advances in Autism* 2016; 2(4): 201–9.

51. Worthington R. What are the key skills that staff require to support adults on the autism spectrum effectively? In *Forensic Update Compendium*. British Psychological Society, 2016: 61–69.

52. Cornet L, Van Gelder J-L. Virtual reality: a use case for criminal justice practice. *Psychology, Crime and Law* 2019; 26(7): 631–47.

Chapter 13

Intellectual Disability: Assessment and Therapeutic Approaches within Forensic Settings

Ken Courtenay and Mhairi Duff

Introduction

Offenders with intellectual disability (ID) may be difficult to identify in criminal justice systems because they may not have been formally assessed or come to the attention of services previously. Episodes of offending behaviour may conceal underlying causes of behaviour, such as the presence of ID. The offender with ID may be skilled in masking their difficulties by imitating others, which helps them pass in the system. The episode of offending behaviour provides an opportunity to identify a cognitive impairment but may be foreshadowed by processing the person through the system. They may pose challenges to personnel, who may not be aware of their cognitive impairments. Assessment of offenders is important to understand the cognitive challenges and adaptive functioning of the person, which could shape appropriate and effective therapeutic interventions [1].

Supporting offenders with ID requires clear understanding of their needs, the nature of the offence and the appropriate environment in which to deliver support. Treatment plans need to focus on the aetiological factors in the offending behaviour in order to ensure effective therapeutic interventions are delivered. The interventions may need to be adapted for the person, considering their cognitive impairment. Assessing and managing comorbid disorders is essential to achieving successful treatment, leading to a reduction in offending behaviour.

This chapter focuses on screening measures for offenders with ID in forensic settings. The support and management of offenders with ID is also discussed, highlighting important aspects of providing effective therapeutic interventions to reduce the risk of further offending.

Assessment of Offenders with ID

Offenders with ID are an especially vulnerable group in the criminal justice system because of their cognitive impairments, challenges in social communication and adaptive skills, which may lead others to take advantage of them. Unfortunately, such impairments are not always easy to detect where difficulties may be subtle, or the person has adapted techniques to function in their environments. Regardless, it is important to detect those offenders who would benefit from comprehensive assessment of their cognitive and adaptive functioning in order to appropriately meet their needs.

Prevalence

The prevalence of ID among prisoners varies across the world. The rate was found to be 7% through a comprehensive study in the UK of 2,439 offenders [2], which compares to a range of 0 to 2.8% across studies through a systematic review involving 10 surveys from four different countries [3]. The prevalence for ID is 2.3% in the general population [4] and refinement of the prevalence rate through repeated assessment in a Norwegian study reported rates of 7–9%, which is over three times that in the general population [5].

There are many aetiological factors suggested for such a high rate, which include social disadvantage, poor educational skills, mental disorder and others. According to Asscher and colleagues, offenders with ID are more likely to have been in the care of children's services in childhood, leave school before 13 years of age, attend a special school for children with educational needs, have lower educational attainment, experience more life events, be in lower paid employment, live in temporary accommodation, receive less support and be more likely to be in prison remand services [6].

Approaches to Assessment

The goal of assessment is a comprehensive objective understanding of the person's cognitive abilities and adaptive functioning. The American Psychiatric Association recommends that formal assessments combine both, since information on adaptive functioning provides a more rounded impression of the performance level of the person [7]. Understanding adaptive functioning should avoid confounders such as language development and educational attainment [8].

Basing a judgement of ID solely on a measure of cognitive functioning, such as intelligence quotient (IQ), and not including assessment of adaptive functioning is erroneous since attainment on standardised intelligence tests could be affected by other factors in the person's developmental period, such as education, childhood trauma, neglect and abuse [9]. It is essential to understand a person's level of adaptive functioning in order to assess against all three criteria of ID. People with mild or borderline ID (one standard deviation below the norm) may adapt well in society and therefore are less likely to be detected in educational, social or custodial settings.

Formal assessment is a comprehensive process conducted by a trained psychologist, taking a holistic perspective of a person's abilities to understand their strengths and to detect areas where support is required. Completing assessments requires resources such as trained personnel, time to conduct assessments and, crucially, to interpret the results, making them meaningful for the person, their supporters and services that support them.

In the UK, the definition of ID follows that of the British Psychological Society where an intelligence cut-off of two standard deviations below the mean of 100 is the cognitive range [10]. Interestingly, in secure settings in the Netherlands, the cut-off is one standard deviation below the mean [11]. Examples of standard assessment tools used in practice are the Weschler Assessment of Intellectual Scale (WAIS-IV) [12] and the Vineland Adaptive Behaviour Scale (VABS) [13].

Screening for ID

Protracted periods in secure settings present an ideal opportunity to assess a person's cognitive and social and adaptive skills. It may not be until a person presents to criminal justice system pathways that staff consider that ID could account for their offending behaviour but it is not always feasible to undertake full formal assessments of offenders in correctional settings because of the demands of security. Therefore, an alternative approach to assessment, which would help to detect offenders who are likely to have cognitive difficulties, is desirable. Screening tools should help to ascertain who among offenders would benefit from full comprehensive assessments.

Offenders with ID present to custodial settings such as police stations, courts or prisons [14]. Often, the barriers to detection of cognitive difficulties include personal and system factors. Among the personal factors is the absence of evidence to suggest or support a diagnosis, high-arousal states or stigma associated with a label of ID. System factors include a lack of awareness among staff, little time to fully assess a person or frequent moves between custodial settings, which hinder comprehensive assessment.

An ideal screening tool should be short, easy to administer and have good specificity to detect the true negative cases and good sensitivity to detect true positive cases. Screening tools that have been developed and validated in community settings include:

- Hayes Ability Screening Index (HASI) [14]
- Wechsler Abbreviated Screening Instrument (WASI) [16]
- Quick Test [15]
- Learning Disabilities in the Probation Service (LIPS) screening tool [16]
- Leicestershire Intellectual Disability Tool (LIDS) [17]
- Learning Disability Screening Questionnaire (LDSQ) [18]
- Screener for Mild Intellectual Disability (SCIL) [11]
- Rapid Assessment of Potential Intellectual Disabilities (RAPID) [19]

The following explores the evidence on those that have been validated among offenders.

Hayes Ability Screening Index

The HASI was trialled in more than 500 offenders in Australia [14, 20]. The index contains self-report questions, spelling sub-test, 'join-the-dots' test and a clock-drawing test. A cut-off score of 84 suggests the presence of ID. The HASI has been assessed against the Kaufmann Brief Intelligence Test (K-BIT) [21] and the VABS [13], where the positive predictive values were 100% with the K-BIT and 82% with the VABS, and therefore is good in identifying true positives. The test takes up to 10 minutes to complete and was designed to be over-inclusive. Criticism of the HASI is that it is too over-inclusive [22] and too sensitive and not specific for ID [5] but the sample sizes in these studies were smaller than the original sample in Australia [20].

Wechsler Abbreviated Scale of Intelligence

The WASI is a shortened version of the Wechsler Adult Intelligence Scale (WAIS) [23]. The WASI is composed of four subtests: vocabulary (31-item), block design (13-item), similarities (24-item) and matrix reasoning (30-item), producing the full scale-IQ score (FSIQ-4). The WASI can be administered in 30 minutes by a qualified psychologist [23].

The WASI-II was developed on a sample of 2,300 people aged 6 to 90 years [24]. Additionally, the WASI-II subtest scores can be substituted for the corresponding subtests on the WAIS-IV, reducing redundancy and administration time when a more comprehensive assessment of intelligence is required. Therefore, after a WASI-II is completed, only six more subtests (rather than 10) from the WAIS-IV are required for completion of the full comprehensive WAIS assessment.

The WASI-II also offers flexible administration options, which include the vocabulary, similarities, block design, matrix reasoning subtests being combined to produce a four-subtest form. It can be administered in just 30 minutes and the two-subtest form, comprised of the vocabulary and matrix-reasoning subtests can be administered in 15 minutes [24]. These two administration options allow the administrator more control of the administration time and depth of the assessment.

Learning Disability Screening Questionnaire

The LDSQ was developed in a community sample of people with ID and not in the criminal justice system [25]. It contains seven items on history and skills that include: reading ability, writing ability, telling the time, living situation, employment history, support at school and contact with ID services.

A study of 83 adults indicated that the LDSQ has good convergent validity with WAIS-IV and discriminated well for ID [26]. Compared with the WAIS-IV, it has a sensitivity of 91% and specificity of 87% [27]. In a sample of 94 offenders, the LDSQ had a sensitivity of 82.3% and specificity of 87.5% that are lower than the values achieved in the community sample [28].

The advantage of the LDSQ is that it can be administered by non-specialists with brief training in using it. This would be especially useful in police custody suites, court liaison and diversion services and in prisons, where staff could use the tool when a person is suspected of having a cognitive impairment.

The LDSQ does not distinguish between severities of ID such as mild and moderate. Its utility is in distinguishing people with ID from those without it [29]. Interestingly, the LDSQ was evaluated for its sensitivity to cultural settings, comparing its applicability in offenders in Norway with offenders in the UK. It was not found to be a valid measure in Norway, possibly because of the differing levels of social support available in various countries, such as employment and contact with services [30].

Adolescent Offenders

The LDSQ has been adapted for use in children and adolescents as the Child and Adolescent Intellectual Disability Screening Questionnaire (CAIDS-Q) and has been validated among young offenders reporting positive predictive values and predicted negative values of 100% [28, 31]. The authors state it does not over-represent the true number of offenders with ID. The evaluation of the tool in adolescents has been limited by the low numbers of young offenders in health services and therefore further evaluation is required.

Other Screening Instruments

The Quick Test [15] is a short test of verbal intelligence using three visual questions. It can be administered within 15 minutes [32] and has good correlation with the WAIS [33]. It has been used in a range of prevalence studies of ID in prisoners [19, 34].

The SCIL was developed in the Netherlands where ID includes people with a full-scale IQ of less than 85 in contrast to definitions used in other countries [11]. It is a 14-item scale containing questions on the level of education, contact with support, preferred reading materials and brief tasks in numeracy and literacy. The SCIL has high specificity and sensitivity [11]. Effective administration relies on a good command of the Dutch language and it can be administered by staff with brief training in using it.

The RAPID [19] is a 15-item self-report screening tool that is designed to be used in high-pressured environments such as prisons and custody settings. It can be administered after brief training to non-specialist personnel. It has not been validated against standard assessment tools.

Adaptive Functioning

According to Gresham and Elliott [35] adaptive functioning is 'the degree to which an individual is able to meet the standards of personal independence and social responsibility expected of their age and cultural group', which is expanded by Soenen [36] to include 'a person's ability to perform the daily activities required for personal and social sufficiency'. The American Psychiatric Association provides clarity on adaptive functioning, describing the three domains of conceptual thinking (language and literacy), social (interpersonal skills) and practical (personal care, use of money) [7]. The importance of understanding adaptive functioning in offenders with ID is that relying on tests of cognitive ability only may underestimate a person's needs [37].

The issue of adaptive functioning in screening for ID has been a challenge for some time and studies have avoided including it as part of the assessment of ID [32]. Uzieblo and colleagues [38] highlight the difficulties in basing an assessment of ID solely on a measure of cognitive functioning and ignoring adaptive functioning, which is a criterion of the definition of ID. Of 37 studies assessing for offenders with ID, only 8 assessed for the three domains of ID, highlighting the importance of critically assessing the evidence on assessment or screening for offenders with ID. There is often a lack of detail evident in the diagnoses of ID among offenders.

Among the tools used to assess adaptive functioning are the VABS [13], Strengths and Disabilities Questionnaire (SDQ) [39], Adaptive Functioning Assessment Test (AFAT) [40] and Adaptive Behaviour Assessment System (ABAS) [41].

The AFAT consists of 46 items covering the four domains of communication, socialisation, independence and occupation. It has been examined for its validity against the Raven's Progressive Matrices as a measure of ID in a prison population [40]. It is a valid and reliable assessment tool of adaptive functioning in prisoners [37]. The advantage of the AFAT is that more reliable diagnoses of intellectual functioning in offenders could be achieved along with providing staff with a greater understanding of the likely specific practical challenges an offender faces in the prison environment.

Management of Offenders with ID

Forensic care involves essentially four phases. Management within each phase depends largely on the purpose and tasks of each. The initial phase of contact with forensic services usually involves liaison with the courts and is for the purpose primarily of assessment and advice to the courts. Depending on the jurisdiction, assessments may be required in relation to competency to stand trial, defences such as diminished responsibility, developmental capacity for mens rea, suggestibility, insanity defences, disposal assessments, and diversionary assessments.

The second phase of contact will generally involve acute management not uncommonly in the context of acute distress or comorbid mental illness. The third phase involves forensic rehabilitation and the final phase, community re-integration. Common to all points of contact are the core principles of forensic mental healthcare and of supporting people with intellectual or developmental disabilities within compulsory care settings.

Whether care is provided in custodial settings, forensic mental health settings or specialised forensic ID settings, the principles of good behavioural management apply. Punishment is ineffective but pervasive. The use of restrictive practices, covert or overt, need to be monitored and reduced, and the safety of the individual, their peers, visitors and staff is paramount [42]. It is important to not lose sight of the forensic nature of the work. Correctional services provide many useful resources to help staff avoid common pitfalls such as 'getting got' and services need to be mindful of the critical importance of good supervision, debriefing and staff support provisions to reduce the risks of vicarious trauma, unconscious bias and burnout, leading to the development of negative cultures of practice (see Table 13.1) [43].

Table 13.1 Risk for staff teams

Overt	Covert
Assaults (verbal/physical)	Getting got
Infections (spitting/biting/body fluids)	False allegations
Workplace hazards (slips/falls/RSI)	Vicarious traumatisation
	Burnout
	Unconscious bias
	Abusive practices developing
	Disciplinary actions
	Deskilling
	Stress
	Maladaptive coping strategies

A common myth for staff beginning work in forensic ID services, particularly those without formal training in working with people with intellectual and developmental disabilities, is that people with ID are not clever. Cleverness is not only linked to cognitive capacity on IQ tests and many people with ID involved in the criminal justice system will lie at the top end of the ID spectrum and will have had to become 'street smart' to survive. Long periods in institutional settings allow time for planning, testing systems for weaknesses and the focus and patience that can be brought to bear can surprise even the most experienced team.

Clear pathways for the functional expression of grievances, mindful role modelling of the behaviours we hope to teach and the provision of robust checks on the integrity of the environment are all necessary elements of safe, functional, forensic care systems. Systems need to manage the risks of false allegations and yet remain open to the real risk of abusive practices occurring [44]. Internal and external audit and monitoring are a necessary part of maintaining positive and safe cultures in what are commonly closed institutions [45].

Purpose of Forensic Rehabilitation Services

Nature abhors a vacuum and the purpose of forensic rehabilitation is not only to reduce or eliminate unsafe offending behaviours but also to understand what causes or perpetuates the behaviours and to find safe replacement skills and adaptive replacement behaviours. Offending behaviours, especially those acts involving child victims or the use of substances, may be suppressed within a forensic environment due to lack of access but have not necessarily been changed even over prolonged periods of care. Systems need to look for and recognise offence replacement and prosocial behaviours as proxy measures of potential positive rehabilitation. The corollary is to recognise offence analogue and offence replacement behaviours as proxy measures of ongoing risk not yet addressed [46].

Specific attention needs to be paid to providing suitably adapted environments, protocols and interventions that are gender specific, where services support male and female service users and meet their cultural and spiritual needs. For instance, in New Zealand, in keeping with most Western cultures, there is an over representation of indigenous Māori within all levels of the criminal justice system, including forensic rehabilitation services and ID forensic care [47].

Needs Assessment

Common to all aspects of residential care, and particularly within inpatient healthcare systems, everyone entering services needs a core baseline assessment that should provide a clear understanding of central issues. These include their degree of ID, areas of cognitive strengths or deficits within their overall level of functioning, aetiology if known, comorbidities (physical, mental health and addictions), risk assessment, communication assessment and sensory assessment.

Targets for forensic rehabilitation need to be specified using one or more of a number of structured needs assessment tools: CANFOR [48], CANDID [49], Level of Service–Care Management Inventory (LS-CMI) [50], DUNDRUM pillars of care [51] and Positive Behaviour Support Plan [52]. Where a non-forensic baseline is selected, this should be supplemented with the additional use of a forensic specific instrument.

Regular scheduled reviews should monitor change against baseline and match the level of forensic need to the appropriate level of forensic secure care and intensity of offence-specific intervention programmes, in line with the principles of the risk–need–responsivity model [53], ensuring offence replacement behaviours are not overlooked (Good Lives Model approach) [54].

Understanding Behaviour and Addressing Violence

A functional assessment targeting specific behaviours of concern is the most effective way of choosing an approach suited to changing behaviours. It is a common error in providing forensic rehabilitation to become side-tracked and focus on institutional problem behaviours rather than on the offending behaviours that brought the person to a forensic level of care in the first place. An example of this is in the focus being on self-injurious behaviour that distresses hospital systems but is rarely the reason why someone is placed in a forensic hospital care. While strategies need to be in place to understand why these behaviours occur and to manage them safely, this should not detract from the need to address the violence towards others or other offending behaviours that may be less problematic in the contained hospital environment

Offending-Specific Interventions

Monitoring Risk of Violence

Monitoring risk is a central activity in forensic settings. Short-term or proximal risk monitoring instruments help maintain awareness of potential increased risk. In mental health, the Dynamic Appraisal of Situational Aggression (DASA) [55] is extensively used and adapting it for ID settings includes less emphasis on symptoms of mental illness and more on environmental stressors [56]. Longer-term measures such as the Essen Climate Evaluation Schema (EssenCES) give a sense of the safety culture within a service, providing subscale measures of 'therapeutic hold', 'patient's cohesions and mutual support' and 'experienced safety' [57].

If not using a specific monitoring instrument, then a structured approach to handover and to reflective nursing practice, monitoring the unit for safety such as that offered under the 'See Think Act' system (Royal College of Psychiatrists), is important [58].

Responding to Behaviour

A structured approach to understanding and responding to challenging behaviours needs to be in place. Positive behaviour support offers one such approach, with an emphasis not on simple behavioural plans but on a functional assessment of the purpose or need the behaviour is serving and a proactive approach to getting these needs met in more functional ways [59]. The emphasis of this approach on avoiding the ineffective and often unethical use of punishment is perhaps its greatest strength, given the almost universal automatic tendency for systems to use punishment if this is not explicitly guarded against. Proactive plans offer interventions designed to reduce the risk of violent events occurring, but reactive strategies are important to identify known setting events, triggers and environmental stressors. Other indicators are signs of increased negative emotions, what to do in a crisis, and how to learn from the incident through a process of debriefing after the event.

Post-Event Management

Dealing with the aftermath of incidents within the forensic setting is important especially where staff or patients cannot be moved easily from the environment for any lengthy period of time. Clear policies on support for staff, respecting the rights of both staff and patients to make a formal complaint to the police about assaults. Clear provisions for debriefing are important and using dialectical behavioural therapy (DBT)-based approaches such as 'What chains' to understand and learn from the event [60]. A process for reconciliation to resolve post-incident 'fallout' and clear the air for continued therapeutic cohabitation amongst peers is also required, as well as supporting staff who may have been victims in the incident.

Pharmacological Approaches to Violent Behaviour

There are no specific licenced medications for aggression. Functional assessment can shed light on comorbidities or symptoms that lead or contribute to violence and can be targeted pharmacologically. The over-use of psychotropic medication in people with ID is well evidenced and over- and under-prescribing of appropriate medication can occur [61]. Clinicians should be clear on the target for medication, set baseline monitoring, avoid polypharmacy (see Table 13.2), go low and slow but be prepared to treat to maximum tolerated doses to get optimal benefit. Note that continued aggression is not only harmful to the victims of aggression but also ultimately to the aggressor, who may suffer prolonged loss of liberty, restrictions on residual liberties and consequences such as criminalisation of behaviours that challenge [62].

Table 13.2 Drugs used in targeting different behaviour

Target behaviour	Drug class
Seizure	Anti-epileptic medication
Fear-driven aggression	Anti-anxiety medication
Compulsive behaviours	Anti-obsessional medication
Psychotic signs	Antipsychotic medication
Impulse control	Attention deficit hyperactivity disorder medication
Over-arousal	Anticonvulsant or anti-anxiety medication

Psychological Interventions

A tiered approach is most easily adapted to the levels of cognitive function and the level of need of individuals. Almost all approaches effective in people without ID are also effective in people with ID. Adaptations may be required to reduce the pace, increase the visual or practical components, reduce the reliance on literacy skills, simplify language or concepts and provide additional 'homework support'.

Social Skills Training

There has been a re-emergence of understanding of the need for the most basic social skills to reduce risk of violence over recent years, after a period in the wilderness. The misinterpretation of the behaviours or intentions of others, lack of awareness of our own verbal and non-verbal communication in social situations, core skills such as use of interpersonal space, managing eye contact, appropriate and inappropriate touch can all make a significant difference to aggressive behaviours [63]. For this reason, it is important to consider the abilities of offenders with ID to relate appropriately to others in a range of settings.

Interpersonal Relationship Skills

Following on from core social skills comes more targeted interpersonal relationship skills training [64]. Such training may involve skills to share living spaces with peers or family or may be more specifically targeted at managing intimate partnerships, if this has been a primary area of violent offending. It is strong on teaching and challenging maladaptive thoughts (attitudes, beliefs, assumptions), feelings and actions.

Emotional Regulation Skills

The development of skills in emotional regulation is essential in that it can help the person recognise emotions, manage anger and other negative emotions, tolerate distress and manage aggression to self and others. Multiple specific adaptations to classic DBT have been tested within forensic ID settings [65, 66].

Anger Management Skills

Skills to manage anger are best used where violence is impulsive rather than instrumental. It forms a core part of DBT training but stand-alone programmes exist. Depending on the level of cognitive function, a manualised approach, such as Novaco taken at a slightly slower pace, has been shown to be effective [67]. Specialist programmes targeting anger management include the Violence Reduction Programme [68], Adaptation for Women [69] and the ManAlive programmes [70].

Sexual Offending

Sexual offending falls into several different subsets and the importance of understanding the nature of the sexual offending is paramount. The aim of interventions is to reduce the risk of future offending behaviour by supporting barriers to offending [71]. Offenders must have access to victims and they must choose to offend. Interference in any or all components of offending reduces the risk of offending occurring.

Targeted sexual offender treatment programmes include therefore educational components on the law, the sanctions and the slightly more subtle issues of consent and coercion.

Skills training will target safe and acceptable social and relationships skills, including social distances, touching, private and public concepts [72]. The next component is identifying and challenging cognitive distortions, being clear about the existence of victims even in non-contact offending such as accessing child pornography. Both a motivational approach, building the barriers to offending, and a practical approach, reducing ways in which the offender creates opportunities for access to unsupervised victims, and learns how to create levels of safety and protection around themselves in order to strengthen external barriers to offending, are needed.

Pharmacological Approaches

There is good indication that surgical and chemical castration can be effective means of reducing sexual offending in some cases [73]. From an ethical, but also from an efficacy perspective, such interventions are most likely to be effective where the desire to adopt these measures is coming primarily directly from the offender themselves [74]. They are also more likely to be effective where a high sexual drive is a strong component of the offending history. High levels of internal motivation to stop the offending behaviours, but difficulty achieving this through choice alone, appear to aid the efficacy. Chemical castration is targeted at reduction or elimination of testosterone but is a reversable option. Compliance can be assured by long-acting agents. Risks include reduction in bone mass density over prolonged periods of use but many other side effects are noted, including weight gain, migraine, gynaecomastia (irreversible) and seizures [75].

Fire-Setting Behaviour

Offending behaviour of fire setting among offenders with ID is a challenge to clinicians supporting offenders because of the risk the behaviour poses to others. Holst and colleagues describe the characteristics of fire setters who mainly have mild ID and histories of engaging in other offending behaviours [76]. Alcohol is associated with up to 25% of arson events. The purpose of clinical management is to address the drivers to the behaviour and to assess the on-going risk of offending. Such drivers include feelings of frustration, anger and distress that they cannot communicate appropriately. Treatment should be based on a clear elucidation of the factors driving the behaviour, such as comorbid mental disorders or difficulties in communicating feelings [77].

Disposal Options

The options available to the criminal justice system in arranging disposal of offenders with ID could be considered limited but have expanded in recent years. From the entry point, court diversion systems exist that can help to identify the offender who could have ID and advise the court accordingly on their fitness to plead [78]. Where a person is not fit to plead, a community or hospital disposal could be arranged. Supporting offenders in the community is preferable to hospital care where the level of risk could be managed safely. Community forensic teams can support local resources to effectively support an offender to live in the community while receiving interventions where necessary.

The standard levels of secure care are available to offenders with ID, from high to low secure [79]. More innovative services are developing, which adopt a 'locked-rehabilitation' model, where people are supported in secure settings but with greater supervised access to the community to assist in their safe reintegration into community living.

For offenders with ID, moving out of the criminal justice system can be a challenge to supporting services [80]. There are a range of systemic challenges to navigate in order for a person to effectively be discharged from secure care, which may not always be achieved and rely on meeting the specific needs of the person in that context.

While it is good practice to commence discharge planning from the time of admission, considering the issues involved in supporting and treating offenders, it is likely that treatment could take protracted periods of time to achieve in secure services. Regardless of this, services should formulate at an early stage of care the likely discharge supports that will be required for the person, whether in the community or elsewhere. The person may require 24-hour support because of the level of risk they pose to, which will depend on their response to treatment. A co-ordinated, multi-agency support approach is likely to be required, involving health services, social care, police and probation services [81]. The success of any support programme depends on the commitment of the agencies providing the support.

Conclusion

Given the prevalence of ID among the offending population, there is a logical pressure to identify those with cognitive impairments, to optimise the support they require while in the criminal justice system. For this reason, and with the demands on services, screening offenders for ID is more feasible than undertaking a fully comprehensive assessment. There is good evidence of the utility and effectiveness of certain cognitive screening tools in prisons and secure hospitals. However, screening for adaptive functioning adds additional useful information on the strengths of a person and areas of functioning where support would be advised. At present, there is not one specific screening tool or battery of tools that are recommended as a gold standard. Therefore, assessors may choose the validated tools that best suit their clinical setting, where people would likely benefit from screening for ID.

Supporting people with ID who offend requires good assessment to help deliver effective and appropriate therapeutic options, whether in inpatient settings or through support in the community. The purpose of treatment programmes is to reduce the likelihood of future offending to lower the risks to others. The environment where treatment is delivered will depend on the level of risk and the nature of the offence and the levels of security required. Staff need to be aware of the impact of the built environment on the response of the person to treatment. Many psychological interventions can be adapted to use with offenders with ID, and clinicians need to be skilled in understanding the subtleties in delivering adapted treatment programmes. Drug therapies can be used along with psychological interventions to treat mental disorders, which should enhance the psychological treatments. Risk assessment and management is crucial to the success of treatment, to ensure the effectiveness of interventions that reduce the risks the person poses.

References

1. Wakeling H, Ramsay L. Learning disability and challenges in male prisons: programme screening evaluation. *Journal of Intellectual Disabilities and Offending Behaviour* 2020; 11(1): 49–59.

2. Murphy GH, Gardner J, Freeman MJ. Screening prisoners for intellectual disabilities in three English prisons. *Journal of Applied Research in Intellectual Disabilities.* 2017; 30(1): 198–204.

3. Fazel S, Xenitidis K, Powell J. The prevalence of intellectual disabilities among 12,000 prisoners: a systematic review. *International Journal of Law and Psychiatry* 2008; 31(4): 369–73.

4. Maulik PK, Mascarenhas MN, Mathers CD, Dua T, Saxena S. Prevalence of intellectual disability: a meta-analysis of population-based studies. *Research in Developmental Disabilities* 2011; 32(2): 419–36.

5. Søndenaa E, Rasmussen K, Palmstierna T, Nøttestad J. The prevalence and nature of intellectual disability in Norwegian prisons. *Journal of Intellectual Disability Research* 2008; 52(12): 1129–37.

6. Asscher JJ, van der Put CE, Stams GJ. Differences between juvenile offenders with and without intellectual disability in offense type and risk factors. *Research in Developmental Disabilities* 2012; 33(6): 1905–13.

7. American Psychiatric Association. *Diagnostic and Statistical Manual of Mental Disorders*, 5th edition: DSM-5. American Psychiatric Association, 2013.

8. Schalock RL, Borthwick-Duffy SA, Bradley VJ, Buntinx WHE, Coulter DL, Craig EM, et al. *Intellectual Disability: Definition, Classification, and Systems of Supports*. American Association on Intellectual and Developmental Disabilities, 2010.

9. Hellenbach M, Karatzias T, Brown M. Intellectual disabilities among prisoners: prevalence and mental and physical health comorbidities. *Journal of Applied Research in Intellectual Disabilities* 2017; 30(2): 230–41.

10. British Psychological Society. Learning disability: definitions and contexts. Available at: www.bps.org.uk/psychologist/defining-learning-disability.

11. Kaal HL, Nijman HL, Moonen XM. Identifying offenders with an intellectual disability in detention in the Netherlands. *Journal of Intellectual Disabilities and Offending Behaviour* 2015. June 9.

12. Hartman DE. Wechsler Adult Intelligence Scale IV (WAIS IV): return of the gold standard. *Applied Neuropsychology* 2009; 16(1): 85–7.

13. Sparrow SS, Cicchetti DV. Diagnostic uses of the Vineland adaptive behavior scales. *Journal of Pediatric Psychology* 1985; 10(2): 215–25.

14. Hayes SC. *Hayes Ability Screening Index: HASI – Manual*. University of Sydney, 2000.

15. Ammons RB, Ammons CH. The Quick Test (QT): provisional manual. *Psychological Reports* 1962; 11(1): 111–61.

16. Mason J, Murphy G. People with an intellectual disability in the criminal justice system: developing an assessment tool for measuring prevalence. *British Journal of Clinical Psychology* 2002; 41(3): 315–20.

17. Tyrer F, McGrother CW, Thorp CF, Taub NA, Bhaumik S, Cicchetti DV. The Leicestershire Intellectual Disability Tool: a simple measure to identify moderate to profound intellectual disability. *Journal of Applied Research in Intellectual Disabilities* 2008; 21(3): 268–76.

18. McKenzie K, Michie A, Murray A, Hales C. Screening for offenders with an intellectual disability: the validity of the Learning Disability Screening Questionnaire. *Research in Developmental Disabilities* 2012; 33(3): 791–5.

19. Ali A, Ghosh S, Strydom A, Hassiotis A. Prisoners with intellectual disabilities and detention status. Findings from a UK cross sectional study of prisons. *Research in Developmental Disabilities* 2016; 53–54: 189–97.

20. Hayes SC. Early intervention or early incarceration? Using a screening test for intellectual disability in the criminal justice system. *Journal of Applied Research in Intellectual Disabilities* 2002; 15(2): 120–8.

21. Kaufman AS. *Kaufman Brief Intelligence Test: KBIT*. American Guidance Service, 1990.

22. Ford G, Andrews R, Booth A, Dibdin J, Hardingham S, Kelly TP. Screening for learning disability in an adolescent forensic population. *Journal of Forensic Psychiatry and Psychology* 2008; 19(3): 371–81.

23. Homack SR, Reynolds CR. *Essentials of Assessment with Brief Intelligence Tests*. John Wiley & Sons, 2007.

24. McCrimmon AW, Smith AD. Review of the Wechsler Abbreviated Scale of Intelligence (WASI-II). *Journal of Psychoeducational Assessment* 2011; 31(3). DOI: https://doi.org/10.1177/0734282912467756.

25. McKenzie K, Paxton D. Promoting access to services: the development of a new screening tool. *Learning Disability Practice* 2006; 9(6): 17–21.

26. McKenzie K, Sharples P, Murray AL. Validating the learning disability screening questionnaire against the Weschler Adult Intelligence Scale. *Intellectual and Developmental Disabilities* 2015; 53(4): 301–7.

27. Paxton D, McKenzie K, Murray G. Putting screening tools to the test. *Learning Disability Practice* 2008; 11(8): 14–18.

28. McKenzie K, Michie A, Murray A, Hales C. Screening for offenders with an intellectual disability: the validity of the Learning Disability Screening Questionnaire. *Research in Developmental Disabilities* 2012; 33(3): 791–5.

29. Murray AL, McKenzie K. The accuracy of the Learning Disability Screening Questionnaire (LDSQ) in classifying severity of impairment: a brief report. *Journal of Intellectual and Developmental Disability* 2014; 39(4): 370–4.

30. Bjørgen TG, Gimse R, Søndenaa E. Selective samples and the accuracy of screening for intellectual disabilities: learning disability screening questionnaire. *Open Journal of Social Sciences* 2016; 4(05): 109.

31. McKenzie K, Paxton D, Murray G, Milanesi P, Murray AL. The evaluation of a screening tool for children with an intellectual disability: the Child and Adolescent Intellectual Disability Screening Questionnaire. *Research in Developmental Disabilities* 2012; 33(4): 1068–75.

32. McBrien J. The intellectually disabled offender: methodological problems in identification. *Journal of Applied Research in Intellectual Disabilities* 2003; 16(2): 95–105.

33. Traub GS, Spruill J. Correlations between the Quick Test and Wechsler Adult Intelligence Scale-Revised. *Psychological Reports* 1982; 51(1): 309–10.

34. Hassiotis A, Gazizova D, Akinlonu L, Bebbington P, Meltzer H, Strydom A. Psychiatric morbidity in prisoners with intellectual disabilities: analysis of prison survey data for England and Wales. *British Journal of Psychiatry* 2011; 199(2): 156–7.

35. Gresham FM, Elliott SN. The relationship between adaptive behavior and social skills: issues in definition and assessment. *Journal of Special Education* 1987; 21(1): 167–81.

36. Soenen S, Van Berckelaer-Onnes I, Scholte E. Patterns of intellectual, adaptive and behavioral functioning in individuals with mild mental retardation. *Research in Developmental Disabilities* 2009; 30(3): 433–44.

37. Ross GE, Hocken K, Auty JM. The reliability and validity of the Adaptive Functioning Assessment Tool in UK custodial settings. *Journal of Intellectual Disabilities* 2020; 24(1): 35–49.

38. Uzieblo K, Winter J, Vanderfaeillie J, Rossi G, Magez W. Intelligent diagnosing of intellectual disabilities in offenders: food for thought. *Behavioral Sciences and the Law* 2012; 30(1): 28–48.

39. Goodman R. The Strengths and Difficulties Questionnaire: a research note. *Journal of Child Psychology and Psychiatry* 1997; 38 (5): 581–6.

40. Smith L. Improving the assessment of intellectual disability (ID) within the UK prison service (who define ID using an IQ below 80). Nottingham Trent University, 2016. Available at: http://irep.ntu.ac.uk/id/eprint/28031/1/LORRAINE.SMITH-2016.pdf.

41. Harrison P, Oakland T. *Adaptive Behaviour Assessment System (ABAS-II)*. The Psychological Corporation, 2003.

42. Higgins L. Secure unit: positive behavioural support and restraint reduction in a unit for offenders with an intellectual disability and/or autism: practice paper. *International Journal of Positive Behavioural Support* 2021; 11(1): 42–54.

43. Carlson JR, Thomas G. Burnout among prison caseworkers and corrections officers. *Journal of Offender Rehabilitation* 2006; 43(3): 19–34.

44. Lawrence D, Bagshaw R, Stubbings D, Watt A. Restrictive practices in adult secure mental health services: a scoping review. *International Journal of Forensic Mental Health* 2021; 13: 1–21.

45. Büsselmann M, Titze L, Lutz M, Dudeck M, Streb J. Measuring the quality of life in forensic psychiatric hospitals. *Frontiers in Psychology* 2021; 12: 701231.

46. Mooney JL, Daffern M. The Offence Analogue and Offence Reduction Behaviour Rating Guide as a supplement to violence risk assessment in incarcerated offenders. *International Journal of Forensic Mental Health* 2013; 12(4): 255–64.

47. Cavney J, Friedman SH. Culture, mental illness, and prison: a New Zealand perspective. In Mills A, Kendall K, eds., *Mental Health in Prisons*. Palgrave Macmillan, 2018: 211–34.

48. Thomas SD, Slade M, Mccrone P, Harty MA, Parrott J, Thornicroft G, Leese M. The reliability and validity of the forensic Camberwell Assessment of Need (CANFOR): a needs assessment for forensic mental health service users. *International Journal of Methods in Psychiatric Research* 2008; 17(2): 111–20.

49. Xenitidis K, Thornicroft G, Leese M, Slade M, Fotiadou M, Philp H, et al. Reliability and validity of the CANDID: a needs assessment instrument for adults with learning disabilities and mental health problems. *British Journal of Psychiatry* 2000; 176(5): 473–8.

50. Andrews DA, Bonta J, Wormith SJ. *Level of Service–Case Management Inventory: LS/CMI*. Multi-Health Systems, 2000.

51. Davoren M, Hennessy S, Conway C, Marrinan S, Gill P, Kennedy HG. Recovery and concordance in a secure forensic psychiatry hospital: the self rated DUNDRUM-3 programme completion and DUNDRUM-4 recovery scales. *BMC Psychiatry* 2015; 15(1): 1–2.

52. Dench C. A model for training staff in positive behaviour support. *Tizard Learning Disability Review* 2005; 10(2): 24–30.

53. Bonta J, Andrews DA. Risk–need–responsivity model for offender assessment and rehabilitation. *Rehabilitation* 2007; 6 (1): 1–22.

54. Ward T, Brown M. The good lives model and conceptual issues in offender rehabilitation. *Psychology, Crime and Law* 2004; 10(3): 243–57.

55. Ogloff J, Dafern M. The dynamic appraisal of situational aggression: an instrument to assess risk for imminent aggression in psychiatric inpatients. *Behavioural Sciences and the Law* 2006; 24(6): 799–813.

56. Barry-Walsh J, Daffern M, Duncan S, Ogloff J. The prediction of imminent aggression in patients with mental illness and/or intellectual disability using the Dynamic Appraisal of Situational Aggression instrument. *Australasian Psychiatry* 2009; 17(6): 493–6.

57. Schalast N, Redies M, Collins M, Stacey J, Howells K. EssenCES, a short questionnaire for assessing the social climate of forensic psychiatric wards. *Criminal Behaviour and Mental Health* 2008; 18(1): 49–58.

58. Chester V, Alexander RT, Morgan W. Measuring relational security in forensic mental health services. *BJPsych Bulletin* 2017; 41(6): 358–63.

59. Sugai G, Horner R. The evolution of discipline practices: school-wide positive behavior supports. *Child and Family Behavior Therapy* 2002; 24(1–2): 23–50.

60. Rizvi SL, Ritschel LA. Mastering the art of chain analysis in dialectical behavior therapy. *Cognitive and Behavioral Practice* 2014; 21(3): 335–49.

61. Sheehan R, Hassiotis A, Walters K, Osborn D, Strydom A, Horsfall L. Mental illness, challenging behaviour, and psychotropic drug prescribing in people with intellectual disability: UK population based cohort study. *BMJ* 2015; 351.

62. Smith P, Waterman M, Ward N. Driving aggression in forensic and non-forensic populations: relationships to self-reported levels of aggression, anger and impulsivity. *British Journal of Psychology* 2006; 97(3): 387–403.

63. Smith RL, Rose AJ, Schwartz-Mette RA. Relational and overt aggression in childhood and adolescence: clarifying mean-level gender differences and associations with peer acceptance. *Social Development* 2010; 19(2): 243–69.

64. Baczała D. Social skills of individuals with intellectual disabilities. *Psycho-Educational Research Reviews* 2016; 5(2): 68–77.

65. Sakdalan JA, Shaw J, Collier V. Staying in the here-and-now: a pilot study on the use of dialectical behaviour therapy group skills training for forensic clients with intellectual disability. *Journal of Intellectual Disability Research* 2010; 54(6): 568–72.

66. Oxnam P, Gardner E. Treatment for emotional difficulties related to offending for people with an intellectual disability. In Lindsay WR, Craig LA, Griffiths D, eds., *The Wiley Handbook on What Works for Offenders with Intellectual and Developmental Disabilities: An Evidence-Based Approach to Theory, Assessment, and Treatment*. Wiley, 2019: 357–72.

67. Taylor JL, Novaco RW, Brown T. Reductions in aggression and violence following cognitive behavioural anger treatment for detained patients with intellectual disabilities. *Journal of Intellectual Disability Research* 2016; 60(2): 126–33.

68. Wong SC, Gordon A. The Violence Reduction Programme: a treatment programme for violence-prone forensic clients. *Psychology, Crime and Law* 2013; 19(5–6): 461–75.

69. Elliott DE, Bjelajac P, Fallot RD, Markoff LS, Reed BG. Trauma-informed or trauma-denied: principles and implementation of trauma-informed services for women. *Journal of Community Psychology* 2005; 33(4): 461–77.

70. Buel SM. Domestic violence and the law: an impassioned exploration for family peace. *Family Law Quarterly* 1999; 33(3): 719–44.

71. Craig LA. Controversies in assessing risk and deviancy in sex offenders with intellectual disabilities. *Psychology, Crime and Law* 2010; 16(1–2): 75–101.

72. Williams F, Mann RE. The treatment of intellectually disabled sexual offenders in the National Offender Management Service: the Adapted Sex Offender Treatment programmes. In Craig LA, Lindsay WR, Browne KD, eds., *Assessment and Treatment of Sexual Offenders with Intellectual Disabilities: A Handbook*. John Wiley & Sons, 2010: 293–315.

73. Gooren LJ. Ethical and medical considerations of androgen deprivation treatment of sex offenders. *Journal of Clinical Endocrinology and Metabolism* 2011; 96(12): 3628–37.

74. Harrison K, Rainey B, eds. *The Wiley-Blackwell Handbook of Legal and Ethical Aspects of Sex Offender Treatment and Management*. John Wiley & Sons, 2013.

75. Daffern M. Anti-libidinal medication use in people with intellectual disability who sexually offend. Available at: www.dhhs.vic.gov.au/sites/default/files/documents/201912/Anti-libidinal%20medication%20use%20in%20people%20with%20intellectual%20disability%20271119.pdf.

76. Holst S, Lystrup D, Taylor JL. Firesetters with intellectual disabilities in Denmark. *Journal of Intellectual Disabilities and Offending Behaviour* 2019; 10(4): 102–18.

77. Alexander RT, Chester V, Green FN, Gunaratna I, Hoare S. Arson or fire setting in offenders with intellectual disability: clinical characteristics, forensic histories, and treatment outcomes. *Journal of Intellectual and Developmental Disability* 2015; 40(2): 189–97.

78. Marshall-Tate K, Chaplin E, McCarthy J, Grealish A. A literature review about the prevalence and identification of people with an intellectual disability within court liaison and diversion services. *Journal of Intellectual Disabilities and Offending Behaviour* 2020; 11(3): 159–69.

79. Devapriam J, Alexander RT. Tiered model of learning disability forensic service provision. *Journal of Intellectual Disabilities*

and *Offending Behaviour* 2012; 3(4): 175–85.

80. Taylor JL, McKinnon I, Thorpe I, Gillmer BT. The impact of transforming care on the care and safety of patients with intellectual disabilities and forensic needs. *BJPsych Bulletin* 2017; 41(4): 205–8.

81. Chester V, Brown AS, Devapriam J, Axby S, Hargreaves C, Shankar R. Discharging inpatients with intellectual disability from secure to community services: risk assessment and management considerations. *Advances in Mental Health and Intellectual Disabilities* 2017; 11: 98–109.

Risk Assessments in People with Neurodevelopmental Disorders

Catrin Morrissey

Introduction

Risk assessment, particularly in relation to risk to others, has become synonymous with forensic clinical approaches. This chapter considers best practice, first in relation to risk-assessment approaches in populations with intellectual disability (ID) and second in relation to those with autism spectrum disorder (ASD). The literature on the former greatly exceeds the latter, although useful guidance is emerging around ASD and forensic risk, which is a developing field. Forensic risk assessment in attention deficit hyperactivity syndrome (ADHD) specifically has, until very recently, been little considered in the literature, but emerging guidance is discussed briefly at the end of the chapter. Understanding of the core diagnostic criteria relating to these three neurodevelopmental conditions is assumed throughout the chapter.

The science of forensic risk assessment has evolved considerably in the last 20 years. This has moved from clinical unstructured approaches, to purely actuarial approaches (where a static risk score based on historical factors predicts the statistical likelihood of offending), to structured dynamic approaches (where variables which relate to risk but are changeable are considered), and combinations of the two. This chapter focuses primarily on the current 'gold standard' methodology which is the structured professional judgment (SPJ) approach.

Risk Assessment in Forensic Populations with ID

There has been a recent increase in research activity and output relating to risk assessment in ID populations. Lofthouse and colleagues [1] systematically reviewed 14 prospective studies of risk-assessment methods applied to people with ID. The studies reviewed used a range of tools, both mainstream and those originally designed for ID. These included the Violence Risk Appraisal Guide (VRAG: actuarial approach), Short Term Assessment of Risk and Treatability (START: dynamic approach); Psychopathy Checklist Revised (PCL-R; SPJ approach), Current Risk of Violence (CUrV: dynamic approach) and the Historical Clinical Risk-20 (HCR-20; SPJ approach). Lofthouse found an average an area under the curve of 0.7 and little difference between the predictive utility of the measures, although actuarial and SPJ measures performed somewhat better than purely dynamic measures. Lofthouse and colleagues concluded that most of these tools did predict future aggression significantly better than chance, but did not go on to recommend specific measures. For the purposes of this chapter the focus will be on clinical utility of the most widely used measures, and on the practical issues for consideration as opposed to research findings. The most commonly used SPJ approaches will be considered primarily in the ID context, although such approaches have equal relevance to risk considerations in ASD and other neurodevelopmental conditions.

Applicability of SPJ Approaches Designed for Mainstream Populations: The HCR-20 V3

The updated Historical–Clinical–Risk Management-20 (HCR-20) Version 3 (V3) [2] risk-assessment scheme and its predecessor HCR-20 Version 2 (V2) is one of the most widely researched SPJ violence risk assessments used in forensic setting worldwide. The scheme takes the assessor through a number of detailed stages, culminating in a risk formulation, an overall risk rating, generation of risk scenarios and a risk management plan. The broad definition of violence in the HCR-20 extends to threatened and attempted violence, and can include sexual and fire-setting offences. Its strength lies in the systematic evaluation of evidence, which is linked to a risk formulation. The evidence in the document can be updated over time and, if completed thoroughly and accurately, can be relied on as a structured summary document for subsequent assessors, saving much trawling though clinical and incident records. As such, it lends itself to settings such as forensic hospitals where patients may remain for lengthy periods of time, often moving between secure settings. These factors make it an attractive option for assessing risk for both inpatients and community forensic patients with ID.

The instrument has a tripartite temporal focus – past, present and future – and includes both static and dynamic risk factors. Ten historical static items (H scale) focus on the past history of problems with violent and antisocial behaviour, relationships and employment. Five clinical items (C scale) highlight current and recent problems with psychosocial, mental health and behavioural functioning. Finally, five future oriented risk management factors (R scale) consider issues such as living conditions, support and access to services. Each item is rated as to whether it is present and relevant. The instrument is not designed to produce summative 'scores'; the authors emphasise that items may have different weight in terms of their relevance in an individual case. Nevertheless, for research purposes, its subscales and total scales have been used quantitatively. The assessment culminates in an overall qualitative risk of serious violence rating (low, medium or high), which research has found to be as predictive as any of the detailed scores.

The HCR-20 V3 is applicable to hospitalised forensic and civil psychiatric populations in the community. The authors of this risk-assessment scheme consider their revised instrument to be sufficiently flexible to be applicable to people with ID in these settings. In particular, the more detailed item descriptors aid accurate coding of both presence and relevance, reducing the need for omitted items for ID cases.

Studies Using the HCR-20 with ID Populations

Notably, in a study scoping the outcome domain for UK forensic ID services, a Delphi survey of clinical staff identified the HCR-20 as the most commonly used risk assessment [3]. Accordingly, since 2004, the applicability and validity of the HCR-20 V2 to ID populations has been considered in research studies conducted in a wide range of clinical settings.

First, Lindsay et al. [4] applied the HCR-20 V2 to 303 individuals with ID in high-, medium-, low- security and community settings. They found that the items had face validity, and could be rated meaningfully, although supplementary guidance for applying the tool to those with ID was later found to be necessary (See Boer et al. [5]). They also found that ratings correlated broadly – as might be predicted – with the level of security. Subsequent studies have established the predictive validity of the HCR-20 in this group. First, a number of studies in different ID settings have established that the HCR-20 predicts inpatient violence. This was found in high-security [6] and, more recently, in medium- and low-security ID populations [7], the latter study finding that it performed as well for ID as it did for a comparison group of mentally disordered offenders without ID. O'Shea et al. [8] nevertheless found the frequency of positive ratings differed across items between the ID and the comparison group, suggesting a somewhat different 'risk profile'.

A small number of studies have assessed whether the HCR-20 predicts a move to a lesser level of security or discharge for ID groups. Morrissey et al. [9] compared 5,000 HCR-20 V2 ratings on patients in different services in a high secure hospital, finding that scores were much less predictive of progress for the ID service patients as compared to those with mental illness and personality disorders. Where predictive validity in relation to violent behaviour in the community is concerned, there is less evidence from the HCR-20. This is likely to be because accurate reoffending data are much less easy to collect than institutional behavioural data collected as part of routine inpatient practice. Nevertheless, in one retrospective study, Gray et al. [10] did find that HCR-20 scores significantly predicted violent reconviction in the community, post discharge from an ID medium secure hospital.

Practical Applicability of the HCR-20 and ID-Specific Guidance

Arguably, group studies examining predictive validity have little bearing on the clinical utility of an instrument for individual cases. While the earlier version of the HCR-20 (V2) began to be used in ID services in the mid-2000s, practitioners found that coding queries frequently arose and so there was a tendency to omit items. As a consequence, ID-specific guidelines were produced to accompany the instrument (outlined by Boer et al. [5]), which paralleled guidelines designed to assist ID clinicians with other clinical assessments, such as the PCL-R for psychopathy [11]. These guidelines address some general principles. First, and crucially, the guidance is only a supplement to the manual, comprising suggestions to conceptualise the items in an ID context, but no change to the flavour or intent of the items is intended. They highlight the fact that the restricted lives of many people with ID reduce opportunities to exhibit some of the behavioural evidence but, conversely, that the nature of ID increases the likelihood that some of the HCR-20 risk factors (such as impulsivity, poor insight and poor response to treatment) are rated as present. Furthermore, they endorse the general principles of the HCR-20 manual that a good clinical interview and thorough collateral file review is necessary, but they emphasise that consultation with significant others is potentially more important when assessing individuals with ID.

Boer et al.'s guidance goes on to address each item in an ID context [5]. They considered issues such as the expectations for employment and relationships in people with ID, and the extent to which such problems should be rated as present when they were in the normal range for a person with ID. They noted that the 'lack of support' item has some unique ID considerations. While the monitored context in which people with ID often live (e.g., supported accommodation) was considered as a potentially protective factor, it is also one where aggressive or even violent behaviour may be more tolerated than in society at large.

It is important to note that the guidelines referred to have not been updated for HCR-20 V3. As noted above, the updated version (published in 2013) certainly made efforts to factor in ID presentations into the manual to a greater extent, making it easier to apply in practice. The manual makes it explicit, for example, that ID (and indeed other neurodevelopmental disorders) is counted as a 'major mental disorder' for Item H6, a factor which was not clear in the previous manual. Because of this, the item will always be coded as 'present' in cases with a diagnosed ID, and the form allows the rater to describe the profile of cognitive and adaptive impairments and their relevance as predisposing risk factors. Similarly, the manual notes that the clinical dynamic item C3, 'Recent problems with symptoms of major mental disorder', will always be coded as present where there are neurodevelopmental disorders which impair functioning to a chronic and unchanging degree. Linked to this, Item C1, relating to recent problems with 'insight' (into either the mental disorder or the need for treatment) is more likely to be an ongoing risk factor in people with cognitive difficulties. Regardless of the inherent capacity to develop insight, or indeed to achieve treatment progress (Item C5), it remains potentially relevant to risk. This said, it is important not to assume a lack of insight based on cognitive ability alone: the key is for the assessor to clarify the relevance of the item to the reoffending risk in that individual. In practice, people with ID are likely to have a higher number of risk factors endorsed as present on the HCR-20 than comparable populations without ID; this is certainly borne out in empirical studies [9, 10, 12].

The V3 historical items (H1 and H2) allow for unconvicted risk behaviours to be recorded in the evidence, unlike many actuarial assessments which rely on charges and/or convictions. Tools that do so are known to be problematic in ID populations where 'offending-like' behaviour is often not processed through the criminal justice system in the way it might be for people without ID. The relationships item (H3) now extends explicitly to non-intimate relationships, which is in line with the previous ID guidance; this is a more meaningful factor for people with ID, where successful intimate relationships are less common and relationships with families and peers are a better indicator of interpersonal functioning. Similarly, the employment item (H4) in V3 now extends to supported activities and education as well as paid employment, in recognition that it is the person's record of ability to sustain occupation of any kind throughout their adult life which is of relevance to risk.

Equally, as observed by Boer et al. [5], the HCR risk management (R) items in V3, focusing on living situation, professional services and availability of support, have direct relevance to people with ID for whom such factors may have a major bearing on risk management. Particular emphasis should be put on the quality and consistency of this support, and the extent to which that decreases the risk. Unlike some contemporary risk tools, the HCR-20 V3 does not focus on such protective factors, which is a potential weakness, but these can be considered in any formulation.

It is important to note that the HCR V3 allows additional items of relevance to be recorded and coded in each of the H, C and R domains under 'Other factors'. This allows ID-specific aspects to be included in the items which are present and relevant to violence risk (e.g., poor processing speed; vulnerability to the influence of others; problems with social understanding).

The formulation approach encapsulated in the HCR-20 allows clinicians to factor aspects of the ID into the explanation of the risk and the factors which precipitate and maintain behaviour. Since it is flexible about the formulation model used, the HCR-20 approach also allows the *function* of the risk behaviour to be considered in terms of the needs met for that individual: notably such functions may well differ in people with ID as compared to those without. The function of behaviour is therefore an important fifth factor to hold in mind when considering the 'four Ps' of predisposing, precipitating, perpetuating and protective factors.

In conclusion, the HCR-20 (and its parallels for sexual offenders Risk for Sexual Violence Protocol (RSVP [13]) and Sexual Violence Risk-20 Version 2 (SVR-20 V2 [14])) is a useful SPJ violence risk assessment when applied to individuals with ID. In practical terms, in the experience of the author, rating of the items per se does not necessarily aid the final risk judgement process, and excessive time should not be spent on determining whether items are present and relevant. The tool's strength lies in its rigour in gathering the evidence for risk, its formulation-based approach, its flexibility in allowing additional ID-related risk items to be incorporated, and the incorporation of risk scenarios and risk management plans. It is considered important that the tool should be applied by clinicians with specific ID clinical expertise, ensuring that the contextual factors relating to the ID and their relevance to risk are carefully weighed up. This includes the important environmental factors relating to care staff and care setting, which should be considered within the R factors. Guidelines which support ID practitioners to think about the contextual evidence may nevertheless have utility, albeit with the usual adherence to the HCR-20 V3 manual. A case example is illustrated in Case Study 14.1.

Case Study 14.1 Brief summary of ID HCR-20

Historical factors (items present and relevant)

P was a 24-year-old man convicted of a serious physical assault on a female, who had rejected his sexual advances, and he was subsequently detained on a civil section. He had relevant historical risk factors of mild ID, with particularly low verbal comprehension (domain score of 50–55) and processing speed (domain score of 55–60), and ADHD, which impaired his decision-making skills and increased his behavioural impulsivity (H6). A victim of adverse childhood experiences (H8), he had had violence modelled to him by his mother and had exhibited physical aggression since childhood (H1) as well as other antisocial and rule-breaking behaviour (H2). He went to a mainstream school with extra support, but because of his ID he had always felt he did not fit in and was particularly resentful that he could not attain an intimate partner like his peers. His ID also extended to poor identification of his emotions, and inhibited his ability to express his feelings verbally because of poor expressive communication skills.

Clinical factors (recent and current)

Clinical or current risk factors included poor insight into his violence risk (C3), present violent ideation as indicated by recent threats towards other peers (C2). His ID, as an ongoing mental disorder, was considered to be relevant to his ongoing risk (C1) particularly his deficits in planning, memory attention and impulse control. Recent incidents of behavioural and affective instability (C3) had led to seclusion on a number of occasions. Treatment compliance was currently poor, in as much as he had refused to participate in anger management work with a psychologist (C5).

Risk management factors

As he was detained in hospital, P's risk management (R) factors, as rated in the current context, were not of concern. However, there was concern that, in future, a robust 24-hour-staffed community setting would be required to manage his behaviour safely (R2). It was anticipated that his communication problems and desire for a partner would lead to additional stressors in the community (R5).

Brief formulation

Main predisposing factors: H1 H2 H6 H8 (as above)

Precipitating factors:

internal: feelings of rejection; feeling under threat; alcohol-related disinhibition

external: situations where others reject P; threats by others

Perpetuating factors: poor emotional recognition and management; lack of secure emotional support outside hospital; behavioural impulsivity and lack of consequential thinking linked to ADHD.

Hypothesised function of risk behaviour: to express feelings of anger and hurt that P could not process emotionally or express verbally

Protective factors: boundaries of hospital setting; staff understanding his triggers

The overall risk of serious or life-threatening physical harm was currently assessed as moderate with imminence as low likelihood.

Risk-Assessment Approaches Designed Specifically for Forensic Populations with ID: the ARMIDILO

There have been a few attempts to develop tools which are specific to people with ID, the most well-developed of which is the Assessment of Risk and Manageability of Individuals with Developmental and Intellectual Limitations who Offend Sexually (ARMIDILO) [15]. This is an SPJ tool which considers actuarial risk approaches as a baseline, and both stable and acute (changing) dynamic factors. It also considers protective factors, giving an overall protective rating. It is particularly useful in that it considers issues of particular relevance to ID clients in its stable/acute environmental factors, including the attitude towards the ID client by the staff, communication and client-specific knowledge among support persons and consistency of supervision and staffing. It is a very useful additional clinical tool for monitoring risk in sexual offenders in the community.

Risk Assessment in Forensic Populations with ASD

While some studies have suggested over-representation of people with ASD in forensic populations, this is by no means a clearly established finding [16]. It is notable that up to three-quarters of people with ASD in secure care have comorbid psychiatric diagnoses, and rates of comorbidities (such as psychosis and personality disorders) have been found to be significant risk factors for criminal convictions in those with ASD [17]. What is commonly agreed by practitioners, however, is that specific aspects of autism often do have a bearing on individuals' vulnerability to offend, and that mainstream risk assessments do not necessarily incorporate all such factors [18, 19].

Applicability of SPJ Approaches Designed for Mainstream Populations: the HCR-20 V3

There are a small number of studies which have explored the utility of SPJ approaches such as the HCR-20 with people who have ASD in hospital settings. In an early screening study, Murphy [18] found that, while some conventional risk factors were present, many of the items had lesser relevance to many of those with ASD (e.g., substance misuse).

More recently, Girardi et al. [20] conducted a retrospective empirical study of the HCR-20 V3 assessing the predictive validity with respect to inpatient violence in a small sample ($n = 22$) of patients in medium and low secure specialist ASD hospital settings. Broadly, they found that the HCR-20 V3 did predict overall and physical violence, with the clinical scale and total score having the highest AUC (over 0.8), suggesting that the tool has validity for use with the inpatient ASD population.

As described above, the HCR-20 V3 does allow for additional risk factors to be added and coded as relevant, which might include specific ASD-related factors. It is nevertheless acknowledged that some ASD-specific difficulties related to risk are not necessarily accounted for or explored in the HCR-20 manual and that these must specifically be considered in formulation, intervention and risk management plans. While some have argued for ASD-specific risk assessments to be developed [19] others have argued that guidelines and frameworks to assist in case formulation with ASD clients alongside the mainstream risk-assessment tools are what is required (e.g., Shine and Cooper-Evans [21]). This is the approach which is advocated here, as opposed to any attempt to create and validate a separate risk assessment for people with ASD. Because of the high comorbidity of ASD with other disorders and the idiosyncrasies of ASD presentation, such a narrow approach is considered neither desirable nor easily achievable. Fortunately, detailed practical guidance for clinicians, which can serve to help them to contextualise factors related to autism when conducting SPJ assessments of risk, have recently been developed by Al-Attar [22, unpublished work, 2020]. The Framework for the Assessment of Risk and protection in offenders on the Autistic Spectrum (FARAS) helps a practitioner to add depth and specificity to standard risk assessments, and is therefore part reproduced and summarised below (with permission of Dr Zainab Al-Attar).

Guidance to Support SCJ Risk Assessment in ASD: the FARAS

The FARAS manual is not a risk-assessment tool, but provides an overview of the key considerations that risk assessors can take into account when carrying out a structured SPJ risk assessment with an offender with ASD. Al-Attar argues that the role of ASD is contextual as opposed to causal to both risk and protective factors. She emphasises that when interviewing offenders with ASD for risk-assessment purposes it is important to examine their ideation, communication and behaviour in the context of each facet of their autistic functioning.

The guidelines are organised through seven sections, which each address an interlinked 'facet' of autism considered of relevance to risk assessments, particularly with respect to delineating the potential functions of behaviour. Each section separately considers risk-relevant issues, protective issues and interviewing considerations. The manual usefully summarises 'tips' to remember for each facet during risk assessment, the relevance of which will of course vary for each individual.

Circumscribed Interests

A defining feature of ASD is intense, absorbing interests, which may be unusual for a person's age or peer group. From a risk perspective a person may:

(a) have a harmless interest which develops into a harmful offshoot (e.g., an interest in pyrotechnics, which is then exploited by others to facilitate bomb making for terrorist purposes)

(b) have a relatively harmless interest which, when acted on more specifically, becomes illegal (e.g., interest in serial killers, progressing to harmful behaviour)

(c) have an inherently harmful or illegal interest (e.g., collecting sexual images of children)

It is considered important to explore the role circumscribed interests play in the pathway to an offence, and the modus operandi of an offence. It is also important to consider whether access to the interests is limited in closed settings, and may re-emerge once external boundaries are removed. Risk management may involve managing the emotional factors that intensify the need to pursue offence-related interests.

Protective considerations of circumscribed interests are that they may be a rich source of esteem and well-being if shaped appropriately, and can be used as a motivational tool in rehabilitation.

In interview, it is considered useful to fully explore aspects of offence-related interests, as well as to identify their function. For example, a possessor of indecent images may be reinforced by the collecting of such images, as opposed to obtaining sexual gratification from them.

Rich Vivid Fantasy and Impaired Social Imagination

Certain individuals with ASD who have offended are known to have a vivid visual memory but impaired social imagination; they can experience vivid fantasy with which they may become preoccupied, which has in turn led to offence-related behaviour. Sources of fantasy can often be visual imagery from films and video games, but if these are harmfully violent/sexual the fantasies are not always adjusted to take into account the individual's usual moral code, or 'real-life' consequences which might arise. Certain setting factors can lead to an enactment of all or part of the fantasy.

Where there is an offence that appears to have been the enactment of a fantasy, risk assessment should involve very detailed analysis of the content of risk-related fantasies and what factors (e.g., low mood; a rejection) might trigger enactment of such fantasies. The function of the person's fantasies should be considered (e.g., negative reinforcement by removing undesirable mood states; positive reinforcement by being paired with masturbation).

Harmless/healthy visual fantasy can be protective in an emotional sense, and help people with ASD cope with stressors. Risk-assessment interviews should therefore explore which fantasies are protective and which are potentially harmful.

Need for Order, Routines and Predictability

Individuals with ASD often have a heightened need for order, predictability, structure and routine. Change can be destabilising, and can be a heightened period of vulnerability for offending for some people with ASD. Alternatively, an offence may be driven by the sense of predictability and order it potentially brings (e.g., endorsing terrorist groups that promise to restore justice and moral order). An individual may escape from the anxiety of social unpredictability by predictable virtual pursuits, which may in turn become the conduit for offending. Finally, impulsive offending can result from a disruption in routine. The role of rules and predictability in past offending behaviour, current functioning and future planning should therefore be considered in a risk assessment of a person with ASD.

Conversely, a person with ASD may thrive in an organised and predictable environment (like prison or secure hospital), which may be a protective factor while in such environments. Clearly explaining prison or hospital rules and license conditions in the community will often help offenders with ASD adhere to them. However, future scenarios with less predictability will ideally need to be anticipated and planned for in collaboration with the person in any risk-management plan.

Obsessionality, Repetition and Collecting

Linked to but distinct from circumscribed interests, individuals with ASD may engage in repetitive behaviours, which can have a compulsive quality to them. They can also find collecting items or information to be highly intrinsically rewarding. It is therefore important that the assessor considers whether obsessional aspects impact the function of the offence, and whether repetitive behaviour increases the risk of harm.

The FARAS notes, by way of example, that in offences of stalking by a perpetrator with ASD the assessor needs to focus not only on the usual cognitive and relational factors but also to explore the sense of compulsion in such cases. Similarly, where people have broken the law by obtaining a large collection of illegal images, assessors may need to explore any possible compulsion to the collecting behaviour. For an offender who collects illegal child images and classifies them with regard to focus on different parts of the body (feet, hands, etc.), each item may have its 'place' in the wider collection as opposed to being intrinsically reinforcing in itself. For the purposes of risk assessment, the number of offence-related images may be relevant to assessing the intensity of the interests, but it may not be a reliable indicator of level of risk. Thus, even when the offence function is found to be sexual, the assessor also needs to explore aspects of offending that satisfy an obsessional need.

When looking at protective factors, obsessiveness and need for repetition are not inherently maladaptive and may serve to meet a range of needs for an individual. Supporting the person to use their intense focus to collect safe items, for example, can provide a safe focus, and appropriate positive reinforcement.

Social Interaction and Communication Difficulties

Social interaction deficits and communication difficulties are a core feature of ASD. For assessors of risk, the direct and indirect role of these difficulties and related stress in the offence pathway need to be explored.

Social and communication difficulties could directly shape risk where an offender's misreading of a social situation was a direct antecedent to the offence, and where the lack of theory of mind is a maintaining factor. An example could include a sexual offender who erroneously assumed that the victim reciprocated his attraction because she was friendly with him and, after sexually touching her, failed to read her distress cues and realise that she was upset. This facet of autism may also have indirect contributions to risk if the offender offends at times of heightened social isolation, dejection and stress (all of which may be shaped by their social and communication impairments).

Conversely, certain aspects of social interaction abnormalities may be protective. Offenders with ASD may be unusually transparent, and appreciative of frank and direct guidance and feedback from professionals, making dialogue with professionals more efficient and genuine. In order to be responsive to the ASD communication style, risk assessors should be direct, literal and specific in their questions and comments and not leave anything to the interviewee's ability to infer or second-guess meaning. In turn, the person with ASD's blunt, graphic offence explanations and forthright comments should not be mistaken for attempts to dominate/control or instil fear and shock. Assessors should try to disentangle which socially inappropriate behaviours are risk-relevant and which are not, and address each separately in their risk-assessment and -management approaches.

Cognitive Styles

There are a number of cognitive difficulties and strengths associated with ASD which, while they may not apply to all individuals with ASD, are worthy of consideration in the process of risk assessment. These are outlined in the FARAS as follows:

- attention to detail and not seeing the 'bigger picture' and context
- frontal-executive impairments: including deficits in attention-shifting and processing simultaneous stimuli
- deficits in theory of mind.

The direct implications of the aforementioned cognitive styles for risk might include, for example, a fixation on the factual and visual details of something (e.g., terrorist materials, firearms) without an appreciation of the wider social context, victim harm and legal implications of the behaviour. Alternatively, reactive aggression may be triggered by someone overloading the individual cognitively or trying to distract their attention away from a task they are intently focused on. Difficulties understanding others' perspectives or understanding that others do not know what is in the offender's mind may exacerbate such situations, and hence a lack of cognitive empathy may be a further risk factor. This said, the FARAS guidelines caution against interpreting the cognitive lack of empathy in ASD as being similar to the lack of emotional empathy seen in psychopathic offenders (see Blair [23] for an explanation of these concepts).

Finally, risk assessors should distinguish cognitive sophistication from social sophistication when evaluating an offender's capability and intent. For example, an offender with exceptional technical or scientific capabilities (due to their ability to see detail and visually process information) may show meticulous bomb-making skills or an ability to source child pornographic images from the dark web, but may not be able to detect when terrorist or paedophile networks exploit them (due to their impaired theory of mind and lack of bigger picture thinking).

Sensory Processing

Autistic individuals may be under- or oversensitive to sensory stimuli in one or more senses (e.g., light/colour, noise, touch/texture/pressure/vibration, smells and taste). They may also have heightened or lowered sensitivity to movement and temperature, and have very high or low thresholds for pain. While *hyper*-sensitivity usually leads an individual to avoid stimuli, *hypo*-sensitivity can lead them to seek out a sensory stimulus. Each can have different forensic risk implications.

It is therefore important to establish an offender's sensory profile (from files/others or by asking them) prior to undertaking an SCJ risk assessment with a person. The risk assessor should explore whether sensory aversions were direct or indirect antecedents to the offence or if the offence behaviour/modus operandi had a sensory reward value.

In terms of protective factors, where less harmful proxies of rewarding offence-related stimuli can be facilitated, this may be appropriate, especially if it diminishes rather than reinforces the need for harmful offence-related stimuli. Case Study 14.2 illustrates an example of using the HCR-20 in a person with ASD.

Case Study 14.2 Brief summary of ASD HCR-20 (see acknowledgments)

Historical factors

Q was an 18-year-old man arrested on suspicion of planning a terrorist attack, and manufacturing explosives and was remanded to prison. He was diagnosed with high functioning autism at age 15. He had no violence history, and few conventional historical risk factors, other than his ASD (coded present and relevant at H6), features of which were directly relevant to risk of harm. These specifically included the facets of circumscribed interests; obsessional behaviour; interpersonal difficulties and poor theory of mind. A specific additional historical risk factor was coded in H for Q's circumscribed interest rooted in a fascination with fireworks from a young age, which diverged into a wider interest and research into explosives, culminating in manufacturing of low-grade explosives and a planned detonation.

Clinical factors (recent and current)

Q was coded as having current problems with insight into his violence risk (C1), as he was currently finding it difficult to understand the violent political agenda of his online 'friends' and why he was deemed to be a risk by the authorities. He was also coded as having violent ideation (C2) since he admitted an all-absorbing visual and sensory fantasy of detonating a high-impact explosive, which he recently discussed with online friends and described to the police. He had sent messages that supported terrorism and urged others to commit terrorist acts (although these seemed to have a rote quality to them). His lack of social imagination did not allow him to think through the true consequences of such an action. Current aspects of his mental disorder (ASD) of relevance to risk were; his repetitive obsessional behaviour patterns in relation to his special interest together with deficits in social interaction and relationships.

Risk management factors (future)

Q lived alone and there was no current scope to monitor his activities, were he to be in the community, other than through surveillance. Future accommodation, support and intervention were unknown, and there were therefore 'possible' future problems with these.

Brief formulation

Predisposing factors: ASD as a developmental disorder confers cognitive differences; longstanding circumscribed offence-related interests in a high-risk area; obsessional features and fantasy life all relate to this diagnosis.

Precipitating factors:

Internal: involvement in online forums where he was reinforced socially and encouraged to undertake actions while not understanding the full intentions of others; intense excitement at the thought of fulfilling fantasies of using the explosives he had developed
External: access to online forums; the presence of others willing to exploit Q's technical skills and interests and reinforce his statements; availability of materials

Perpetuating factors: ongoing lack of insight; ongoing obsessive interest in explosives and explosions; ongoing lack of consideration of consequences of behaviour (related to lack of social imagination)

Function of risk behaviour: to achieve excitement and intrinsic reinforcement fulfilling the fantasy linked to his special interest. A possible secondary function was to obtain approval and some social contact from others.

The overall risk of serious or life-threatening physical harm was currently assessed as high, with a high degree of imminence, were he unsupervised in the community.

Guidance to Support SCJ Risk Assessment in ADHD: the FARAH

The prevalence of ADHD in offender populations is known to be high [24], and the disorder may be comorbid to either ASD or ID or both. Yet empirical studies relating to forensic risk and assessment of that risk in people with ADHD specifically are almost non-existent, and until recently there has been little consideration of specifically contextualising risk with an understanding of that disorder. However, Al-Attar (2021) [25] has recently produced useful parallel guidance to the FARAS in the form of the Framework for the Assessment of Risk and Protection in Offenders with Attention Deficit Hyperactivity Disorder (FARAH). As with the FARAS, this is not a risk-assessment tool but takes the form of comprehensive clinical guidelines for risk assessors to use alongside mainstream risk assessments such as the HCR-20 V3, and as an aid to formulation. The FARAH is structured around 12 items, which comprise first, four core diagnostic features of ADHD (e.g., difficulty with organising, planning and prioritising), a further four features commonly associated with ADHD (e.g., binging on instant reward activities) and, finally, four 'secondary sequelae', which may arise from ADHD (e.g., alcohol and drug use).

Elements of the FARAH guidance relating to the first four core diagnostic features and their potential link with risk are outlined here for illustrative purposes.

Difficulties Regulating Attention

The impact of attentional deficits on prosocial goal achievement across all areas of life may be significant in offenders with ADHD. While most prosocial goals may demand some tasks which require sustained attention and delayed rewards, by contrast many antisocial goals may appear to offer immediate reward and intense experiences, which hold attention for short periods. Alternatively, individuals with ADHD and attention deficits may become disruptive, to avoid having to remain in environments which cause them to become distracted or dysregulated. Clearly, both these aspects of functioning related to attention deficits can have relevance to the risk formulation.

Difficulties with Organising and Planning Multiple or Complex Tasks

Symptoms of ADHD include neurocognitively driven difficulties in organising tasks and activities, and the ability to multitask and switch between goals and tasks may be impaired

Disorganisation and a chaotic approach to life goals can lead to loss of financial, practical social and emotional capital and leave needs which may be met more easily through criminal behaviour, where there is a focus on a 'minute-by-minute' approach to life. Criminal lifestyles may in the short-term place less strain on the person with ADHD, which offers some explanation as to why they may be attractive to the person. Risk reduction may therefore be attained by supporting development of skills in self-organisation.

Impulsivity, Short-Term Reward Seeking and Risk Taking

The FARAH notes that the neurocognitive and motor symptoms of ADHD may lead to decisional emotional and behavioural impulsivity, whereby an individual can act without consideration of the risks or consequences and find it difficult to inhibit their behavioural response where there is an immediate reward. This group of symptoms can fuel risk taking and seeking of immediate gratification, which is clearly linked to a range of types of addiction and criminal behaviour. Habitual impulsive seeking of such immediate rewards can lead to a significant area of criminogenic risk, which becomes self-maintaining. Furthermore, peers may deliberately exploit the risk-taking tendency to encourage a person with ADHD to commit crimes. It is further noted that this aspect of ADHD is relevant to treatment response in that individuals may quickly abandon rehabilitation goals which do not offer immediate resolution of their difficulties, lessening the likelihood of successful intervention as a protective factor.

Motor Hyperactivity and Restlessness

The final core diagnostic feature of ADHD that may affect risk is motor hyperactivity and restlessness, which is also linked to feelings of boredom. The FARAH notes that restlessness can further lead to agitation, irritation and a heightened need for stimulation when bored, which can – as with the last item – create the preconditions for offending behaviour. Examples of the consequences of these feelings may include reactive aggression and, as such, motor hyperactivity should be considered alongside the factors above when considering the function of risk-related behaviour in a person with ADHD.

While the clinical utility of the FARAH guidance for risk assessors has yet to be fully evaluated, in the course its development the guidance has been peer reviewed by experts in the ADHD field and it promises to be a helpful resource for interviewing and risk formulation.

Conclusion

Successful approaches to risk assessment in neurodevelopmental disorders are those which contextualise SPJ risk assessment in relation to the neurodevelopmental disorder and its individual characteristics, preferably utilising supplementary guidance to mainstream risk assessments, similar to those described in this chapter. A focus on risk formulation, with careful attention paid to the function of the behaviour in the context of the neurodevelopmental condition, is advocated.

A final note of caution should be that attributing *all* aspects of risk to a person's ID, ASD or ADHD is as inappropriate as ignoring those factors in a risk assessment. All risk assessment requires a holistic approach, and careful use of current SPJ methodologies facilitate this with people with neurodevelopmental disorders.

Acknowledgement

I am grateful for permission provided by Dr Zainab Al-Attar to summarise the FARAS and FARAH and to utilise aspects of a case study.

References

1. Lofthouse R, Golding L, Totsika V, Hastings R, Lindsay W. How effective are risk assessments/measures for predicting future aggressive behaviour in adults with intellectual disabilities (ID)?: a systematic review and meta-analysis. *Clinical Psychology Review* 2017; 58: 76–85.

2. Douglas KS, Hart SD, Webster CD, Belfrage H. *HCR-20V3: Assessing Risk of Violence – User Guide*. Mental Health, Law, and Policy Institute, Simon Fraser University, 2013.

3. Morrissey C, Geach N, Alexander RT, Chester V, Devapriam J, Duggan C, et al. Researching outcomes from forensic services for people with intellectual or developmental disabilities: a systematic review, evidence synthesis and expert and patient/carer consultation. *Health Services and Delivery Research* 2017; 5(3).

4. Lindsay WR, Hogue TE, Taylor JL, Steptoe L, Mooney P, O'Brien G, et al. Risk assessment in offenders with intellectual disability: a comparison across three levels of security. *International Journal of Offender Therapy and Comparative Criminology* 2008; 52(1): 90–111.

5. Boer DP, Frize, M, Pappas, R, Morrissey, C, Lindsay, WR. 2010. Suggested adaptations to the HCR-20 for offenders with intellectual disabilities. In Craig LA,

Lindsay WR, Browne KD, eds., *Assessment and Treatment of Sexual Offenders with Intellectual Disabilities: A Handbook*. John Wiley & Sons, 2010: 177–92.

6. Morrissey C, Hogue T, Mooney P, Allen C, Johnston S, Hollin C, et al. Predictive validity of the PCL-R in offenders with intellectual disability in a high secure hospital setting: institutional aggression. *Journal of Forensic Psychiatry and Psychology* 2007; 18(1): 1–5.

7. Fitzgerald S, Gray NS, Alexander RT, Bagshaw R, Chesterman P, Huckle P, et al. Predicting institutional violence in offenders with intellectual disabilities: the predictive efficacy of the VRAG and the HCR-20. *Journal of Applied Research in Intellectual Disabilities* 2013; 26(5): 384–93.

8. O'Shea LE, Picchioni MM, McCarthy J, Mason FL, Dickens GL. Predictive validity of the HCR-20 for inpatient aggression: the effect of intellectual disability on accuracy. *Journal of Intellectual Disability Research* 2015; 59(11): 1042–54.

9. Morrissey C, Beeley C, Milton J. Longitudinal HCR-20 scores in a high-secure psychiatric hospital. *Criminal Behaviour and Mental Health*. 2014; 24(3): 169–80.

10. Gray NS, Fitzgerald S, Taylor J, MacCulloch MJ, Snowden RJ. Predicting future reconviction in offenders with intellectual disabilities: The predictive

efficacy of VRAG, PCL-SV, and the HCR-20. *Psychological Assessment* 2007; 19 (4): 474.

11. Morrissey, C. Guidelines for assessment of psychopathy in offenders with intellectual disabilities. 2006. Available at: www.seman ticscholar.org/paper/Assessment-of-psychop athy-in-offenders-with-Morrissey/2322ae4fe d59bbd7cee27258a0afc36b867ae31b.

12. Morrissey, C, Hobson, B, Faulkner E, James T, et al. Outcomes from a high secure forensic service: findings and challenges. *Advances in Mental Health and Intellectual Disabilities.* 2015; 9: 116–23.

13. Hart S, Krop P.R, Laws DR, Klaver J, Logan C, Watt KA. *The Risk for Sexual Violence Protocol (RSVP): Structured Professional Guidelines for Assessing Risk of Sexual Violence.* The Institute Against Family Violence, 2003.

14. Boer, DP, Hart SD, Kropp, PR Hart SD, Webster, CD. *Manual for Version 2 of the Sexual Violence Risk-20.* Protect International Risk and Safety Services Inc., 2017.

15. Boer DP, Haaven JL, Lambrick F, Lindsay WR, McVilly K, Sakdalan J, et al., ARMIDILO-S manual: web version 1.0. 2012. Available at: www.armidilo.net/index .html.

16. Allely CS. A systematic PRISMA review of individuals with autism spectrum disorder in secure psychiatric care: prevalence, treatment, risk assessment and other clinical considerations. *Journal of Criminal Psychology* 2018; 5: 1.

17. Långström N, Grann M, Ruchkin V, Sjöstedt G, Fazel S. Risk factors for violent offending in autism spectrum disorder: a national study of hospitalized individuals. *Journal of Interpersonal Violence* 2009; 24 (8): 1358–70

18. Murphy D. Risk assessment of offenders with an autism spectrum disorder. *Journal of Intellectual Disabilities and Offending Behaviour* 2013; 4(1–2): 33–41.

19. Westpahl, A, Allely, C. The need for a structured approach to violence risk assessment in autism. *Journal of the American Academy of Psychiatry and the Law* 2019; 47(4): 437–9.

20. Girardi A, Hancock-Johnson E, Thomas C, Wallang PM. Assessing the risk of inpatient violence in autism spectrum disorder. *Journal of the American Academy of Psychiatry and the Law* 2019; 47(4): 427–36.

21. Shine J, Cooper-Evans S. Developing an autism specific framework for forensic case formulation. *Journal of Intellectual Disabilities and Offending Behaviour* 2016; 7(3): 127–39.

22. Al-Attar Z. Development and evaluation of guidance to aid risk assessments of offenders with autism. 2018. Unpublished MA dissertation: Sheffield Hallam University.

23. Blair RJR. Responding to the emotions of others: dissociating forms of empathy through the study of typical and psychiatric populations. *Consciousness and Cognition* 2005; 14(4): 698–718.

24. Young S. The identification and management of ADHD offenders within the criminal justice system: a consensus statement from the UK adult ADHD Network and criminal justice agencies. *BMC Psychiatry* 2011; 11: 32.

25. Al-Attar Z. ADHD as a context for risk, protection and responsivity in offenders: Introducing the FARAH guidance. National Autistic Society, Autism, Learning Disabilities and the Criminal Justice System Conference (virtual event), September 23, 2021.

Chapter 15

Assessment and Treatment of Young Offenders

Louise Theodosiou and Rachel Elvins

Introduction

The UK has a strong tradition of creating principles that enshrine the needs of children and young people (commonly referred to as CYP). The 1908 Children Act applied to all parts of the UK and mandated that the courts should seek to educate rather than punish young offenders, and that their hearings should be held separately to that of adults. In the past century, Scotland has followed a different journey to England, Wales and Northern Ireland; the ground-breaking Kilbrandon Report [1] was key in the development of the children's hearing system [2]. This system is 'centred on the welfare of the child' in which children and young people who offend and those in need of care and support are managed within the same system. However, in England, Wales and Northern Ireland, children and young people who have been charged with an offence will be seen within a youth court.

The complexities of providing comprehensive care to vulnerable children and young people and offering them the life opportunities that they need has been brought into sharp focus by the coronavirus (COVID-19) pandemic, which has highlighted and heightened disparities in living standards. A body of fictional works from *Oliver Twist* [3] to *Trainspotting* [4] has detailed the links between poverty, early adversity, mental health needs, substance misuse and contact with the criminal justice system. Research has evidenced that young offenders have higher rates of childhood adversity, learning needs, developmental disorders, traumatic brain injuries, substance use disorders, physical and mental health needs [5]. To quote from the Kilbrandon Report [1]: 'From the earliest age of understanding, every child finds himself part of a given family and a given environment – factors which are beyond his or society's power to control. During childhood the child is subject to the influences of home and school. Where these have for whatever reason fallen short or failed, the precise means by which the special needs of this minority of children are brought to light are equally largely fortuitous'.

The paradigm shift that followed Kimberlé Crenshaw [6] articulating the concept of intersectionality has reverberated through the health and social care literature. Intersectionality addresses the fact that people who are minorities within minorities experience a cumulative disadvantage. To fully assess and therefore treat young offenders, there has to be an acknowledgement of the reasons why socio-economic, demographic, developmental, mental health and physical health needs may be unmet. This must of course address the reluctance that some young people may feel to engage with mental health and youth justice services.

Children and young people encounter the youth justice system at a number of different junctures; they may be at risk of offending, engaged in a community order or within the secure estate. A number of tools are available to undertake a comprehensive assessment of health, social care and educational needs. Guidance is available to support the engagement of young offenders with healthcare, education and training as described below.

The Demographics of Young Offenders in the UK

The Youth Justice Board [7] reports that the number of children and young people who received a caution or a sentence in England and Wales has fallen significantly in the past decade (82%). The same is true of first-time entrants to the youth justice system (84%). However, the length of the average custodial sentence has increased in this time frame. Furthermore, the numbers of incidents of self-harm involving children and young people in custody and the rates of restrictive physical interventions are the highest in the past five years. Experimental statistics released by the Youth Justice Board [8] note the high numbers of children and young people working with youth justice services who have mental health needs, speech, language and communication difficulties, learning needs and those using substances. The bulletin also notes the high proportion of children and young people who have accommodation needs and those who have been looked after within the social care system. The paper notes the increased complexity and vulnerability of young offenders, which underscores the importance of ensuring that a comprehensive assessment is offered in a way that children and young people can engage with.

Finally, it is of note that the ethnicity of children and young people in England and Wales who are in custody has changed in the past decade [7]. The proportion of children and young people who identify as being from Black, Asian and minority ethnic backgrounds has risen from 28% in 2010 to 51% in 2020.

The proportion of girls within the youth justice system has fallen in the past decade [7]. While sexual orientation is not reported within the UK statistics for youth justice, it is important to note that a report from the USA [9] notes that lesbian, gay, bisexual and transsexual youth are over-represented within the US justice system. Finally, the Ministry of Justice [10] reported that there were 125 adult transgender prisoners in the year 2016–2017.

Contact with the youth justice service can provide an opportunity for a comprehensive assessment that may previously have been lacking from a child's life. The UK's National Institute for Health and Care Excellence (NICE) [11] notes the fact that young offenders are a group at risk of drug misuse and are also more likely than their peers to have missed early childhood vaccinations, to have moved through a range of educational settings and to live within reconstituted families [12]. Furthermore, a meta-analysis of psychiatric comorbidity in the UK custody system identified that 11% of boys and 29% of girls had a diagnosable depressive disorder [13]; while a longitudinal study of male offenders revealed that adolescent substance misuse and depressive symptoms correlated strongly with adult substance misuse [14]. Furthermore, McKinlay et al. [15] noted that 79.6% of young Scottish males believed that alcohol use had contributed to their offending. This was echoed in the Youth Justice Board [8] bulletin reporting on children and young people sentenced in England and Wales between April 2018 and March 2019. The report noted that 71% had mental health needs, while 75% reported substance misuse and 71% had needs relating to speech, language and communication. Chronic high-level offenders were found to be particularly at risk of developing depression and drug use in adulthood. An association between antisocial behaviour and self-harm has also been demonstrated; a study identified that 1 in 10 offenders reported self-harm in the preceding month [16]. Predictors of an increased risk include previous attempts, prolonged low mood, attention deficit hyperactivity disorder (ADHD), impulsivity and substance misuse [17, 18].

An updated systematic review [19] examined data from 19 countries relating to adolescents in detention facilities from January 1999 to October 2019. The authors emphasise the heterogeneity of study design, interviewers and diagnostic instruments used in the studies. However, it is interesting to note that 2.7% of boys and 2.9% of girls were diagnosed with psychosis, while 10.1% of boys and 25.8% of girls were diagnosed with a major depressive disorder. When looking at ADHD, 17.3% of boys and 17.5% of girls in custodial settings met the criteria for this condition. Finally, 8.6% of boys and 18.2% of girls were diagnosed with post-traumatic stress disorder (PTSD).

Physical health needs are also likely to be higher and to be unmet [20], with higher rates of poor oral and respiratory health, often connected to smoking, and higher rates of sexually transmitted diseases.

Assessing the Needs of Young Offenders

In England and Wales, the age of criminal responsibility is 10 years old [21]. However, it is of note that, in Scotland, the age of criminal responsibility will be increased to 12 years old. The concept of early intervention has become a mainstay of all aspects of children's well-being and healthcare needs [22]. Looking specifically at routes into youth justice [23], it is important to note that children and young people with unmet neurodevelopmental needs are more likely to be in contact with the youth justice system. Other chapters in this book address the treatment of specific conditions including specific neurodevelopmental disorders and comorbid mental health needs. This chapter addresses core principles of assessment and treatment in young offenders, with reference to substance use and mental health needs.

NHS England [24] describes the liaison and diversion services that work with the police and courts. As this may be the first contact that a young offender has with justice services, the assessment of immediate health needs, such as the risk of suicide, is essential. Such services are required to have a good working knowledge of local mental health services, and of course the Mental Health Act 1983 [25].

The Crime and Disorder Act 1998 [26] led to the development of specific youth justice teams in England and Wales. These teams have at their heart the principles of 'child first'; workers are encouraged to prioritise the best interest of the child and understand their strengths and capabilities. Teams are multidisciplinary in nature, with youth justice workers and staff who have been seconded in, for example from the police, social care, education and healthcare. When young people first come into contact with the youth justice system, comprehensive assessments are undertaken. The Youth Justice Board [27] notes that the primary purpose of this assessment is to detail the factors that would impact on the likelihood of further offending behaviour. However, as noted previously, this process provides an opportunity for a comprehensive assessment that children may not previously have enjoyed.

Before the pandemic, young offenders in the community were generally seen in specific bases, accessible by public transport, with opportunities to engage in one-to-one work. Principles of privacy and confidentiality were maintained. Since the COVID-19 pandemic, many community services have been offering their services via video or telephone. However, as noted by Hampson [28], young offenders are more likely than their peers to struggle to retain mobile phones and tablets. Thus, they may be dependent upon parents or carers if attending phone or video appointments. They are also more likely to live in families with limited internet access; thus, the current lack of internet cafes and libraries is more likely to impact on their contact with services.

Within the UK, a number of tools to have been developed over the years to standardise the assessments undertaken by youth justice workers, including Asset, Onset, mental health screening questionnaire interview for adolescents (SQUIFA) and the mental health screening interview for adolescents (SIFA). These have now been replaced by the Youth Justice Board's AssetPlus [27]. The AssetPlus provides a proforma which can be used to develop an understanding of the strengths and needs of the young person and thus support the youth justice worker to develop a network of professionals around the young offender. It explores the young person's social circumstances including parenting and social care history, learning and educational history, physical and mental health and substance misuse. The offending behaviour, engagement and potential for change are also explored. One of the key potential advantages of the AssetPlus is the fact that it can be dynamically updated to monitor changes in the young person. The tool is also designed to be used with young offenders in both community and secure settings. This means that information can be shared as the young person moves from one part of the youth justice environment to another. Finally, it is of note that the Lammy Report [29] identified that children and young people from Black, Asian and minority ethnic backgrounds do not trust the justice system. The report calls for more work to be done to develop culturally sensitive ways of explaining legal rights and options to defendants.

The AssetPlus is designed to work with the Comprehensive Health Assessment Tool (CHAT) [30]. There are versions available for youth justice workers to use in the community and in custodial settings [31, 32]. The neurodevelopmental and traumatic brain injury section, which includes screening for speech and language difficulties, learning disability, autism spectrum disorder and traumatic brain injury, has been validated in a pilot study [33]. The implementation of the CHAT has been accompanied by the delivery of training to staff working in a range of youth justice services.

When a young person enters the secure estate in the UK, the CHAT reception screen is administered to identify needs that should be addressed immediately, such as drug withdrawal, acute suicidal ideation or diabetes mellitus. The Youth Justice Board [34] details the deaths of 15 boys in custody, all of which appear likely to have been due to suicide. Adolescents may have been managing anxiety or distress with alcohol or drugs, which may come to light during the early stages of incarceration [35]. Dame Carol Black [36] notes the vulnerability of children and young people in relation to substance misuse, and identifies that one in four young people report seeing illegal drugs for sale on social media. Furthermore, a report addressing children and young people [37] admitted into secure settings from April 2014 to March 2016 identified that 45% reported substance use. The National Treatment Agency for Substance Misuse [38] essential elements document advised that all young offenders should be screened for substance misuse; the timescale is not specified, but the document advises that those with identified needs should be assessed within 5 working days and treated within 10 working days.

Finally, the HM Inspectorate of Probation [39] report noted that social media forms a large part of young people's lives, and that the range of ever increasing platforms available provide a means for children and young people to plan and incite offences. The National Crime Agency [40] notes that around 60% of hackers begin to engage in hacking before they reach the age of 16. The paper posits that children and young people with autistic spectrum conditions may be over-represented in this cohort.

Consent and Engagement

If the AssetPlus identifies factors which require further assessment from another professional, the CHAT [41] manual provides guidance on the process of gaining consent from young people over 16; ensuring that the young person is capable of understanding the decision to be made, is acting voluntarily and has enough information to make the decision. For children under 16 who do not want to involve their parents/carers, their capacity for consent should be assessed, however it is important to consider gaining guidance from safeguarding leads.

Treatment, interventions and Service Models for Young Offenders

The past two decades has seen increasing awareness of the need to provide consistent yet innovative models of healthcare to young offenders. Khan and Wilson [42] note that community healthcare support for young offenders is not delivered to a consistent model. Some services employ healthcare professionals from a physical health background while others employ mental health professionals. They also identify a range of different models of healthcare delivery: the 'lone health practitioner model', 'foot in–foot out model', 'virtual locality health team', 'outreach consultative team model', 'external young offending team (YOT) health one-stop-shop', 'health team within a YOT', 'YOT teams with no recorded health input'.

Dent et al. [43] detail the different models of forensic child and adolescent mental health services (FCAMHS) for young offenders, once again noting their heterogeneity.

Healthcare professionals working with young offenders have the opportunity to provide advocacy and support to some of the most vulnerable children and young people. As noted previously, there is evidence to suggest that the cohort of children and young people within youth justice have higher rates of learning needs, mental health needs and speech and communication needs, while also experiencing higher rates of family difficulties, care outside the family and non-engagement with education [8]. Furthermore, Black, Asian and minority ethnic children and young people are over-represented within this cohort. Lammy [29] suggests that youth justice services need to engage local communities by working with community groups and offering appointments in non-traditional spaces.

Within the community, young offenders encounter a range of professionals, including the police, staff in court, lawyers and youth justice workers in community youth offending services. In addition to the liaison and diversion services described previously [24], court services will often have strong links with both specialist FCAMHS services and the healthcare staff working in community youth offending services.

Gibson and Evennett [44] note the connection between children and young people not attending appointments and greater social deprivation. They urge the use of the term 'was not brought' rather than 'did not attend'. Healthcare professionals working in youth justice settings have an opportunity to provide a positive experience of healthcare; they can offer guidance on ways to engage children and young people with speech and communication needs, they can liaise with primary care, they can provide an understanding of mental health needs and can support children and young people to engage with the wider child and adolescent mental health services.

Dent et al. [43] describe the mental health settings where young offenders can be placed. For those with the highest level of mental health needs, for example psychosis, forensic adolescent inpatient settings are available. For other young offenders, a range of services has developed. Specialist FCAMHS teams are available, often providing a range of services, including 'in reach' to young offenders in custody, and training, liaison and specialist second opinion services for general CAMHS teams.

Custodial youth justice settings may have specialist healthcare environments where young offenders with physical and mental health needs can be supported. There will be in reach from primary care and CAMHS, in many places this in reach is provided by FCAMHS. As noted previously, all young offenders entering custody will be screened for healthcare emergencies, such as thoughts of suicide, or diabetes, and will of course have ongoing care. This will range from dental care through to sexual health and the treatment of mental health needs such as depression. The CHAT was designed with custodial and community branches to enhance the transition of care across these two settings.

NICE [45–47] provides guidance to support children and young people to reduce drug use and for over 16 year olds who need to detoxify from heroin use. Intervention is often provided by specialist trained drug workers; however, the guidance emphasises the importance of all staff working with children and young people being mindful of the possibility of substance misuse. The guidance recommends that questions should be asked in a non-judgemental way, and that treatment can be provided through information sharing and skills training to children and young people and their parents and carers. It is important to understand the context within which a young offender is using alcohol, cigarettes or drugs; explore whether drugs are used with peers or alone and consider the overall mental health of the young person. NICE [48] notes that ADHD can be a risk factor for substance misuse and increase the likelihood of conditions such as depression and anxiety. Thus, to fully treat a young offender who is using substances, it will be important to understand their mental health needs. See Case Study 15.1 for an example of community-based teamwork.

Case Study 15.1 Example of a community-based team

One of the chapter authors (LT) provides input to a community healthcare team working across a large English city within the 'Foot in–Foot out' model [42]. In this model, clinicians are based between a community youth offending service and a general CAMHS. As noted by Khan and Wilson [42], clinicians benefit from the ongoing skills sharing with CAMHS colleagues, and the formal and informal support. LT provides supervision and consultation to three highly skilled clinicians, who in turn offer supervision and consultation to youth justice workers and direct clinical care to young offenders who are referred to them. The clinicians are based for part of the week within the youth offending service offices. This has led to the development of strong professional relationships with youth justice workers, thereby enabling ongoing consultation whenever needed, rapid offering of appointments when young offenders are very distressed or agitated and, of course, the opportunity for joint appointments. The latter can be very important when working with young offenders who struggle to trust professionals and have formed good working relationships with youth offending workers. The clinicians are able to start working with young offenders before they leave custodial settings and have a good working relationship with the local FCAMHS.

Intagliata described the core purpose of case management as service users being 'provided with whatever services they need in a co-ordinated, effective, and efficient manner' [49]. The fact that many young offenders have limited family support, a history of non-engagement with education and communication difficulties makes the role of the CAMHS case manager particularly important. The three clinicians within this specialist team liaise with families, carers, education, primary care and mental health services, ensuring that physical and mental health needs can be met, sometimes for the first time.

Transition into Adult services

As noted, young offenders have high levels of complex needs, as illustrated by Case Study 15.2. Thus, healthcare workers should ensure that they are following local and national guidance in relation to transition. Multi-agency input may be required to ensure that young adults will have accommodation, ongoing training and education opportunities, healthcare input and financial

---

Case Study 15.2 Philomena's journey towards transition

Thank you to the young person who consented for her story to be told anonymously (her name and key details have been changed) and nurse practitioner Jo Marshall for writing it).

Philomena's mother was a looked-after child and Philomena was born when her mother was 15. Philomena was removed at age 7, following non-accidental injuries, and placed with her aunt. In 2014, the placement broke down, and Philomena was passed between several family members, who were believed to give her drugs and alcohol.

Philomena presented at accident emergency in 2015 (age 15). She was noted to be suicidal and low in mood, she had taken an overdose in the past and concealed it, she also disclosed a history of cutting her legs. Philomena was discharged to her grandmother's house and referred to CAMHS. She was offered three appointments, all three of which she missed, and her case was closed. At the time Philomena was open to a multi-agency service working with children at risk of sexual exploitation, and a service supporting children and young people who are using drugs and alcohol.

Philomena was initially accommodated in a children's home in 2016. Following this, she experienced five placement breakdowns due to giving other residents spice, and hazardous smoking of spice in her room, which caused a fire. In 2017, she was placed in a different city due to lack of suitable placements available closer to her home; at this time her social worker also changed. Philomena lived out of area for six months; during this time there was a high level of missing-from-home incidents and in increase in spice use. She reported feeling abandoned and forgotten about. There were concerns around her vulnerability; she was found unconscious at a train station with facial injuries and intoxicated with spice. Philomena continued to work with the initial substance use service, who offered an inpatient detoxification which she declined.

Philomena moved back to her home city later in 2017 and was referred to the specific CAMHS/youth justice service, following a conviction for robbery. Philomena engaged well with the assessment and disclosed one ounce per week of spice use. She reported a history of self-harm, and was noted to be frequently missing from home. She described pervasive low mood for two years, and agreed to weekly appointments to monitor mental state. An appointment was arranged with the psychiatrist in the CAMHS/youth justice service two weeks later and Philomena was offered anti-depressant medication. Philomena was also offered an urgent general practitioner review due to the effects of smoking spice.

Funding for a placement was agreed until Philomena's eighteenth birthday, a new Barnardo's worker was allocated to her at the end of 2017. However, no planning for transition to adulthood was completed. Philomena had difficulty registering with a new general practitioner as the surgery wanted photo identification and proof of address. A referral was made to adult mental health services in early 2018 and there was also agreement by children's services to fund an additional three months in placement due to lack of planning for post 18 years of age. Health needs do not change on reaching an eighteenth birthday and the young person may be vulnerable to becoming homeless without the right support and transition planning.

support. This is particularly important in cases such as Philomena's, where the young person has needs in relation to social care, attachment, mood disorders and substance use. NICE [50] provides guidance for young people transitioning with health or social care needs. Philomena required joined up care that offered her support as she moved into adult life (see Case Study 15.2).

Conclusion

Young offenders including those with neurodevelopmental impairments are a vulnerable group of young people. Ideally, their well-being needs will be identified at an earlier age with the advent of increasing awareness in education of the impact of adverse childhood events. However, there is much work to be done. The impact of COVID-19 is starting to become clearer. Families seen in child and adolescent mental health settings report an impact on finances, relationships, access to food, technology and adult supervision. There is a responsibility for all adults working with children to look for early signs of adverse childhood events. Furthermore, adults working with young offenders must emphasise that the professional networks supporting them can provide opportunities to address unmet needs in relation to education, health and well-being. Contact with the youth justice system can provide a final chance to engage with systems, address any identified neurodevelopmental impairments, physical health needs and re-engage with education and training.

References

1. Scottish Government. The Kilbrandon Report. 2003. Available at: www.gov.scot/pu blications/kilbrandon-report/pages/4.

2. Scottish Government. The children's hearings system in Scotland: training resource manual, volume 2. 2013. Available at: www.gov.scot/binaries/con tent/documents/govscot/publications/ad vice-and-guidance/2013/04/training-resource-manual-volume-2-childrens-hearings-handbook/documents/0041942 0-pdf/00419420-pdf/govscot%3Adocum ent/00419420.pdf.

3. Dickens C. *Oliver Twist*. Richard Bentley, 1837–1839.

4. Welsh I. *Trainspotting*. Secker & Warburg, 1993.

5. Hughes N, Williams H, Chitsabesan P, Davies R, Mounce L. Nobody made the connection: the prevalence of learning disability in young people who offend. 2012. Available at: www.childrenscommis sioner.gov.uk/publication/nobody-made-t he-connection.

6. Crenshaw K. Demarginalizing the intersection of race and sex: a black feminist critique of antidiscrimination doctrine, feminist theory and antiracist politics. (University of Chicago Legal Forum 1989, Issue 1, Article 8). Available at: https://chi cagounbound.uchicago.edu/cgi/viewcon tent.cgi?article=1052&context=uclf.

7. Youth Justice Board/Ministry of Justice. Youth justice statistics 2019–20 England and Wales. Available at: https://assets .publishing.service.gov.uk/government/uplo ads/system/uploads/attachment_data/file/95 6621/youth-justice-statistics-2019-2020.pdf.

8. Youth Justice Board/Ministry of Justice. Assessing the needs of sentenced children in the youth justice system. 2020. Available at: www.gov.uk/government/statistics/asse ssing-the-needs-of-sentenced-children-in-the-youth-justice-system.

9. Center for American Progress, Movement Advancement Project and Youth First. UNJUST: LGBTQ youth incarcerated in the juvenile justice system. Available at: www.lgbtmap.org/file/lgbtq-incarcerated-youth.pdf.

10. Ministry of Justice. Prisoner transgender statistics: March to April 2016. Available at: https://assets.publishing.service.gov.uk/go vernment/uploads/system/uploads/attach

ment_data/file/567053/prisoner-transgender-statistics-march-april-2016.pdf.

11. National Institute for Health and Care Excellence. Drug misuse prevention: targeted interventions. NICE guideline [NG64]. 2017 Available at: www.nice.org.uk/guidance/ng64.

12. British Medical Association. Young lives behind bars: the health and human rights of children and young people detained in the criminal justice system. Available at: www.bma.org.uk/media/1861/bma-young-lives-behind-bars-2014.pdf.

13. Fazel S, Khosla V, Doll H, Geddes J. The prevalence of mental disorders among the homeless in Western countries: systematic review and meta-regression analysis. PLoS Medicine 2008; 5(12): e225.

14. Wiesner M, Windle M. Young adult substance use and depression as a consequence of delinquency trajectories during middle adolescence. Journal of Research on Adolescence 2006; 16: 239–64.

15. McKinlay W, Forsyth A, Khan F. Alcohol and violence among young male offenders in Scotland (1979–2009). Available at: www.sps.gov.uk/Corporate/Publications/Publication-2677.aspx.

16. Chitsabesan P, Kroll L, Bailey S, Kenning C, Sneider S, MacDonald W, et al. Mental health needs of young offenders in custody and in the community. British Journal of Psychiatry 2006; 188: 534–40.

17. Sanislow C, Grilo C, Fehon D, Axelrod SR, McGlashan TH. Correlates of suicide risk in juvenile detainees and adolescent inpatients, Journal of the American Academy of Child and Adolescent Psychiatry 2003; 42(2): 234–40.

18. Putnins L. Correlates and predictors of self-reported suicide attempts among incarcerated youths. International Journal of Offender Therapy and Comparative Criminology 2005; 49(2): 143–57.

19. Beaudry G, Yu R, Långström N, Fazel S. An updated systematic review and meta-regression analysis: mental disorders among adolescents in juvenile detention and correctional facilities. Journal of the American Academy of Child and Adolescent Psychiatry 2021; 60(1): 46–60.

20. Department of Health. Healthy children, safer communities: a strategy to promote the health and wellbeing of children and young people in contact with the youth justice system. Available at: www.ryantunnardbrown.com/wp-content/uploads/2012/11/HCSC-strategy1.pdf.

21. Gov.UK. Age of criminal responsibility. Available at: www.gov.uk/age-of-criminal-responsibility.

22. Department of Health. Future in mind. Available at: https://assets.publishing.service.gov.uk/government/uploads/system/uploads/attachment_data/file/414024/Childrens_Mental_Health.pdf.

23. Hughes N, Chitsabesan P. Supporting young people with neurodevelopmental impairment. 2015. Available at: www.crimeandjustice.org.uk/sites/crimeandjustice.org.uk/files/Supporting%20young%20people%20with%20neurodevelopmental%20impairment.pdf.

24. NHS England. Liaison and diversion standard service specification 2019. Available at: www.england.nhs.uk/wp-content/uploads/2019/12/national-liaison-and-diversion-service-specification-2019.pdf.

25. Mental Health Act 1983. Available at: www.legislation.gov.uk/ukpga/1983/20/contents.

26. Crime and Disorder Act 1998. Available at: www.legislation.gov.uk/ukpga/1998/37/contents.

27. Youth Justice Board. AssetPlus model document. 2014. Available at: https://assets.publishing.service.gov.uk/government/uploads/system/uploads/attachment_data/file/364092/AssetPlus_Model_Document_1_1_October_2014.pdf.

28. Hampson C, Youth justice in a pandemic: the situation in England and Wales. Available at: https://blogs.lse.ac.uk/socialpolicy/2020/07/24/youth-justice-in-a-pandemic-the-situation-in-england-and-wales.

29. Gov.UK. Lammy review: an independent review into the treatment of, and outcomes

for Black, Asian and minority ethnic individuals in the criminal justice system. 2017. Available at: www.gov.uk/government/publications/lammy-review-final-report.

30. Chitsabesan P, Lennox C, Theodosiou L, Bailey S, Shaw J. The development of the comprehensive health assessment tool for young offenders within the secure estate. *The Journal of Forensic Psychiatry and Psychology* 2014; 25: 1–25.

31. Bailey S, Shaw J, Tarbuck P, et al. Mental health care pathways for juveniles and young persons in the criminal justice system. 2008 Department of Health, London (unpublished).

32. Lennox C, Theodosiou, L. Comprehensive health screening and assessment for young people in the secure estate. 3rd EFCAP Congress. 7–9 March 2012, Berlin.

33. Chitsabesan P, Lennox C, Williams H, Tariq O, Shaw J. Traumatic brain injury in juvenile offenders: Findings from the comprehensive health assessment tool study and the development of a specialist link worker service. *Journal of Head Trauma Rehabilitation* 2015; 30(2): 106–15.

34. Youth Justice Board. Deaths of children in custody: action taken, lessons learnt. 2014. Available at: https://assets.publishing.service.gov.uk/government/uploads/system/uploads/attachment_data/file/362715/deaths-children-in-custody.pdf.

35. Kroll L, Rothwell J, Bradley D, Bailey S, Harrington RC. Mental health needs of boys in secure care for serious or persistent offending: a prospective, longitudinal study. *Lancet.* 2002; 359(9322): 1975–9.

36. Black C. Review of drugs: evidence relating to drug use, supply and effects, including current trends and future risks. 2020. Available at: https://assets.publishing.service.gov.uk/government/uploads/system/uploads/attachment_data/file/882953/Review_of_Drugs_Evidence_Pack.pdf.

37. Youth Justice Board. Key characteristics of admissions to youth custody: April 2014 to March 2016. Available at: https://assets.publishing.service.gov.uk/government/uploads/system/uploads/attachment_data/file/585991/key-characteristics-of-admissions-april-2014-to-march-2016.pdf.

38. National Treatment Agency for Substance Misuse. Young people's substance misuse treatment services: essential elements. 2005. Available at: www.drugsandalcohol.ie/6223/1/documental_2657_en.pdf.

39. HM Inspectorate of Probation. The work of youth offending teams to protect the public. 2017. Available at: www.justiceinspectorates.gov.uk/hmiprobation/wp-content/uploads/sites/5/2017/10/The-Work-of-Youth-Offending-Teams-to-Protect-the-Public_reportfinal.pdf.

40. National Crime Agency. The cyber threat to UK business. 2017. Available at: www.nationalcrimeagency.gov.uk/who-we-are/publications/178-the-cyber-threat-to-uk-business-2017-18/file.

41. Offender Health Research Network. Manual for the Comprehensive Health Assessment Tool (CHAT): young people in the secure estate. Available at: https://sites.manchester.ac.uk/hjrn/.

42. Khan L, Wilson J. *You Just Get on and Do It: Healthcare Provision in Youth Offending Teams.* Centre for Mental Health, 2010.

43. Dent M, Peto L, Griffin M. Forensic child and adolescent mental health services (FCAMHS): a map of current national provision and a proposed service model for the future. Final Report for the Department of Health. 2013. Available at: www.sph.nhs.uk/wp-content/uploads/2017/07/FCAMHS-Report-24-Jan-2013-Final-Version.pdf.

44. Gibson J, Evennett J. Child not brought to appointment. *British Journal of General Practice* 2017; 67(662): 397.

45. National Institute for Health and Care Excellence. Drug misuse in over 16s: psychosocial interventions. Clinical guideline [CG51]. 2007. Available at: www.nice.org.uk/guidance/cg51/resources.

46. National Institute for Health and Care Excellence. Drug misuse in over 16s: opioid detoxification. Clinical guideline [CG52]. 2007. Available at: www.nice.org.uk/guidance/cg52/resources.

47. National Institute for Health and Care Excellence. Vaccine uptake in under 19s. Quality standard [QS145]. 2017. Available at: www.nice.org.uk/guidance/qs145/chap ter/Quality-statement-5-Checking-immunisation-status-of-young-offenders-and-offering-outstanding-vaccinations.

48. National Institute for Health and Care Excellence. Attention deficit hyperactivity disorder: diagnosis and management. NICE guideline [NG87]. Available at: www.nice.org.uk/guidance/ng87.

49. Intagliata J. Improving the quality of community care for the chronically mentally disabled: the role of case management. *Schizophrenia Bulletin* 1982; 8(4): 655–74.

50. National Institute for Health and Care Excellence Transition from children's to adults' services for young people using health or social care services. NICE guideline [NG43] 2016. Available at: www.nice.org.uk/guidance/ng43.

Criminal Justice Pathways and Neurodevelopmental Disorders

Andrew Forrester, Iain McKinnon and Samir Srivastava

Introduction

In healthcare, it is now standard practice to use a pathways approach to design, organise and deliver services. Care pathways approaches first appeared in the 1970s, then were implemented in the 1980s, and in the decades that followed they have developed considerably and reshaped the way in which we conceptualise healthcare provision [1, 2]. According to the widely accepted definition described by Vissers and Beech, care pathways operate at five distinct levels, each of which are necessary to the overall provision of optimal care. These five levels include: care planning at an individual level; organising and planning care for groups of patients in so-called care pathways; planning the delivery of clinical and non-clinical staff and associated resource, including equipment and clinics; planning for patient volume and the interventions they require; and long-term, or strategic, planning for organisations [1, 3]. As these concepts have continued to develop, pathways, which are often summarised in easily understood flowcharts, have become a standard way to consider the delivery of care in specific clinical areas. The UK's National Institute for Health and Care Excellence (NICE), for example, has produced such pathways for a wide range of conditions and services, from clinical issues as diverse as acne, delirium and varicose veins, to service-related issues such as safe staffing for nurses and workplace health. Clinical pathways similarly exist for a wide range of mental health conditions, such as anxiety, attention deficit hyperactivity disorder (ADHD), learning disabilities, and schizophrenia, and one particular service area – the health of people in the criminal justice system – has been allocated their own guidelines in recognition of the special circumstances arising in the criminal justice system, and the existing evidence base within this specialist field [4, 5].

Therefore, there is now clear recognition that the delivery of healthcare services in the criminal justice system itself is a specialist area, with sufficient differences from generic service provision to generate specific pathway requirements. While this is, in and of itself, helpful within the field, it is also the case that the apparent journeys taken by people through services as they enter, navigate and exit criminal justice systems do not easily lend themselves to pathways thinking. This is because people generally enter the criminal justice system via community settings, such as the street or their homes, before they then arrive in police custody, are dealt with through the court system, enter prison if sent there on remand or after receiving a sentence, and may then be released back to the community, often under the management of probation services. This movement, or journey, through the system, can be thought of as a pathway in which each distinct element requires its own set of procedures for clinical assessment and intervention [5, 6].

However, this criminal justice system pathway is not a unitary phenomenon; it is not as seamless as it first appears, nor as neat as a diagrammatic flowchart may make it appear.

This is because the precise routes taken by people as they journey through the criminal justice system can vary considerably. For example, they may have contact with police in the street following an incident, but not be arrested, or they may enter police custody only to be released, while others may go on to be formally charged. Then, some may be bailed, while others go on to attend court, where they could be released, convicted or remanded into prison custody, and some may be diverted to hospital care, or to other alternatives to custody. They may remain in prison while on remand (pre-trial) and unconvicted, after conviction while awaiting sentencing or while serving a subsequent prison sentence. And, of course, they can be released if, for example, charges are dropped, or a community sentence is applied. Finally, some may then be released to the community and come under the management of probation services, while others may undergo further charges, or simultaneously await trial for one offence, while serving a sentence for another. In summary, there are myriad potential routes that individuals may take through the criminal justice system, even though these routes exist within an over-arching framework, or skeleton, that is provided by a contextual pathway such as that outlined in Figure 16.1.

Yet despite these variegated journeys taken by people entering the criminal justice system, it would be refreshingly simple if we only had to consider movement through the system itself as sufficient evidence of a pathway. Instead, however, we also must think of the particular health and social care needs of individuals, and bear in mind the need for different interventions depending upon the presenting clinical need (see Case Study 16.1). For

Pathways

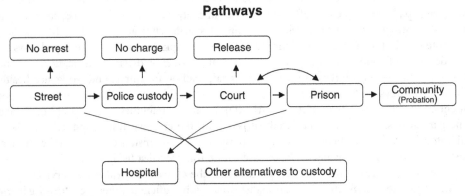

Figure 16.1 Potential routes in the criminal justice system.

Case Study 16.1

A 23-year-old man was arrested for shoplifting and taken into police custody. While there, he was formally charged with an offence of shoplifting and transferred to a lower magistrates' court to be further dealt with. During this process, he was identified as presenting with a learning disability necessitating the support of an appropriate adult while he was questioned in police custody. Although he was fit to plead, his condition also adversely impacted upon his effective participation in the court process. After allowances were made for this, he pleaded guilty as charged and received a community order, to be managed under an officer of probation. He was therefore released from court and returned to the community, under the specific requirements of his community order.

example, acute alcohol withdrawal or serious head injuries can be life threatening, and may therefore require immediate intervention, while others with chronic but stable conditions may only require that this is recorded, and their treatment continued in the community if not sent to prison [7]. However, throughout the criminal justice system, people often present with relatively high levels of clinical complexity and comorbidity, meaning that an extra layer of vigilance is necessary to ensure identification [8]. For that purpose, specific screens are recommended at points of entry into police custody and prisons, so that clinical conditions can be identified and then managed accordingly [9, 10]. For prisons in particular, such screens are a core minimum international standard, and simply must be offered [11].

In considering how best to apply clinical pathways and their associated standards within the criminal justice system, it is necessary to consider the overall numbers involved. Internationally, almost 12 million people are said to be detained in prisons, their total number having increased by around a quarter (25%) since the year 2000. The vast majority (93%) are men, although the population of female prisoners has been increasing at a faster rate. There are very substantial difference across regions of the world, with a global average imprisonment rate of 152 per 100,000 people. Up to a third of the world's total prison population are detained on a remand, or pre-trial, basis, meaning that they have not been found guilty, and very many people are held in unsuitable and overcrowded conditions [12].

Among this population, levels of mental health conditions are considerably higher than they are in the general population, and prisoners also present with increased levels of harm, including self-harm, suicide and violence [13]. Although there are limitations to our knowledge regarding the specific prevalence of neurodevelopmental conditions, the literature indicates that between 0.5% and 1.5% of prisoners present with intellectual disability (ID) [14]. The journeys taken by many of these people as they pass through the criminal justice system are essentially unknown and largely undescribed, however we do know that substantial diagnostic comorbidity – including major mental illness and substance use disorders – is present [15, 16]. There is a high estimated prevalence of ADHD, identified in over a quarter (25.5%) of incarcerated populations [17]. This group also presents with increased rates of comorbid psychiatric disorders, compounding the difficulties they experience [18]. Less is known about the prevalence of autism spectrum disorder (ASD) amongst people in the criminal justice system [19], screening projects having suggested both very low levels [20] and much higher levels [21]. Although we do not know the specific prevalence of ASD amongst people in prison, or the wider criminal justice system, at the moment, we do know that they may experience difficulty coping at each stage of their journey through the system, and this area is therefore one in which greater academic attention is now urgently required [22].

Although all the various neurodevelopmental conditions are considered together for the purposes of this chapter, and within the context of the journeys people take through the criminal justice system, it is important to acknowledge that they are, of course, very distinct conditions. A full description of these disorders is beyond the remit of this piece, and can easily be found elsewhere, but it does not take much imagination to realise, for example, that a person with ID may present with a range of issues that can be most unlike those presented by an individual with ADHD. While there is, of course, some diagnostic cross-over and co-occurrence between these conditions, care pathways need to be sufficiently robust, yet sufficiently nuanced, to identify differences between conditions, and between individuals, then manage them accordingly [2, 23]. Tailoring such services to the presentation and needs of each individual is challenging, given volume considerations within the criminal justice system, yet ensuring the implementation of a systematic operational approach to the identification and management of people with mental health conditions is the aim, whether they present with mental illness, a wider range of mental health conditions or specific neurodevelopmental conditions [24, 25].

Having therefore identified the aim, the remainder of this chapter is devoted to considering how to achieve it within the criminal justice system. Internationally, this is very much still a piece of work in progress, and while it seems that nowhere has yet got this completely right, it is also apparent that there are considerable differences in approach between countries and regions of the world. While holding this global context in mind, it is now important to consider parts of the criminal justice system in turn, to attempt to understand what we currently know, and what we do not, then try to use what knowledge we do have for the betterment of care pathways in this specific field.

Police Custody

As in other parts of criminal justice system, the available literature describes high levels of morbidity amongst people who enter police custody, but with one key difference – at the point when they enter the criminal justice system, this population is more likely to present with acute health conditions necessitating urgent intervention. These presentations have the potential to run the full gamut of conditions, from acute medical conditions such as head injuries or stab wounds, to more chronic physical health conditions such as asthma or epilepsy [7]. They may also include substance use disorders – such as acute intoxication, dependence or withdrawal, which can complicate the process of clinical assessment – and many present with mental health conditions, with suicidality in 16–18% of cases [7, 26, 27]. Significant numbers present with ID, likely between 4% and 7% [26, 28, 29], while rates of ADHD have been estimated as similar to prison samples, at 23.5% [29].

There is therefore an exceptional need to be vigilant when first assessing, or screening, this group; however, the literature regarding police healthcare screening is presently limited and, where screening mechanisms do exist, they may be unfit for purpose [30]. Yet it is clear that full operational clinical pathways cannot function without high-quality screening, for which there is good research evidence at the point of entry to the criminal justice system, and screening for ID in particular is known to be beneficial [31]. Therefore, the ability to adequately screen is presently a significant limitation to care pathways planning in police custody, not just for people with neurodevelopmental conditions, but across the whole range of clinical conditions. It is an area that requires urgent research prioritisation [32].

Mental health services operate in police custody in different ways across the world; however, in some countries, so-called liaison and diversion services are now in place. In England and Wales, these services operate in police custody and the lower magistrates' courts, and their aim is to identify people with mental health and neurodevelopmental conditions, liaise widely with other involved organisations and individuals (e.g., community mental health teams, general practitioners, voluntary sector agencies, families). Thereby they both obtain information to fully inform their assessment and communicate information to the court about the presenting conditions and any risk they may present, and divert people away from the criminal justice system where this is appropriate [33]. Diversion is an activity that is potentially wide in scope; for those presenting with acute conditions, it may involve compulsory admission to secure hospitals, while for others it may involve diversion away to community sentences, including community orders incorporating mental health

---

Case Study 16.2

A 52-year-old man arrived in police custody, where he was to be questioned regarding an alleged rape. He was seen by mental health services and identified as presenting with both ID and co-occurring ASD. He had been known to specialist services for most of his life. Despite his ID, he was found fit for interview, and he was questioned by police officers in the presence of an appropriate adult. During the interview, he made a number of statements indicating his guilt. Later, during the court process, a clinical psychologist acting as an expert witness found that he was highly suggestible and compliant at interview. This meant that the police interviews, which had been an important part of the prosecution case made against him, could not be used. The charges were dropped and he was released from court.

---

treatment requirements, drug treatment requirements or other probation requirements [34]. However, although there is increasing understanding of the effectiveness of mental health services [35], it remains the case that relatively little is known about the presentations of people with neurodevelopmental conditions within them. Yet within police custody, in particular, a number of issues arise that are of potential concern, including questions about mental capacity and fitness to be detained, fitness for interview and, in some cases, problems arising from suggestibility and compliance (see Case Study 16.2). Fitness for interview may require careful examination and documentation [36], not least because information obtained as a result of these interviews may be used during the process of prosecution, including subsequently during a criminal trial [37]. Similarly, issues relating to interrogative suggestibility and compliance may arise when some people with neurodevelopmental conditions and associated vulnerabilities yield under questioning. Suggestibility has been defined as 'the extent to which, within a closed social interaction, people come to accept messages communicated during formal questioning, as the result of which their subsequent behavioural response is affected', while compliance has been defined as 'the tendency of the individual to go along with propositions, requests or instructions, for some immediate instrumental gain' [38, 39].

Overall, although it is apparent that mental health services in police custody have improved over the last decade or more, at least in some jurisdictions it remains the case that much needs to be done to improve the identification and management of people with neurodevelopmental conditions at the point when they enter the criminal justice system. Nonetheless, from the perspective of care pathways, the introduction of services, and the resulting improved liaison, does at least mean that those presenting with the highest risk are more likely to receive care. These services are not yet sufficiently nuanced to cater in full for the wide range of neurodevelopmental conditions that may present, and further work – both research and service development – is now required to move this forward.

Court

In most jurisdictions, court systems are organised into lower and upper courts, with the lower courts dealing with the majority of – usually lower-level – criminal charges, and the upper courts dealing with the smaller number of more serious charges. For the purposes of this chapter, while we are considering pathways in the criminal justice system, we will mainly refer to the lower, or magistrates' courts. That is not because presentations in the upper, or Crown, courts are unimportant, but rather because the work done in these settings is mainly the result of expert witness assessments, and they are not the places of first presentation within the criminal justice system.

In some jurisdictions, mental health services have been developed in lower court settings [40]. In England and Wales, in particular, these services are designed to be continuous with the liaison and diversion services operating in police custody, to ensure service integration and the best possible communication [33]. These services also encounter high levels of psychiatric morbidity [41], and of neurodevelopmental disorders where specific screening takes place [42], which is perhaps unsurprising given that they receive much of their population directly from police custody. However, specialist service provision for people with neurodevelopmental conditions is few and far between, with variations between jurisdictions, and it is therefore likely that many such people go unidentified as they pass through the courts [43].

Yet, as in police custody, a number of important issues arise in court settings, many of which are relevant to people with neurodevelopmental conditions – including the effective participation of vulnerable accused persons, fitness to plead (which technically only becomes an issue later in the upper courts but can nonetheless be identified and planned for early) and arrangements for disposal and diversion [44, 45]. While effective participation and fitness to plead can become issues in cases in which mental capacity is reduced or absent, such as those involving some people with ID, it is necessary to consider presentations on a case-by-case basis to determine how best to proceed. From a clinical perspective, mental state assessment, informed by background clinical review, and an assessment of mental capacity when required, are key components of these determinations; yet they can be difficult to complete in full when appropriate specialist expertise is not available. Similarly, diversion away from custody requires first that the relevant individual's underlying neurodevelopmental condition has been appropriately identified and, second, that receiving services exist which are willing to receive the diversion, whether in hospital or community settings (see Case Study 16.3). Despite progress, many of these areas remain challenging, and it is still the case that we simply do not currently know what journeys most people with neurodevelopmental conditions take as they travel through the courts. Although there is early evidence that the use of specialist services can assist with the identification of conditions, and perhaps ultimately with encouraging alternatives to custodial remands, this remains an area in which much more needs to be done before we can be confident that our services are as effective as they should be [43, 46].

Case Study 16.3

A 32-year-old woman attended the magistrates' court, charged with assault. She had a known history of ID and dependence upon alcohol and multiple substances. In the community, she had been coerced into prostitution, and she had not engaged with clinical services that could have offered her support. At court, she was thought to have sufficient mental capacity to make major decisions; however, she was very vulnerable and at risk of further harm in the community. She was bailed to supported accommodation, to be reviewed by primary care and appropriate voluntary sector services. Finally, the case was disposed of via a community order, which allowed her to be supported using a framework including a drug rehabilitation requirement and specified accommodation.

Prison

Given the high levels of mental health and neurodevelopmental conditions amongst prisoners [13, 14, 16, 17], it is important to ensure that appropriate interventions and services are available for the purposes of identification, assessment and clinical management. In clinical pathways terms, the point of entry into prison, at prison reception, is the first point at which identification becomes possible, and it is internationally accepted that screening must be done at this point [12, 13]. This should ideally include screening for neurodevelopmental conditions, because we know that such screening is necessary for recognition [47]. After screening has been completed, clinical pathways models become relevant, with one such model – the STAIR (screening, triage, assessment, intervention and reintegration) model– describing the various stages of health engagement for prisoners [24, 25]. Although this model was not designed for people with neurodevelopmental conditions, the stages described apply equally to this population. After screening has been done, it is operationally necessary to review the result and subject them to a form of triage, to determine who will then require specialist assessment. Then, once a full assessment has been completed, it is possible to plan treatments and interventions, and later, at the point of release from prison, planning for community reintegration takes place.

However, while this theoretical pathway sounds relatively smooth, and understanding how it might apply to people with neurodevelopmental conditions appears straightforward, it is also important to consider the relative under-supply of services for people with neurodevelopmental conditions in prisons. We do not know how many prisons provide specialist clinics for ID, ASD or ADHD, or how these specialist services interact with other primary or secondary care services in these settings. However, the available literature, combined with our own clinical knowledge, leads us to the view that these specialist services are likely provided on a patchy basis, probably dependent upon local interests and other factors, and service evaluations and descriptions are hardly available [48]). Instead, we think it is likely that much of this care is picked up by generic services that lack specific knowledge in this area. While all of this is hardly conducive to the best possible pathways care, and it is not in keeping with the underpinning principle of equivalent care for prisoners, we do know that the aim of service provision should be to deliver the best quality care on a multidisciplinary basis, and that this should include medication when required, regular clinical support and psychological interventions if indicated [49, 50]. At present, it is the case that considerable amounts of clinical need remain unmet, thereby limiting the utility and application of pathways approaches in this field.

When implemented, these multidisciplinary care arrangements need to take into account a number of issues of potential relevance to people with neurodevelopmental conditions in prisons. Bullying is common in prisons, but often hidden, and people with neurodevelopmental conditions are particularly at risk [51]. Gang activity is also prevalent, often relating to the supply of drugs within an illicit internal market, and coercive activities relating to this supply and demand can involve vulnerable people [52] (see Case Study 16.4). Much of daily life in prison requires self-advocacy, or standing up for yourself, whether it involves keeping a place in the rowdy medication queue, or ensuring that you receive your allocated gym, shower or telephone time – and, in such circumstances, many vulnerable people can struggle and be left behind [15, 53]. Clinically, proper account needs to be taken of coexisting conditions and vulnerabilities, which are common and may include other mental health and neurodevelopmental conditions, substance use disorders and self-harm

Case Study 16.4

A 46-year-old man with ID was sentenced to 15 years for offences of rape and false imprisonment. After spending an initial period on remand, he was transferred to another prison to serve his sentence. While there, he was coerced into giving his medication to another prisoner. Fearing for his safety, he felt unable to reveal this information. His mental state deteriorated, such that he became seriously depressed and attempted suicide.

or suicidality [54]. And finally, special approaches to prisoner discipline, including the giving or removal of privileges, or segregation, should not be used for people who are thought to be 'at risk' in prisons [55]. Yet very little is presently known about the characteristics of people who are subject to these conditions, and we cannot be fully assured that people with neurodevelopmental conditions are not swept up in them from time to time. Therefore, this is a further area in which more research is required if we are to have optimal clinical pathways within our prisons.

Conclusion

Although we now know a great deal about how to best provide joined-up services within criminal justice settings, it has too often been the case that service provision has lagged behind the theory. We know, for example, that screening plays a key role within the criminal justice system, particularly in police custody and at prison reception, and we understand that multidisciplinary and specialist care is the best way to ensure quality provision. However, we have yet to resolve basic screening requirements in some parts of the criminal justice system, particularly in police custody, multidisciplinary teams are often not fully provided, and specialist care for people with neurodevelopmental conditions cannot presently be assured. At a very basic level, we need to understand what services are provided, and where, and what level of expertise they offer. If we do this, then start to ensure that specialist services for people with ID, ASD and ADHD are planned and organised within the criminal justice system, then we will be able to ensure clinical and care pathways that are fit for purpose. Until such times, it is unfortunately the case that we can only provide these services for an unrepresentative number of people, while the journeys taken by many others remain essentially unknown and unreferenced.

References

1. Schrijvers G, van Hoorn A, Huiskes N. The care pathway: concepts and theories: an introduction. *International Journal of Integrated Care* 2012; 12: e192.

2. Kinsman L, Rotter T, James E, Snow P, Willis J. What is a clinical pathway? Development of a definition to inform the debate. *BMC Medicine* 2010; 8(1): 1–3.

3. Vissers J, Beech R. *Health Operations Management*. Routledge, 2004.

4. National Institute for Health and Care Excellence. Physical health of people in prison. Available from: www.nice.org.uk/guidance/ng57.

5. National Institute for Health and Care Excellence. Mental health of adults in contact with the criminal justice system. Available from: www.nice.org.uk/guidance/ng66.

6. Forrester A, Hopkin G. Mental health in the criminal justice system: a pathways

approach to service and research design. *Criminal Behaviour and Mental Health* 2019; 29(4): 207–17.

7. McKinnon IG, Thomas SD, Noga HL, Senior J. Police custody health care: a review of health morbidity, models of care and innovations within police custody in the UK, with international comparisons. *Risk Management and Healthcare Policy.* 2016; 9: 213.

8. Fazel S, Baillargeon J. The health of prisoners. *Lancet* 2011; 377(9769): 956–65.

9. McKinnon I, Grubin D. Health screening in police custody. *Journal of Forensic and Legal Medicine* 2010; 17(4): 209–12.

10. Martin MS, Colman I, Simpson AI, McKenzie K. Mental health screening tools in correctional institutions: a systematic review. *BMC Psychiatry* 2013; 13(1): 275.

11. United Nations. United Nations standard minimum rules for the treatment of prisoners (the Nelson Mandela Rules). 2015. Available at: www.unodc.org/docu ments/justice-and-prison-reform/Nelson_ Mandela_Rules-E-ebook.pdf.

12. United Nations Office on Drugs and Crime. Data matters. Available at: www.unodc.org/ documents/data-and-analysis/statistics/Dat aMatters1_prison.pdf.

13. Fazel S, Hayes AJ, Bartellas K, Clerici M, Trestman R. Mental health of prisoners: prevalence, adverse outcomes, and interventions. *Lancet Psychiatry* 2016; 3(9): 871–81.

14. Fazel S, Xenitidis K, Powell J. The prevalence of intellectual disabilities among 12 000 prisoners: a systematic review. *International Journal of Law and Psychiatry* 2008; 31(4): 369–73.

15. Jones G, Talbot J. No one knows: the bewildering passage of offenders with learning disability and learning difficulty through the criminal justice system. *Criminal Behaviour and Mental Health* 2010; 20: 1.

16. Hassiotis A, Gazizova D, Akinlonu L, Bebbington P, Meltzer H, Strydom A. Psychiatric morbidity in prisoners with intellectual disabilities: analysis of prison survey data for England and Wales. *British Journal of Psychiatry* 2011; 199(2): 156–7.

17. Young S, Moss D, Sedgwick O, Fridman M, Hodgkins P. A meta-analysis of the prevalence of attention deficit hyperactivity disorder in incarcerated populations. *Psychological Medicine* 2015; 45(2): 247–58.

18. Young S, Sedgwick O, Fridman M, Gudjonsson G, Hodgkins P, Lantigua M et al. Co-morbid psychiatric disorders among incarcerated ADHD populations: a meta-analysis. *Psychological Medicine* 2015; 45(12): 2499–510.

19. Underwood L, Forrester A, Chaplin E, McCarthy J. Prisoners with neurodevelopmental disorders. *Journal of Intellectual Disabilities and Offending Behaviour* 2013; 4(1/2): 17–23.

20. Robinson L, Spencer MD, Thomson LD, Stanfield AC, Owens DG, Hall J, et al. Evaluation of a screening instrument for autism spectrum disorders in prisoners. *PLOS One.* 2012; 7(5): e36078.

21. Underwood L, McCarthy J, Chaplin E, Forrester A, Mills R, Murphy D. Autism spectrum disorder traits among prisoners. *Advances in Autism* 2016; 2(3): 106–17.

22. Robertson CE, McGillivray JA. Autism behind bars: a review of the research literature and discussion of key issues. *Journal of Forensic Psychiatry and Psychology* 2015; 26(6): 719–36.

23. Dewey D. What is comorbidity and why does it matter in neurodevelopmental disorders?. *Current Developmental Disorders Reports* 2018; 5(4): 235–42.

24. Forrester A, Till A, Simpson S, Shaw J. Mental illness and the provision of mental health services in prisons. *British Medical Bulletin* 2018; 127: 101–9.

25. Simpson AIF, Gerritsen C, Maheandiran M, Adamo V, Vogel T, Fulham L. A systematic review of reviews of correctional mental health services using the STAIR framework. *Frontiers in Psychiatry* 2018; 12: 747202.

26. Samele C, McKinnon I, Brown P, Srivastava S, Arnold A, Hallett N, et al. The prevalence of mental illness and unmet

needs of police custody detainees. *Criminal Behaviour and Mental Health* 2021; 31(2): 80–95.

27. Forrester A, Samele C, Slade K, Craig T, Valmaggia L. Suicide ideation amongst people referred for mental health assessment in police custody. *Journal of Criminal Psychology* 2016; 6(4): 146–56.

28. Forrester A, Samele C, Slade K, Craig T, Valmaggia L. Demographic and clinical characteristics of 1092 consecutive police custody mental health referrals. *Journal of Forensic Psychiatry and Psychology* 2017; 28 (3): 295–312.

29. Young S, Goodwin EJ, Sedgwick O, Gudjonsson GH. The effectiveness of police custody assessments in identifying suspects with intellectual disabilities and attention deficit hyperactivity disorder. *BMC Medicine* 2013; 11(1): 248.

30. McKinnon IG, Grubin D. Health screening of people in police custody: evaluation of current police screening procedures in London, UK. *European Journal of Public Health* 2013; 23(3): 399–405.

31. McKinnon I, Thorp J, Grubin D. Improving the detection of detainees with suspected intellectual disability in police custody. *Advances in Mental Health and Intellectual Disabilities* 2015; 9(4): 174–85.

32. Noga HL, Walsh EC, Shaw JJ, Senior J. The development of a mental health screening tool and referral pathway for police custody. *European Journal of Public Health* 2015; 25(2): 237–42.

33. NHS England and NHS Improvement. Liaison and diversion standard service specification 2019. Available at: www.eng land.nhs.uk/wp-content/uploads/2019/12/national-liaison-and-diversion-service-specification-2019.pdf.

34. Department of Health. The Bradley Report: Lord Bradley's review of people with mental health problems or learning disabilities in the criminal justice system. Available at: https://lx.iriss.org.uk/sites/default/files/resou rces/The%20Bradley%20report.pdf.

35. Scott DA, McGilloway S, Dempster M, Browne F, Donnelly M. Effectiveness of criminal justice liaison and diversion services for offenders with mental disorders: a review. *Psychiatric Services* 2013; 64(9): 843–9.

36. Gudjonsson G. 'Fitness for interview' during police detention: a conceptual framework for forensic assessment. *Journal of Forensic Psychiatry* 1995; 6(1): 185–97.

37. Stark M, Rix K. Fitness to be interviewed and fitness to be charged. In Stark M, eds., *Clinical Forensic Medicine*. Springer, 2020: 393–420.

38. Gudjonsson GH, Clark NK. Suggestibility in police interrogation: a social psychological model. *Social Behaviour* 1986; 1: 83–104.

39. Gudjonsson GH. *The Psychology of Interrogations and Confessions: A Handbook*. John Wiley & Sons Ltd, 2003.

40. James DV. Court diversion in perspective. *Australian and New Zealand Journal of Psychiatry* 2006; 40(6–7): 529–38.

41. Shaw J, Creed F, Price J, Huxley P, Tomenson B. Prevalence and detection of serious psychiatric disorder in defendants attending court. *Lancet* 1999; 353(9158): 1053–6.

42. Chaplin E, McCarthy J, Marshall-Tate K, Ali S, Xenitidis K, Childs J, Harvey D. Evaluation of a liaison and diversion court mental health service for defendants with neurodevelopmental disorders. *Research in Developmental Disabilities* 2021; 1(119): 104103.

43. McCarthy J, Chaplin E, Hayes S, Søndenaa E, Chester V, Morrissey C, et al. Defendants with intellectual disability and autism spectrum conditions: the perspective of clinicians working across three jurisdictions. *Psychiatry, Psychology and Law* 2021; 2: 1–20.

44. Gerry F, Cooper P. Effective participation of vulnerable accused persons: case management, court adaptation and rethinking criminal responsibility. *Journal of Judicial Administration* 2017; 1: 265–75.

45. Brown P. Unfitness to plead in England and Wales: historical development and contemporary dilemmas. *Medicine, Science and the Law* 2019; 59(3): 187–96.

46. Forrester A, Hopkin G, Bryant L, Slade K, Samele C. Alternatives to custodial remand for women in the criminal justice system: a multi-sector approach. *Criminal Behaviour and Mental Health* 2020; 30(2–3): 68–78.

47. Murphy GH, Gardner J, Freeman MJ. Screening prisoners for intellectual disabilities in three English prisons. *Journal of Applied Research in Intellectual Disabilities* 2017; 30(1): 198–204.

48. Patel R, Harvey J, Forrester A. Systemic limitations in the delivery of mental health care in prisons in England. *International Journal of Law and Psychiatry* 2018; 1; 60: 17–25.

49. National Institute for Health and Care Excellence. People with learning disabilities. Available at: www.nice.org.uk/guidance/population-groups/people-with-learning-disabilities.

50. Young S, Gudjonsson G, Chitsabesan P, Colley B, Farrag E, Forrester A, et al. Identification and treatment of offenders with attention-deficit/hyperactivity disorder in the prison population: a practical approach based upon expert consensus. *BMC Psychiatry* 2018; 18 (1): 1–6.

51. Ireland J. *Bullying Among Prisoners: Innovations in Theory and Research* Willan Publishing, 2005.

52. Maitra DR. 'If you're down with a gang inside, you can lead a nice life': prison gangs in the age of austerity. *Youth Justice* 2020; 20(1–2): 128–45.

53. Maxwell Y, Day A, Casey S. Understanding the needs of vulnerable prisoners: the role of social and emotional wellbeing. *International Journal of Prisoner Health* 2013; 9(2), 57–67.

54. McCarthy J, Chaplin E, Forrester A, Underwood L, Hayward H, Sabet J, et al. Prisoners with neurodevelopmental difficulties: vulnerabilities for mental illness and self-harm. *Criminal Behaviour and Mental Health* 2019; 29 (5–6): 308–20.

55. National Offender Management Service. Service specification for prison discipline and segregation: segregation of prisoners. Available at: https://assets.publishing.service.gov.uk/government/uploads/system/uploads/attachment_data/file/278911/2014-01-14_Segregation_of_Prisoners_Specification_P2_2.pdf.

The Mental Health Act and Other Relevant Legislation in Relation to Neurodevelopmental Disorders in the UK

Harm Boer, Eleanor Brewster and Ryan McHugh

Introduction

In the UK, different sources of law are relevant to people with intellectual disability (ID) and autism spectrum disorder (ASD), including international treaties (in particular the European Convention on Human Rights (ECHR)), acts of Parliament (statute law) including the Mental Health Act 1983 (England) [1], the Mental Health (Care and Treatment) (Scotland) Act 2003 [2], the Mental Capacity Act 2005 [3], codes of practice and common law.

England and Wales

Under King Edward II, an Act, De Prerogativa Regis, introduced a form of guardianship and allowed the king to take the possessions of people with ID, with an obligation to look after their affairs. In the past 250 years there have been more than 35 Acts of Parliament dealing with services for the mentally ill [4].

The Royal Commission on the Care and Control of the Feeble-minded in 1908 proposed a number of different classes of people of unsound mind to be placed under the general protection and supervision of the central authority including 'persons mentally infirm', 'idiots', 'imbiciles', 'feeble-minded' and 'moral imbiciles' [5]. Separate legislation for 'mental defectives' followed in the form of the Mental Deficiency Acts of 1913 and 1927.

In the 1950s advances in psychotropic medication in part led to the Percy Report [6] had the potential effect of decriminalising mental disorder. This included the introduction of Mental Health Review Tribunals, allowing the admission of mentally disordered offenders to hospital as an alternative to imprisonment and allowing the transfer of mentally disordered prisoners from prison to hospital [7].

The Mental Health Act 1983 (MHA) still has many of the basic principles of the Mental Health Act 1959 and has further safeguards for people with a mental disorder. The Act includes the phrase 'arrested or incomplete development of mind', which was derived from the Mental Deficiency Acts of 1913 and 1927. It was accepted by Parliament that people with learning disability may require detention in hospital as an alternative to imprisonment [7]. 'Arrested or incomplete development of mind' came to mean mental handicap in the MHA and 'learning disability' in the 2007 amendment of the MHA, in which it is used and defined.

The MHA contained two categories of arrested or incomplete development of mind, namely 'severe mental impairment' and 'mental impairment' and these phrases were replaced by 'learning disability'. Learning disability is defined in the MHA (as amended

2007) as 'a state of arrested or incomplete development of the mind which includes significant impairment of intelligence and social functioning'. In a further change introduced by the 2007 amendments, the definition of medical treatment was revised to include psychological treatment and treatment no longer needs to be under medical supervision.

Before the changes introduced to the MHA in 2007 [8], which came into force in November 2008, there had been a discussion as to whether it was correct for someone with a learning disability to come under the mental health legislation unless they also have a mental illness [9, 10]. The (English) MHA Code of Practice [1] (2015, paragraph 20.14, which shows professionals how to carry out their responsibilities under the MHA) recommends that unless in emergency it is not good practice to diagnose a person as having a learning disability associated with abnormally aggressive or seriously irresponsible behaviour without an assessment by a consultant psychiatrist in ID and a formal specialist psychological assessment, as part of a multidisciplinary team assessment, and in consultation with a relative, advocate or supporter of the person.

The definition of a mental disorder in the MHA is broad and includes ASD (without the need to specify abnormally aggressive or irresponsible behaviour).

Part II of the MHA

Part II of the MHA relates to the detention of patients in hospitals for the treatment of a mental disorder. Applications for Sections 2 and 3 are usually made by an approved mental health practitioner and require the written recommendation of two doctors. The definition of hospital for this purpose includes National Health Service (NHS) inpatient units, which can be a general or a mental health service, but also registered private or independent hospitals. Although it is the most used detention power [11], Section 2 is not often used in forensic services, but most secure units have a number of patients on section 3, particularly patients who have been referred from non-forensic hospital units or direct from the community, as opposed to court orders (see below).

Section 2 Admission for Assessment

Section 2 provides the power to admit and treat a patient who has or is thought to have a mental disorder in hospital for up to 28 days. The patient can be given treatment for a mental disorder with or without his or her consent.

Section 3 Admission for Treatment

Section 3 enables detention and treatment of a patient in hospital for up to six months and can be renewed (for six months, and then yearly). The patient can be given treatment for a mental disorder with or without his or her consent.

There are two community sections, guardianship (Section 7) and community treatment order (CTO) (Section 17A–G).

Guardianship

Guardianship is used as an alternative to admitting people to hospital and to enable discharge from hospital, particularly where the focus is on welfare rather than treatment, and there is little risk of the patient needing to be admitted to hospital against his or her will.

Community Treatment Order (Section 17A–G)

A CTO is a community-based section and is used when the responsible clinician needs the authority to recall the patient to hospital. A CTO can only be applied for if the patient is on a treatment order without restriction, such as Section 3 or 37. The effect is that the patient is not discharged from the original section, but the section is suspended and retriggered if the patient is readmitted.

Although CTOs appear to have been intended for patients who discontinue their medication on leaving the hospital, they have been used for patients with ID who, without such an order, would disengage from aftercare.

Part III of the MHA

Part III of the MHA deals with the circumstances in which patients may be admitted to and detained in hospital or received into guardianship on the order of a court, or may be transferred to hospital or guardianship from prison on the direction of the Secretary of Justice [12]. These are called sections relating to courts and prisons or forensic sections [13]. The court can only order admission to hospital under the MHA if the (alleged) offence is publishable by imprisonment. There does not need to be a connection between the disorder and the crime.

Section 3 Hospital Order

Section 37 can be imposed if the patient is convicted of an offence punishable with imprisonment (by the magistrates' court or Crown Court), or if the court is satisfied that he or she has committed the act or offence the patient has been charged with (by the magistrates' court) for a period of up to six months. This is renewable, initially for six months, and then for periods of a year. The patient suffers from a mental disorder of a nature or degree which makes it appropriate for him or her to be detained in hospital for treatment. Appropriate medical treatment must be available, and the court has to be of the opinion that this is the most suitable method of dealing with the patient. Two doctors are required to give oral or written evidence.

Section 37/41 Hospital Order with Restriction

Section 41 is a further order by the Crown Court to restrict the patient's discharge, transfer or his or her leave from hospital, unless agreed by the Secretary of State. The restriction is without limit of time. A judge can impose this further order 'when it appears to the court, having regard to the nature of the offence, the antecedents of the offender and the risk of his committing further offences if set at large, that it is necessary for the protection of the public from serious harm so to do'.

The main ways for the section to end is through discharge by a tribunal or by the Ministry of Justice. Most patients on Section 37/41 are conditionally discharged (at least initially). Once conditionally discharged, the patient has a medical and a social supervisor, and there are conditions attached to the discharge (such as where to reside, to agree to take medication, to abstain from alcohol and drugs, etc.).

Patients on Sections 47 and 48 also usually have a restriction order attached (Section 49). For patients on a restriction order (Sections 41 and 49), the responsible clinician cannot grant leave from hospital, transfer the patient to another hospital or unit, outside the boundaries of the hospital or unit named in the order, or discharge the patient.

Permission for leave outside the hospital grounds must be sought from the Ministry of Justice. Leave within the hospital grounds can be granted by the responsible clinician. This can cause problems; for instance, if the patient is formally admitted to a particular unit within the hospital, it may be difficult to determine what the hospital grounds are, and where possible it may be worth considering whether to request (in reports to the court when recommending a hospital order, and in transfer requests to the Ministry of Justice) that the patient is detained in the hospital rather than an individual unit, as this may help with ground leave and with transfer between hospital units where appropriate.

Patients who are in the community on a conditional discharge may be readmitted to hospital as an informal patient, but they may also be recalled by the Ministry of Justice, in which case he or she again becomes a restricted patient.

Patients who are detained in England or Wales under the Criminal Procedure (Insanity and Unfitness to Plead) Act 1991 [14] when found to be unfit to plead and found to have done the act(s) they have been charged with, can be detained as if they are under a Section 37 or Section 37/41 (hospital order with or without restriction).

Section 38 Interim Hospital Order

An interim hospital can be used to detain a patient who is convicted, initially for up to 12 weeks, renewable monthly for up to a maximum of one year. Either the magistrates' court or Crown Court can make the order for an offence punishable by imprisonment. The patient must have a mental disorder and there should be reason to suppose that the mental disorder from which he or she is suffering from is such that it may be appropriate for a hospital order to be made. The oral or written evidence from two doctors is needed, and the patient can be given treatment for a mental disorder with or without his or her consent.

Interim hospital orders can be surprisingly useful for those people with mild learning disability for whom a prison sentence would not be unthinkable, and where it is not initially clear whether he or she would cooperate with psychological treatment in order to reduce the risk of future offending.

Section 45A Hospital and Limitation Direction

Section 45A is also called a hybrid order and was added to the MHA for England and Wales in 1997, but it has been rarely used [13]. It is used when the Crown Court is considering making a Section 37 hospital order and allows a patient to be given both a prison sentence and a hospital order with restriction, at the same time. The patient is admitted to hospital, and if the responsible clinician decides that treatment is no longer needed or if treatment proves unsuccessful, the patient can be transferred (remitted by the Secretary of State) back to prison to serve the rest of his or her sentence. In hospital, the order has the same effect as Section 47/49. This 'power' was designed for patients whose responsibility for his or her actions, while diminished, remains high [12]. If the patient is still in hospital at the time of the automatic release day, the patient stays in hospital, but there will no longer be input from the Ministry of Justice, and the responsible clinician can discharge the patient. On discharge or release from prison, supervision is by the probation service.

Section 47 Transfer from Prison to Hospital

Section 47 enables the transfer of a sentenced prisoner to hospital, initially for up to six months, and has the same effect as a Section 37 hospital order once the patient is in hospital.

The order is nearly always made with a restriction order attached, and is then known as Section 47/49, and should the patient no longer require treatment in hospital, or no effective treatment can be given, the patient is usually returned to prison. If the patient is still in hospital when his or her sentence has expired, the restriction ends and, if the patient continues to be detained, the term 'notional hospital order' is sometimes used. This means that the patient is still under Section 47 (but not 49), and this has the same legal effect as a Section 37 hospital order [12' 15].

Section 48 Removal to Hospital of Unsentenced Prisoners

Section 48 refers to a transfer of an unsentenced prisoner. It requires recommendations from two doctors that the patient has a mental disorder which means that he or she should be in hospital for treatment, that there is an urgent need for treatment and that this treatment is available in hospital. In nearly all cases this is made with a restriction and is then known as Section 48/49.

Hospital Managers

Patients who are detained under the MHA have the right to appeal to hospital managers and to the First-tier Tribunal, also known as the Mental Health Tribunal. At a hearing, three hospital managers must agree in order for a patient to be discharged from hospital.

Tribunals

The First-tier Tribunal consists of a judge, a medical member and a specialist (lay) member. Most patients detained in a hospital (on Sections 2, 3, 37, 47 and 48), on a CTO, on a guardianship order or on a conditional discharge have a right to appeal.

The patient should be discharged by the Tribunal under Section 73 of the MHA if the he or she does not suffer from a mental disorder (in case of a patient with ID, this means that the ID is not associated with abnormally aggressive or seriously irresponsible behaviour); or the mental disorder is not of a nature or degree which makes it appropriate for him or her to be detained in hospital; or it is not necessary for the health or safety of the patient or for the protection of others that he or she should receive such treatment; or appropriate treatment is not available. A patient on a Section 41 restriction order should be given a conditional discharge if these conditions are met, but it remains appropriate for the patient to remain liable to be recalled to hospital for further treatment and given an absolute discharge if this condition is met.

In terms of outcomes, the Tribunal can make an adjournment, for instance if more information is needed; a discharge, a deferred discharge and a conditional discharge (for restricted patients). A patient may be discharged from his or her section and opt to stay in hospital as an informal patient. Zigmond and Brindle [15] give some helpful thoughts on writing reports and giving evidence.

Parole Boards

Patients under a Section 45A hybrid order or a Section 47 hospital transfer, who have received a life or indeterminate sentence, will need authorisation by the parole board before they can be released into the community. In such cases, if the Tribunal has recommended a conditional discharge (and the patient is eligible for parole) the parole board meets at the hospital and may allow the patient to be discharged into the community.

The Human Rights Law, Deprivation of Liberty and Liberty Protection Safeguards

The Deprivation of Liberty Safeguards (DoLS) were introduced in England and Wales following the Bournewood case [16]. DoLS have been incorporated in the Mental Capacity Act 2005 since 2008. Under DoLS, an independent assessor can authorise depriving a person of their liberty in a hospital or care home if granted by a supervisory body for the purpose of care and treatment if the patient (amongst others) is over 18, has a mental disorder, lacks capacity regarding the decision to accept care or treatment, is not under the MHA, and the deprivation of liberty is in his or her best interest or to prevent harm. There is a right to appeal to the High Court of Justice.

Liberty Protection Safeguards were introduced in the Mental Capacity (Amendment) Act 2019 [17], received Royal Assent on 19 May 2019, but at the time of writing a date for full implementation had not yet been agreed. This will have the effect of extending the settings in which safeguards are applicable from hospitals and care homes to supported living settings, and to reduce the number of assessments from six to three (capacity assessment, medical assessment and necessary and proportionate assessment). Local authorities and NHS bodies will be 'responsible bodies' under the Liberty Protection Safeguards.

Responsible bodies will organise the assessments needed under the scheme and ensure that there is sufficient evidence to justify a case for deprivation of liberty.

Conditional Discharge of Patients Who Lack Capacity

In November and December 2018, the Supreme Court handed down judgements in the MM [18] and PJ [19] cases. The effect of the MM case is that the Tribunal or the Ministry of Justice cannot impose a condition on a conditionally discharged patient which would amount to detention or a deprivation of liberty. Similarly, the Court stated that a Tribunal cannot impose conditions in a CTO which effectively deprive a patient of his or her liberty. For this purpose, deprivation of liberty is defined as 'under continuous supervision or control and not free to leave' (Lady Hale in the 'Cheshire West' case, in 2014 [20]).

Before 'Cheshire West' it was sometimes possible to argue in tribunals that although, if discharged, it would be necessary for the protection of others that he or she continue to be escorted by members of staff in the community, this would in practice not be a problem as the patient would be escorted in the community for reasons other than for the protection of others. Such reasons could include physical and cognitive disabilities. However, 'Cheshire West' made it clear that the purpose of the restrictions, the nature or extent of the patient's disability or care needs, their contentment or acquiescence and the quality of the care being provided are not relevant to the question of whether there is an objective deprivation of liberty.

If a patient lacks capacity to consent to his or her care, where he or she lives or treatment, it may be possible to conditionally discharge a patient under a DoLS or under an order of the Court of Protection.

The Mental Health Casework Section of the HM Prison and Probation Service provided guidance in January 2019 on patients who cannot be discharged, but whose risks can be safely managed in the community, and proposed that long-term leave under Section 17(3) of the MHA be considered.

MHA Codes of Practice

Wales and England have different Codes of Practice [1, 21]. The Welsh assembly made changes to the MHA in 2011 and 2012, including a duty to carry out mental health assessments and a statutory requirement to appoint a care coordinator with defined responsibilities.

White Paper

In January 2021, the government published the white paper reforming the MHA in response to the independent review of it, delivered by Sir Simon Wessely in 2018. In this document, the government accepted and proposed to take forward most of the recommendations of the independent review. The main change affecting people with ID ('learning disability') and ASD is that neither ID nor ASD would be considered to be a mental disorder for which someone can be detained for treatment under Section 3 of the MHA, which would mean that people with ID (whether or not they have abnormally aggressive or seriously irresponsible behaviour) and ASD could not be detained for longer than 28 days (under Section 2), and could not continue to be detained unless there is a co-occurring mental health condition. This change however will not apply to those detained under Part III of the MHA.

Scotland

Scotland has a distinct legal system. There are three areas of statute in Scotland which may be relevant to people with neurodevelopmental disorders and forensic presentations. While it is not the role of this chapter to comprehensively describe all relevant legislation, a summary of the main statutory provision is useful. These are:

The Mental Health (Care and Treatment) (Scotland) Act 2003 [2]

The Adults with Incapacity (Scotland) Act 2000 [22]

The Adult Support and Protection (Scotland) Act 2007 [23].

The Mental Health (Care and Treatment) (Scotland) Act 2003 allows for the compulsory treatment in hospital or the community of people with a mental disorder. Broadly, the Act can be invoked in cases where there is a mental disorder, the presence of significant risk to the person or others and where treatment is available that would prevent a deterioration in that person's condition or alleviate its symptoms or effects. The Act can either be used on a civil basis, in cases where a person has significantly impaired decision-making ability, or in criminal cases, where this criterion is not required. Regardless, the order must be deemed to be necessary. Orders can be made for up to 72 hours, up to 28 days and up to 6 months.

In Scotland, mental health orders are considered and determined by the Mental Health Tribunal, which allows scrutiny of orders, and provides patients with a right to appeal against orders, or to seek direction or the use of a 'recorded matter' if a required aspect of treatment is not being provided [24].

The Adults with Incapacity (Scotland) Act 2000 exists to enable decisions to be made around the well-being (including medical treatment) and financial affairs of people who lack capacity to make their decisions in those areas, either by reason of mental disorder, or an inability to communicate. Amongst other functions, this act enables guardianship powers, so that a named person, on behalf of the person who lacks capacity, can make decisions. It also describes Section 47 certificates, used in documenting capacity for consent to medical treatment for people with impaired capacity.

The Adult Support and Protection Act (Scotland) 2007 is designed to offer protection to adults who are unable to safeguard their own interests and are at risk of harm (including self-harm and neglect) because they are affected by disability, mental disorder, illness or physical or mental infirmity

The Act requires councils and various public bodies to work together to support and protect adults who are unable to safeguard themselves, their property and their rights.

Principles

These legislative instruments are based on stated principles, which generally are to be observed by people undertaking functions under the act. This provides clarity, and a rationale for dealing with uncertainty. Table 17.1 details some commonalities between the principles of these Acts, and Case Study 17.1 illustrates their use (note this does not represent a real patient).

Table 17.1 Commonalities between the principles of the three acts in Scotland

	Mental Health (Care and Treatment) (Scotland) Act 2003	Adults with Incapacity (Scotland) Act 2000	Adult Support and Protection (Scotland) Act 2007
Provide benefit that could not be achieved without the intervention		Y	Y
Least/minimal restriction	Y	Y	Y
Taking account of past and present wishes	Y	Y	Y
Taking account of nearest relative/carer/welfare guardian	Y	Y	Y
Participation and exercising skills	Y	Y	Y
Providing information to enable participation	Y		Y
Not being treated any less favourably than another adult/ someone who is not a patient would be in a comparable situation	Y		Y
Having regard to the persons abilities, background and characteristics	Y		Y
Providing the maximum benefit to the patient	Y		

Table 17.1 (cont.)

	Mental Health (Care and Treatment) (Scotland) Act 2003	Adults with Incapacity (Scotland) Act 2000	Adult Support and Protection (Scotland) Act 2007
Take account of the range of options available in the patient's case	Y		
Except for decisions about medical treatment, taking into account the needs and circumstances of the carer	Y		
Considering the right of the patient to confidentiality, and also the right of the carer to have a carer's needs assessment	Y		
Have regard to the importance of the provision of appropriate services to the person, who is, or has been subject to an order, including continuing care, where the person is no longer subject to the certificate or order (reciprocity)	Y		
Not making a decision is still considered to be taking a decision bound by the principles of the act	Y		
Safeguard and secure the welfare of any involved child	Y		
Ensure that the function is discharged in a manner which encourages equal opportunities and the observance of the equal opportunities requirements	Y		

Review of Legislation

There have, in the last few years, been a series of reviews of the relevant Acts as described in the section above on the proposed white paper in 2021 for England and Wales and as discussed below on the independent review of the Mental Health (Care and Treatment) (Scotland) Act 2003.

Case Study 17.1 Example of Scottish legislation

Mr Lowe is a 42-year-old Scottish man with a mild learning disability (full scale intelligence quotient (IQ) 64), ASD and a past diagnosis of psychosis. He had received care from learning disability services for a number of years, and prior to admission was living in a care home. He had threatened a worker when he felt that she had been 'cheeky' to him. He had begun to refuse care. He had thrown objects from his window at some local children and made comments suggestive of mental illness. The police attended and requested a mental health assessment. A hospital admission was arranged under a short-term detention. The care home gave notice that they would not be able to support Mr Lowe in the future.

It was apparent that further assessment and stabilisation in an inpatient environment would be required, and to allow detailed future planning. A hospital-based CTO was applied for by Mr Lowe's mental health officer, based on two medical reports, one by his consultant (the 'responsible medical officer') and one by his general practitioner (GP). Mr Lowe rejected the offer of legal support and did not appear to understand the role that a solicitor could have. The Mental Health Tribunal for Scotland appointed a 'curator ad litem' (a legal representative appointed to safeguard Mr Lowe's best interests) and the curator arranged an independent medical report.

The tribunal considered whether the criteria for detention were met. There was no dispute as to the legal criteria, and so a CTO was agreed.

Mr Lowe remained in hospital and, while he made some progress, the CTO was extended, at 6 months, and again at 12 months. It became the view of the responsible medical officer that Mr Lowe could move to a community accommodation, but a lack of suitable options meant that he remained in hospital. Two years later there was another tribunal, as a tribunal review is mandatory at two-year intervals. A curator ad litem was again appointed. They raised a concern about whether Mr Lowe would face a lengthy wait for a suitable community accommodation to be identified and asked the tribunal to make a 'recorded matter' asking the social work department to investigate future accommodation options. The tribunal made a recorded matter, asking parties to work together to determine suitable community options.

In 2018, there was a consultation around potential reform of the Adults with Incapacity (Scotland) Act 2000 [25]. This included looking at ways to potentially alter and increase the range of options and scrutiny available with guardianship orders.

An independent review of the Mental Health (Care and Treatment) (Scotland) Act 2003 ran from 2018, with a final report produced in December 2019 [26]. This recommended that learning disability and autism be removed from the Act, and also that Scotland should work towards compliance with the United Nations Convention on the Rights of Persons with Disabilities, removing compulsory treatment on the basis of disability. It recommended supporting access to positive rights, including independent living, and proposed a human-rights-based system for all decision making, including human rights assessment to ensure human rights were promoted and protected. Proposals were also made around strengthening rights to advocacy and around the introduction of a disability model to the criminal justice system in order to ensure fair access to trials, fairness in responsibility, fair punishment and fair access to support and treatment.

It was decided to incorporate both of the aforementioned works into an overarching review of mental health and incapacity laws, the Scottish mental health law review, which produced its final report in Autumn 2022 [27].

Neurodevelopmental Conditions: Some Relevant Aspects of Scottish Law

A topic of debate, and one of the driving factors for the independent review of the Mental Health (Care and Treatment) (Scotland) Act 2003 was the ongoing inclusion of ID and ASD as types of mental disorder. The key question was whether someone should be able to potentially meet the legal criterial for detention in hospital, on the basis of having ID or ASD (in addition to the other legal criteria – i.e., the presence of significant risk to self or others, the availability of treatment to prevent a deterioration in that person's condition or alleviate its symptoms or effects, that the person has significantly impaired decision-making ability and that the order is deemed to be necessary).

The criteria for detention in Scotland are therefore broader than in England, where learning disability can only be used as a mental disorder if it is 'associated with abnormally aggressive or seriously irresponsible conduct'. While the number of people detained solely on the basis of learning disability or ASD in Scotland is low [28], it raises questions not just about what is right for the patients in that group, but also wider questions of principle.

One argument for inclusion ID and ASD in the Act was that it aids access to treatment. It has been the experience in other jurisdictions that exclusion of ID can lead to a 'legislative gap' [29], limiting options for addressing risk.

The ability to detain people on the basis of ID and ASD when others without those diagnoses and otherwise identical presentations has caused some concern about discrimination based on diagnosis. It has also been suggested that the ability to detain people with ID on the basis of that diagnosis has contributed to delayed hospital discharge. The argument goes that if a person with ID is in hospital, subject to a CTO, that provides a mechanism for authorising that person's stay in hospital. If, on the other hand, ID was not a legal basis for detention in hospital, the person could no longer be lawfully there and this in turn would aid in efforts to secure a discharge.

Northern Ireland

Northern Ireland existed as a political entity from 1921 until 1972. It then experienced a period of direct rule from Westminster due to the 'Troubles', before devolution led to the formation of the Northern Ireland assembly in 2000. The mental health legislation has usually followed that of England and Wales reasonably closely.

Six district asylums were built at end of nineteenth century and managed by the Lunacy Inspectorate. The vast majority of patients were never discharged. The Mental Treatment Act (NI) 1932 was based on the work of the MacMillen Commission in 1924, which had recommended early treatment, treatment without certification or fear of detention and a standard method of funding. Voluntary admissions and temporary admissions to gain treatment were allowed for the first time. This was replaced by the Mental Health Act (NI) 1948. The mentally handicapped received recognition for the first time and services were to be developed for their care. Muckamore Abbey Hospital was established as a 'special care colony' in 1958, with 600 beds initially.

Mental Health Act (NI) 1961 had a focus on community care and established the Mental Health Review Tribunal, allowing appeal of detention. This was superseded by the Mental Health (NI) Order 1986 [30], which introduced the role of the approved social worker as a protective measure for the patient.

Mental Health (NI) Order 1986

The Mental Health (NI) Order 1986 makes provision for the detention, guardianship, care and treatment of patients suffering from mental disorder and for the management of the property and affairs of such patients. A mental disorder is defined as 'mental illness, mental handicap and any other disorder or disability of mind'. It covers all forms of mental ill health and disability except those conditions which are excluded: personality disorders, promiscuity, sexual deviancy and dependence on alcohol or drugs.

Those with ID are considered under three categories:

- Mental handicap, defined as a state of arrested or incomplete development of mind, which includes significant impairment of intelligence and social functioning.
- Severe mental handicap, defined in the same way as mental handicap except that severe replaces significant. The distinction between the two categories is one of degree and it is entirely a matter for clinical judgement.
- Severe mental impairment is an additional sub-category where severe mental handicap must be associated with abnormally aggressive or seriously irresponsible conduct. It was introduced to ensure that mental handicap can never by itself be sufficient grounds for long-term detention in hospital.

Article II: Compulsory Admission to Hospital or Reception into Guardianship

The Order allows for the compulsory detention for assessment up to 14 days. The application is made by a doctor (usually the patient's GP) and their nearest relative or an approved social worker. After 14 days, the consultant psychiatrist can recommend further detention for treatment and, at that time, can treat against the patient's wishes. Those patients with a mental handicap can be detained for assessment (up to 14 days) but cannot be detained for treatment or placed under guardianship unless they have a severe mental handicap or severe mental impairment.

Guardianship is to primarily ensure that patients receive the care and protection they need rather than medical treatment. A guardianship application may be made if the person is suffering from mental illness or severe mental handicap (medical ground) and it is necessary in the interests of the welfare of the patient that they should be so received (welfare ground). The guardian has the power to determine where the patient should live and that they should attend specified appointments, including medical, occupational and training. The guardian can also require access to the patient for any doctor, social worker or other person specified by the guardian.

Article III: Powers of the Court

If someone with ID is found not fit to plead and to have committed the act by a trial of the facts, there are four options for disposal:

(1) Absolute discharge.
(2) Guardianship. The patient must satisfy the medical and the welfare grounds and the court must be satisfied that it is the most suitable method of dealing with the case.
(3) Supervision and treatment order. This allows the treatment in the community of the patient for a minimum of one year up to three years. The patient is required to attend regular appointments with their approved social worker, consultant psychiatrist and any treatment recommended by them.

(4) Hospital order. The court can recommend a transfer to hospital for treatment with or without restriction. The patient must have a mental illness or severe mental impairment. If the case is unclear, an interim hospital order can be used to determine the suitability of a hospital order (initially 12 weeks, up to a maximum of 6 months).

The courts can also remand an accused person to hospital for assessment for 28 days up to a maximum of 12 weeks. The Order also allows for the transfer of sentenced prisoners for periods of treatment.

Difficulty of Use of Order in ID

In practice, those with mild ID (mental handicap) were detained if their behaviour was considered to be abnormally aggressive or seriously irresponsible. This was challenged at several mental health review tribunals and led to some judicial reviews of the tribunal decisions. In the wake of this, the definitions were applied more stringently, which, in practice, made the detention of those with mild ID (assessed IQ > 55) impossible unless they also had a mental illness. This had significant implications for those detained under hospital orders as they often had mild ID and no comorbid mental illness.

The Royal College of Psychiatrists – NI Division issued a consensus statement in 2005 drawing from the judgement of Mr Justice Weatherup [31] who had stated that 'there is a real difference between test intelligence and world intelligence'. The College commended a holistic approach, taking into account social functioning and not just relying on the measured IQ.

Mental Capacity Act NI 2016

In the early 2000s, the Bamford Review began an examination of law, policy and provisions affecting people with mental health needs and learning disabilities. The Review recommended a comprehensive reform of mental health and capacity laws in Northern Ireland [32]. A draft proposal for legislative reform – the Mental Capacity Bill – was eventually passed and received Royal assent in 2016 [33]. The Northern Ireland Department of Health has been working on a phased implementation and, once the Act is fully implemented, the Mental Health (NI) Order 1986 will be repealed.

Northern Ireland has opted for a form of 'fusion legislation' [34], bringing together capacity and mental health law across medical specialities. It applies in all circumstances where a person's autonomy might be compromised on health grounds. It acknowledges the importance of recognising 'parity of esteem' between mental and physical illness. The aim is to treat mental and physical illness equally under the law, with the objective of reducing stigma associated with separate mental health legislation.

The first phase of the Mental Capacity Act NI 2016 implementation programme was commenced on 2 December 2019. This involved the introduction of the DoLS. An application for a DoLS authorisation is only required when a person is deprived of his or her liberty, as opposed to having his or her freedom restricted. In short, the deprivation of liberty has to be necessary to protect a person from harm, be proportionate and be in his or her best interests. The criteria for determining whether there has been a deprivation of liberty is whether the person in question is under continuous supervision and control, and whether he or she is free to leave. This draws on the 'acid test' set out by Baroness Hale in Cheshire West [20].

The Mental Capacity Act NI 2016 will have significant implications for the care of those with ID as the DoLS apply to a large proportion of the population with ID. As the Act was only implemented in December 2019, the coronavirus pandemic has led to significant delays in its application to practice specifically in the general hospitals.

References

1. Mental Health Act 1983. Available at: www.legislation.gov.uk/ukpga/1983/20/contents.

2. Mental Health (Care and Treatment) (Scotland) Act 2003. Available at: www.legislation.gov.uk/asp/2003/13/contents

3. Mental Capacity Act 2005. Available at: www.legislation.gov.uk/ukpga/2005/9/contents.

4. Zigmond AS. Medical incapacity act. *Psychiatric Bulletin* 1998; 22: 657–8.

5. Report of Royal Commission on the Care and Control of the Feeble-minded, 1908. Available at: www.ncbi.nlm.nih.gov/pmc/articles/PMC2437104.

6. Report of the Royal Commission on the Law Relating to Mental Illness and Mental Deficiency (Percy Commission), 1957. Available at: https://navigator.health.org.uk/theme/percy-commission.

7. Bluglass R. The Mental Health Act 1983. In Bluglass R, Bowden P, eds., *Principles and Practice of Forensic Psychiatry*. Churchill Livingstone, 1990, chapter XIII.

8. Mental Health Act 2007. Available at: www.legislation.gov.uk/ukpga/2007/12/contents.

9. Parker C. The Mental Health Act 1983: the impact of the changes introduced by the Mental Health Act 2007 on people with learning disabilities. *Tizard Learning Disability Review* 2008; 13: 38–43.

10. Hollins S, Lodge KM, Lomax P. The case for removing intellectual disability and autism from the Mental Health Act. *British Journal of Psychiatry* 2019; 215: 633–5.

11. Health and Social Care Information Centre. Inpatients formally detained in hospitals under the Mental Health Act 1983, and patients subject to supervised community treatment: uses of the Mental Health Act: Annual Statistics, 2015/16. Available at: https://digital.nhs.uk/data-and-information/publications/statistical/inpatients-formally-detained-in-hospitals-under-the-mental-health-act-1983-and-patients-subject-to-supervised-community-treatment.

12. Jones RM. *Mental Health Act Manual*. Sweet & Maxwell, 2019.

13. Richards S, Mughal AF. *Working with the Mental Health Act*. Matrix Training Associates, 2010.

14. Criminal Procedure (Insanity and Unfitness to Plead) Act 1991. Available at: www.legislation.gov.uk/ukpga/1991/25/contents.

15. Zigmond T, Brindle N. *A Clinician's Brief Guide to the Mental Health Act*. Royal College of Psychiatrists, 2016.

16. *HL v The United* Kingdom [2004] 40 EHRR 761.

17. Mental Capacity (Amendment) Act 2019, Available at: www.legislation.gov.uk/ukpga/2019/18/contents,

18. *Secretary of State for Justice v. MM* [2018] UKSC 60.

19. *PJ v. Welsh Ministers* [2018] UKSC 66.

20. *Cheshire West and Chester Council and Central v. P* [2011] EWCA Civ 1257.

21. Welsh Government. Mental Health Act 1983: code of practice. Available at: https://gov.wales/mental-health-act-1983-code-practice.

22. The Adults with Incapacity (Scotland) Act 2000. Available at: www.legislation.gov.uk/asp/2000/4/contents.

23. The Adult Support and Protection (Scotland) Act 2007. Available at: www.legislation.gov.uk/asp/2007/10/contents.

24. The Mental Health Tribunal for Scotland (practice and procedure) (No. 2) rules. 2005.

Available at: www.legislation.gov.uk/ssi/200
5/519/contents/made.

25. Scottish Government Health and Social
Care Directorates. Adults with incapacity
(Scotland) Act 2000: proposals for reform.
Available at: www.gov.scot/publications/a
dults-incapacity-scotland-act-2000-
proposals-reform.

26. Rome A. Evans C. Webster S. Independent
review of learning disability and autism in
the Mental Health Act. 2019. Available at:
https://webarchive.nrscotland.gov.uk/2020
0313213229/https://www.irmha.scot/wp-
content/uploads/2020/01/IRMHA-Final-
report-18-12-19-2.pdf.

27. Scott J. Scottish mental health law
review. Available at: www.mentalhealth
lawreview.scot.

28. Scottish Government Health and Social Care
Directorates. Learning disability and autism
provision in the Mental Health (Scotland)
Act 2003: findings from a scoping exercise
2017. Available at: www.gov.scot/publica
tions/review-learning-disability-autism-
mental-health-scotland-act-2003-findings.

29. McCarthy J, Duff M. Services for adults
with intellectual disability in Aotearoa New
Zealand. *BJPsych International* 2019; 16:
71–3.

30. Mental Health (NI) Order 1986. Available
at: www.legislation.gov.uk/nisi/1986/595.

31. Weatherup J. Neutral Citation No. [2003]
NIQB35. Available at: www.judiciaryni.uk
/judicial-decisions/2003-niqb-63.

32. Department of Health. *The Bamford
Review of Mental Health and Learning
Disability (Northern Ireland):
A Comprehensive Legislative Framework.*
Department of Health, 2007.

33. Department of Health and Social Services
and Public Safety, Northern Ireland,
Department of Justice. Draft Mental
Capacity Bill (NI): Principles Framework.
2015. Available at: www.niassembly.gov.u
k/globalassets/documents/raise/publica
tions/2015/hssps/6315.pdf.

34. Dawson J, Szmukler G. Fusion of
mental health and incapacity legislation.
British Journal of Psychiatry 2006; 188:
504–9.

Chapter 18

Fitness to Plead and Neurodevelopmental Disorders

Penelope Brown, Salma Ali and Elizabeth Harris

Introduction

People with neurodevelopmental disorders such as intellectual disability (ID), autistic spectrum disorder (ASD) and attention deficit hyperactivity disorder (ADHD) face particular challenges when they come into contact with the criminal justice system. Difficulties understanding and navigating the complexities of the system contribute to poor outcomes, not least during court proceedings where the individual must enter a plea, and guilt and punishment are determined. Symptoms such as communication deficits, stereotypical behaviours, restlessness and lack of theory of mind can impact on appearance and behaviour in court, as exemplified by the case of Daniel (Case Study 18.1), and may not reflect what the person is actually thinking or feeling. The abstract nature of court, widespread use of complex legal jargon and lack of explanation about the legal process can lead to unfair trials and, at worst, an innocent individual being found guilty of a crime they did not commit. In some jurisdictions, especially England and Wales, it is standard practice to place the accused in a dock, often behind a glass screen, which not only increases jury perceptions of guilt but also reduces effective communication between defendant and legal counsel [1]. For individuals with underlying cognitive and communication impairments, the outcomes can be devastating.

The relationship between neurodevelopmental disorders and offending behaviour is complex, but it is generally established that they are over-represented in individuals in custodial settings, especially ADHD and ID [2, 3]. Lack of awareness and understanding of

---

Case Study 18.1 Daniel – How engagement and perceptions can affect sentencing

Daniel has been charged with burglary, possession of a bladed article and assaulting a police officer, following an incident in his neighbourhood, alongside two co-defendants. He is 19 years old, unemployed, and his case is being heard at the Crown Court. He was remanded to prison after his first hearing and now sits in the dock, behind a glass screen, flanked by two security officers, while his solicitor and barrister sit some distance away in the well of the court. His solicitors have discussed the case with him, but he does not appear interested in what they have to say. He tells them he is not guilty, stating 'I never meant to hurt anyone'. For this reason, he also believes that he will not be punished and will be allowed to go home at the end of it all. He looks down at his feet and fiddles with his hands throughout the hearing. When asked to speak, he does not make eye contact and mumbles under his breath. He shows no emotion when the charges are read to him and at one point appears to laugh when the victim's injuries are described. He is found guilty by the jury and receives a custodial sentence, with the judge citing his membership of a group, possession of a weapon and lack of remorse as factors considered in the sentencing decision.

underlying mental health conditions leads to prejudicial perceptions of guilt and detrimental outcomes [4]. Inconsistent training about neurodevelopmental disorders amongst criminal justice and health professionals compounds the problem [5]. This population of vulnerable offenders are disadvantaged as a result, and without specialist support and intervention there are serious questions about how well they are served by criminal justice processes [6–8] as illustrated in Case Study 18.1.

In this chapter we outline the legal frameworks surrounding fitness to plead and the right to a fair trial, before considering how neurodevelopmental disorders can impact an individual's ability to effectively participate at court. We explore how neurodevelopmental disorders and ID can be identified and assessed in criminal defendants and outline current measures for improving the court system for this vulnerable group of defendants.

Fitness to Plead and the Right to a Fair Trial

Under Article 6 of the European Convention on Human Rights (ECHR), every individual has the right to a 'fair and public hearing by an independent and impartial tribunal' [9]. Many justice systems are grounded on English common law and follow an adversarial contest between the prosecution, acting on behalf of the state to ensure justice is met in the public interest, and the accused, often represented by legal counsel. For a criminal trial to be fair, due process must be followed and the accused person, or defendant, must be able to understand what they have been charged with, be able to follow the legal procedures involved in establishing their innocence or guilt and be able to actively participate in the criminal justice process, including collaborating with legal counsel. This is often referred to as 'fitness to plead'. Subjecting an individual to a trial when they are not able to defend themselves or participate effectively, for example due to mental illness, neurodevelopmental disorder or young age, has been described by the legal philosopher Anthony Duff as a 'travesty' because 'we would be attempting to treat as a rational agent, answerable for his actions, someone who cannot answer for them' [10].

In cases where there is doubt about fitness to plead, defendants undergo a mental health assessment and are assessed for fitness to plead according to a legal test. The exact criteria for fitness to plead vary across jurisdictions but generally originate from English law. In England and Wales, the current test outlining what is needed to be considered to be fit to plead is often referred to as the Pritchard test or Pritchard criteria. This was defined in 1837 following the case of *R* v. *Pritchard* [11], a deaf and mute defendant on trial for bestiality. Although able to enter a written plea, Judge Baron Anderson questioned Pritchard's ability to stand trial on the basis that he lacked the 'sufficient intellect' for a fair trial [12]. Anderson stated an individual should be deemed fit to plead if they are able to:

(1) plead the indictment with understanding
(2) follow the proceedings
(3) challenge a juror
(4) understand the evidence.

In 1853, a fifth criterion was added in the case of *R* v. *Davies* [13], which outlined the ability to instruct counsel. This set of criteria is still in use today within the England and Wales Crown Courts, and has been expanded to consider the ability to give evidence in one's own defence [14, 15], as outlined in Box 18.1.

Box 18.1 Unfitness to plead tests in common law jurisdictions: the UK, the USA and Australia

England and Wales (Pritchard criteria, as laid out in *R* v. *Marcantonio*)

A person is unfit to plead if on the balance of probabilities any one of these is beyond their capability:

(1) understanding the charges
(2) deciding whether to plead guilty or not
(3) exercising the right to challenge jurors
(4) instructing solicitors and counsel
(5) following the course of proceedings
(6) giving evidence in one's own defence.

Scotland (as laid out in the Criminal Procedure (Scotland) Act 1995 and the Criminal Justice and Licensing (Scotland) Act 2010)

A person is unfit for trial if it is established on the balance of probabilities that the person is incapable, by reason of a mental or physical condition, of participating effectively in a trial ... (with) regard to the ability of the person to

(1) understand the nature of the charge
(2) understand the requirement to tender a plea to the charge and the effect of such a plea
(3) understand the purpose of, and follow the course of, the trial
(4) understand the evidence that may be given against the person
(5) instruct and otherwise communicate with the person's legal representative
(6) any other factor which the court considers relevant.

Australia (as laid out in the Presser test)

To be fit to plead an accused must have sufficient mental or intellectual capacity to understand the proceedings and to make an adequate defence, according to the following abilities:

(1) an understanding of the nature of the charges
(2) an understanding of the nature of the court proceedings
(3) the ability to challenge jurors
(4) the ability to understand the evidence
(5) the ability to decide what defence to offer
(6) the ability to explain his or her version of the facts to counsel and the court.

United States of America (as laid out in Dusky the criteria)

Competence to stand trial considers whether the defendant has:

(1) sufficient present ability to consult with his lawyer with a reasonable degree of rational understanding
(2) whether he has a rational as well as factual understanding of the proceedings against him.

When concerns are raised about a defendant's fitness to plead, clinicians must independently assess the defendant, using the Pritchard criteria, before presenting their results as evidence to a judge [16]. The final arbiter of fitness is the judge. If found unfit, a separate 'trial of the facts' takes place whereby a jury decide whether the defendant committed the act or omission for which they were charged. The trial of the facts is not considered a criminal trial and cannot result in a finding of guilt or criminal conviction. However, if the accused is found to have done the act, there are three possible options for disposal: hospital order, a supervision order or absolute discharge [17]. In each case, the defendant is diverted from the Criminal Justice System.

In the justice system, the law and procedures relating to fitness to plead run alongside the related framework of 'effective participation'. This has been explicitly considered in the High Court in terms of the minimum requirements for a trial to be fair according to ECHR Article 6 [18]. It is considered to encompass a broader range of issues going to the heart of mounting an effective defence and holds that defendants must not only be physically present in their trials but also play an active role and have reasonable opportunity to make the relevant representations [16]. It recognises that vulnerable defendants and children need to be treated carefully in court and may require reasonable adjustments and additional support in order to take part in their trials [19, 20]. In recent years, attempts have been made to bring together the concepts of fitness to plead and effective participation [21], but the relationship between the two legal frameworks is imprecise and there is concern that the current procedures relating to fitness to plead are incompatible with Article 6 rights [22].

International Fitness to Plead laws

The law on fitness to plead in other adversarial jurisdictions such as the USA, Canada and Australia has broadly evolved from the system in England and Wales, but with some variability across states, including within those jurisdictions. In Australia, the leading test for whether the defendant should be found fit to stand trial is laid out in *R* v. *Presser* [23], in which the judge held that there should be a presumption of fitness and based the test for fitness on the criteria laid out by Baron Alderson in the Pritchard criteria (see Box 18.1).

The Presser test has been widely adopted across Australian state jurisdictions as incorporating the minimum requirements for a fair trial, but there remains inter-state variability in terms of procedures when the defendant is found unfit [24]. In most states there are special hearings akin to the trial of the facts to consider whether the accused is in fact innocent of the charges. The consequences of being found unfit also varies across Australian states, and broadly includes custodial or non-custodial supervision orders.

In the USA, fitness to plead is more commonly referred to as competence to stand trial, or competence to proceed. The main standard for competence is laid out in the Dusky criteria (see Box 18.1) [25]. Unlike the Pritchard and Presser tests, Dusky explicitly considers a defendant's decision-making abilities alongside foundational abilities relating to participation in court procedures (such as understanding the charges and instructing counsel) and requires the defendant to have both a rational and factual understanding of the proceedings [26]. Like Australia, the legal processes surrounding competency to stand trial varies across states, but unlike other jurisdictions there is no trial of the facts. Instead, there is a greater focus on 'restoration of competence', usually comprising inpatient or community treatment and education to better prepare defendants to be able to participate in their own trials [27]. If competence is restored, the case may proceed. If it is agreed the defendant cannot be restored, the government must dismiss the charges and there is no exploration of whether they are innocent or guilty.

Modernising Fitness to Plead

In recent years there has been international concern that current procedures relating to fitness to plead are unfit for purpose and do not adequately safeguard the rights of vulnerable defendants, including those with developmental disorders [22, 24, 28–30]. One of the main criticisms, identified both by the Law Commission of England and Wales [31] and the Victorian Law Reform Commission in Australia [30], is that there is too strong a focus on 'sufficient intellect' within the Pritchard and Presser tests respectively. Unlike the Dusky criteria in the USA, these tests are seen to assess a defendant's cognitive abilities in relation to court procedures without necessarily considering decision-making abilities, something that medical and legal professions have become increasingly concerned with in recent years. Decisional capacity, referred to as mental capacity or simply 'capacity', is a concept which is heavily intertwined with autonomy and is central to modern psychiatric practice. In England and Wales, the Mental Capacity Act 2005 [32] introduced a statutory framework for assessing whether individuals have the mental abilities to make decisions in relation to a number of civil issues, including consenting to medical treatment or writing a will, but does not apply to criminal proceedings. It is suggested that the Pritchard criteria set a threshold for unfitness to plead much higher than that for mental incapacity, raising concerns that individuals found fit do not in reality have the capacity to decide how to plea, and too many vulnerable defendants are slipping through the net [22, 33–35]. Other British jurisdictions and Crown dependencies such as Scotland and the Channel Islands, respectively, explicitly consider decision-making capacity in their tests for fitness to plead, which aligns with the closely related concept of 'effective participation' at court [29, 36, 37].

Other criticisms of the current procedures relate to the practical application of the law. First, lack of systematic screening for mental disorder in defendants can lead to vulnerable individuals not being identified and sent for assessment in the first place. This is especially true for neurodevelopmental difficulties, which are not always picked up by existing services that focus on identifying defendants presenting with severe mental illness [38]. Second, studies have found that when defendants are assessed for fitness to plead, the professionals involved are inconsistent in their application of the legal criteria [39, 40]. In a qualitative study involving senior criminal barristers with experience in unfitness to plead, Rogers and colleagues [41] criticised the modern-day irrelevance of some of the criteria (especially the need to challenge the jurors) and highlighted the subjective and unreliable application of the criteria by professionals. The jury is often swayed by the defendant in the witness box, with likeability and eloquent presentation thought to influence the jury's perception. In addition, suggestibility is not accounted for despite it being an important vulnerability that may influence the reliability of answers during questioning [42]. Memory impairments (in relation to mental health disorders or cognitive impairments) are also not acknowledged, despite the potential to place an individual at a significant disadvantage during trial. In particular, the reduced ability to recall information discussed during the trial may place a defendant at a disadvantage.

Recommendations from this study were broadly incorporated into the Law Commission's final recommendations for reforming fitness to plead in England and Wales [43]. The report includes proposals to unite the concepts of decision-making capacity and effective participation into the law, widen screening programmes to identify mental disorder in defendants and standardise the psychiatric assessment of fitness to plead. A new statutory test for 'capacity to participate effectively' has specifically been proposed [21], yet these recommendations have not yet been brought into law and the Pritchard criteria continue to lay out the legal threshold for unfitness.

Despite lack of statutory changes, in recent years there has been a widespread roll-out of liaison and diversion services in police stations and courts, which aim to identify vulnerable defendants at an early stage in the criminal justice system [44]. A study examining criminal justice liaison services across a number of jurisdictions underscores the need for these services to focus on neurodevelopmental disorders as the first step in ensuring adequate support can be provided at court [38]. In some parts of the world, for example North America, the use of standardised measures of fitness (or competency to stand trial) is already commonplace both in clinical practice and in research [45–47]. In response to the Law Commission's consultation, Brown and colleagues have developed a standardised instrument for assessing fitness to plead in England and Wales, which considers both the Pritchard criteria as well as decision-making capacity, and is designed to be used as an adjunct to clinical assessments considering fitness to plead [48]. This has been validated in individuals with mild ID as well as those with ASD [49] and is likely to apply in other common law jurisdictions with a similar legal standard of fitness.

Fitness to Plead and the Right to Legal Capacity

In addition to improving the identification and assessment of vulnerable individuals at court, there has been a shift to better support individuals through trials to enable them to take part and defend themselves rather than simply being diverted. This aligns with concurrent developments in human rights law, which challenge procedures relating to fitness to plead across the world. The United Nations Convention on the Rights of Persons with Disabilities (UNCRPD) requires member states to 'recognize that persons with disabilities enjoy legal capacity on an equal basis with others in all aspects of life' (Article 12(2)) and 'take appropriate measures to provide access by persons with disabilities to the support they may require in exercising their legal capacity' (Article 12(3)) [50]. Given findings of unfitness are primarily only available to those lacking mental abilities, fitness to plead procedures potentially result in the denial of legal capacity on an equal basis with others for this group of defendants. Indeed, depriving an individual of their entitlement to exercise legal capacity by not allowing them to enter a plea due to intellectual and mental disability has been found to be a violation of their UNCRPD rights [51–53]. There have even been suggestions that laws considering fitness to plead, resulting in declarations of unfitness and diversion from trial, should accordingly be abandoned altogether [54, 55]. Findings of unfitness and diversion from trial should certainly be seen as a last resort, although the Law Commission of England and Wales acknowledges 'there will be a small group of defendants who will be unable to participate effectively in trial, whatever the level of support provided to them'.

Before we turn to methods employed to support individuals with neurodevelopmental disorders at court, we first explore in greater depth how different disorders impact on fitness to plead.

Fitness to Plead and ADHD

ADHD is a neurodevelopmental disorder characterised by patterns of inattention, hyperactivity and impulsivity. The worldwide prevalence of ADHD in children is estimated to be 8–12% [56]. Although previously considered a childhood disorder, it has recently been understood that ADHD persists into adulthood in approximately 50–75% of cases [57], resulting in an estimated adult prevalence of 2.5–4% [58]. It is divided into three subtypes: inattentive, hyperactive–impulsive and combined.

ADHD has commonly been associated with delinquent behaviour and is viewed as a risk factor for criminality. The presence of ADHD in childhood has been found to increase the risk of arrest by twofold, and conviction and incarceration by threefold [59]. Furthermore, individuals who had ADHD in childhood are more likely to have a younger age of first offence and higher rates of recidivism. The relationship between ADHD and criminality is complicated by common comorbidities, in particular conduct disorder [60], low academic performance, and substance misuse [61], all of which are in themselves strong predictors of offending.

The prevalence of ADHD at all stages in the criminal justice system is higher than in the general population. Studies in London, England have found 23.5% of detainees at police stations detainees report current ADHD symptoms, with 32.1% screening positive for childhood ADHD [62]. In criminal defendants, adult ADHD has been estimated in 13–20% of individuals attending court [63], and within incarcerated populations it is estimated at 25.5% [2]. A review of international studies in male prisoners across eight countries found 71% had symptoms of childhood ADHD and 45% had current symptoms [64].

Despite studies finding high levels of ADHD throughout the criminal justice system, it has been suggested that it is often missed in practice, especially in older offenders and those with the hyperactive–impulsive subtype, possibly as comorbid behavioural issues mask the underlying symptoms [65]. However, ADHD symptoms are known to impact on an individual's ability to navigate the criminal justice system and participate in their trials, as evidenced in the case of Billy-Joe Friend (see Case Study 18.2) [66].

Numerous empirical studies have outlined the impact ADHD may have, both in police interviews and in the courtroom. False confessions and 'don't know' answers are more common in defendants with ADHD symptomatology [42, 67], adversely affecting any subsequent court proceedings. Suggestibility is also more common in individuals with ADHD than healthy controls, and compliance (which is associated with a reduced reliability of answers in interrogation [68, 69] is also closely linked with current ADHD symptoms. Defendants with ADHD are more likely to employ maladaptive coping strategies during

Case Study 18.2 Fitness to plead, ADHD and the case of Billy-Joe

Billy-Joe Friend was 15 years old when accused, alongside his brother, of killing a friend at a party. During the first two police interviews, he exercised his right to silence. In his third interview, he obliged, although it was later acknowledged that some of his answers were lies. This was used against him during trial, where the issue of fitness to plead was not raised. A pre-trial psychological assessment suggested that his low intelligence quotient (IQ) of 63, poor attention control and distractibility may impair his ability to give evidence. Despite this, the judge concluded that the jury could draw adverse inferences from his failure to provide evidence, should they choose. He was found guilty of murder.

His case was subsequently appealed in the light of a new diagnosis of ADHD. Although his inattention was considered at trial, it was not highlighted in terms of his ability to participate effectively. Furthermore, his impulsivity was not acknowledged, despite it being a potential contributor to the lies told at interview. His conviction was subsequently overturned on the basis that his ADHD would have impacted his ability to participate in trial, and the jury should not have drawn adverse inference from his silence [4].

periods of stress, including escape–avoidance, confrontation and poor planned problem solving [70]. Furthermore, individuals with attention problems are less likely to request support and advice from others, which may impact on their ability to work with counsel. They may also struggle to cope with other aspects of the courtroom process [71], such as sustaining attention for long periods of time, while also being able to answer questions and focus on evidence exhibits.

Despite high levels of ADHD in criminal defendants, it is rare that individuals found unfit have a diagnosis of ADHD [72]. However, as noted above, ADHD symptoms can profoundly impact a defendant's abilities at court and it is likely that it is not routinely identified. In younger defendants, symptoms can be particularly problematic. There are no formal procedures for finding individuals unfit to plead at youth courts in England and Wales, but in exceptional circumstances the court has the power to stay proceedings if the defendant is found unable to participate effectively. In the *Crown Prosecution Service* v. *P* case, the district judge in England highlighted the impact ADHD symptoms had on a child defendant as follows: '(P) would not be capable of understanding the nature of court proceedings. He would not be able to concentrate on the evidence and argument in a court room. His memory capacity was so impaired that he would not remember what had gone before. He would not understand much of what was going on during the proceedings' [73].

It is essential that professionals at court are aware of ADHD symptoms and how these can impact effective participation and fitness to plead. ADHD is a treatable condition and, once identified, medication and behavioural interventions can be initiated to support the defendant in managing their symptoms during courtroom proceedings. Special measures can also be put in place, such as providing intermediaries who support defendants before and during the proceedings, making reasonable adjustments such as frequent breaks or short and simple questioning styles and providing psychological support to help them cope with the stress and anxiety of the trial [66]]. Furthermore, further guidance for support and rehabilitation, should the individual be convicted, can be provided.

Fitness to Plead and ASD

The impairments which characterise ASD – social communication and interaction, restricted, repetitive patterns of behaviour, interests or activities in addition to a limited theory of mind – mean that people on the autistic spectrum see and make sense of the world differently to their neurotypical counterparts, which can have a significant impact on a wide variety of situations [74–76]. Such difficulties affect different people in different ways in spite of differing levels of intellectual functioning, with some being more able in particular areas than others [77]. It is important to remember that autism exists on a spectrum. Those who are functioning at a higher intellectual level are likely to have difficulties that are not obvious or easily distinguishable.

There has been increasing consideration given to examining the specific core features of ASD and how they may contribute to offending behaviour, and in turn may be highlighted as risk factors to offending in this population [78–81]. Reasons for entry into the criminal justice system can vary significantly [82], and subsequent concerns for this group are raised during court proceedings [5], and especially considering their fitness to plead [38]. Features of ASD can disadvantage defendants in the courtroom in numerous ways. Lack of empathy and remorse, appearing cold and calculating, inappropriate facial expression, odd speech patterns and deficits in reciprocal communication, can all impact on the evaluation of a defendant's guilt by the jury and influence sentencing decisions by judges [4]. Like ADHD, ASD can affect the ability of a defendant to provide an accurate or reliable account of an event [83]. Being mindful of the difficulties that individuals with ASD experience and how this can impact on their ability to enter a plea, will assist accurate assessment. For example, the unfamiliar, formal and often noisy surroundings of custodial environments are likely to increase stress and anxiety, which can negatively impact on communication, both verbal and non-verbal. A person with ASD may have trouble understanding the interviewer, particularly if the questions are complex, indirect and use metaphors, idioms or colloquialisms [84]. Where possible, unnecessary use of jargon, legal or otherwise, should also be avoided. It is noteworthy that it is possible for the interviewer to misinterpret where inappropriate facial expressions, particularly smiling or laughter (which can often be responses to anxiety) or incongruent vocal tone, are observed alongside responses. Delays in processing speech, selective mutism or simple 'stage fright' are also easily misinterpreted as wilful. The difficulties outlined earlier mean that there are significant differences in the way that people with ASD present [74], and therefore approaches to assessment should be tailored to the individual's presentation and ability. For example, if the defendant has significant sensory issues, the environment should be considered [85], and other reasonable adjustments to facilitate assessment should be introduced against that backdrop. Ground rules hearings are also used to set parameters regarding the fair treatment of vulnerable defendants (as well as witnesses) and occur at the start of a trial to ensure agreement about how questions should be asked, how many breaks should be offered and other adjustments needed to ensure the trial is fair [86].

Furthermore, it is important to be aware that, given their often very concrete way of thinking, people with ASD can misinterpret rules and relationships. Rigidity can mean that they stick to (and believe in) a story once it is in their head, and underlying all of these difficulties is the risk that they may not be recognised as a vulnerable adult, particularly if they are functioning higher intellectually. Consequently, such defendants may not be adequately protected by the Pritchard criteria, which emphasise the cognitive abilities of a defendant. A well-developed understanding of right and wrong, and of the nature of the court and its proceedings, may be insufficient when legal issues become complex [87, 88]. Defendants may be compromised further by an inability to present themselves effectively.

It is generally agreed that the courts require more knowledge about ASD in order to influence sentencing decisions in a timely manner [88–90]. Doing so may enable those on the autistic spectrum to be dealt with during criminal proceedings more appropriately, and issues around fitness to plead can be identified and addressed earlier. Studies have suggested the numbers of defendants found unfit to plead in England and Wales is so low that questions arise as to whether current procedure for determining fitness and identifying defendants who are unfit may not be fit for purpose in the first place [28, 41]. It is therefore likely, given the spectrum of difficulty, that defendants with ASD are even less likely to be identified as needing a fitness to plead assessment, and supported appropriately at trial. Screening at court for ASD is not well established and, even where it is in place, some people remain unidentified [38, 91].

Notwithstanding, it is not the case that every defendant with ASD will have difficulty in court, but where legal proceedings are necessary, identification and acknowledgement of the various vulnerabilities a person with ASD can have should be considered and investigated as part of the assessment. Once identified, reasonable adjustments can be implemented to mitigate against communication difficulties, thus facilitating proceedings in a way that benefits both the defendant and the court.

Fitness to Plead and ID

As is the case with ASD, there is little research specifically examining the impact on ID and fitness to plead. The broad concept of fitness to plead and inconsistencies in the application of the Pritchard criteria in clinical assessment has led to a likely under-identification of defendants who might otherwise be considered unfit to plead [31]. Of note, a large proportion of defendants found unfit are reported to have a diagnosis of mental impairment [72] and the tests for fitness to plead in certain jurisdictions such as Australia and England and Wales are seen to better consider intellectual abilities over other symptoms of mental illness [40]. This may be due in part to the lack of knowledge about the specific cognitive abilities that underpin the Pritchard criteria [48, 49] and there is little evidence that robust psychological assessment has been adopted to determine the specific nature of cognitive ability in relation to fitness to plead cases.

Difficulties in understanding and following evidence in court are likely to place a greater demand on a number of different cognitive capacities. A good understanding of complex language and the ability to process, assimilate and understand often abstract concepts draw on previously learned semantic knowledge and common-sense reasoning. Additionally, verbal information delivered in a court setting is stressful and likely to place a greater demand on working-memory abilities (holding information in mind) and processing-speed abilities (the ability to process large amounts of information quickly and efficiently), in order to formulate a response. Comprehension and reasoning ability about the information during the course of the proceedings is also necessary to provide an adequate response.

Evidence from the international arena has highlighted the need to incorporate cognitive assessment in fitness to stand trial cases. For example, White et al. [92], in a review 328 expert reports, found 65 were conducted by psychologists, who reported the presence of ID in 50.7% of reports. A further 13.8% of reports were classified as having borderline/below average intellectual functioning. The authors highlighted the importance of specifically understanding cognitive functioning when determining fitness to stand trial, and in particular attention and memory. In an earlier study examining a Scottish sample, Brewster et al. [93] concluded that evidence of ID should be sufficient to consider an assessment for fitness to plead.

It is highly likely that a significant number of defendants with ID are erroneously considered fit to plead, or at the very least their disorders are not adequately identified or supported at court. The absence of an empirical basis for the clinical assessment of fitness means that clinical and legal judgments of defendants remain critically uninformed [41]. The onus therefore remains on both legal and healthcare professionals based in court to identify defendants with ID, who have difficulties understanding and communicating. If permitted and appropriate, they can then be referred on for a formal fitness to plead assessment, and recommendations should be made for a cognitive assessment to establish the level of cognitive functioning at the outset. This assessment can inform further assessment and appropriate application of the Pritchard criteria.

Utilising liaison and diversion services [44] can assist in such situations, particularly where there may be questions and concerns around a defendant's presentation. Often, a behavioural presentation related to poor understanding and ID is mistaken for a mental health presentation. This can mean that such defendant's needs are not adequately met and, therefore, they may be disadvantaged without specialist support [6, 7, 94, 95]. Improvements to professional training can help address this gap in knowledge. Providing defendants with ID with reasonable adjustments to enable them to participate more effectively in proceedings will go some way to meeting their needs and ensuring access to equitable criminal justice outcomes. For example, employing the services of an intermediary might be preferred, although availability and experience of intermediaries varies across jurisdictions [96]. The following adjustments could also be considered:

- Place a seat next to the defence counsel instead of in the dock. This will help reduce overall stress levels and improve the defendant's understanding and meaningful participation. If the defendant requires extensive explanation and repetition, this can be facilitated easily.

- Regular breaks can provide opportunities for the defendant to consult with counsel and obtain clarification to maximise understanding. They can also help manage heightened anxiety and stress.

- Utilise short sentences and simple language that is free from jargon should, at all times. Check in with the defendant to clarify their understanding.

- Refrain from the use of abstract concepts altogether; utilise examples to fully explain information

Case Study 18.3 illustrates how Daniel, as described earlier in Case Study 18.1, would have a different outcome if his needs were identified.

Case Study 18.3 How neurodevelopmental disorder can be identified and supported to improve outcomes

The case of Daniel could look very different if his difficulties were identified as symptoms of mental disorder and supports were put in place to enable him to better engage in his trial. Here we consider a different outcome to his case.

Daniel has been charged with burglary, possession of a bladed article, and assaulting a police officer, following an incident in his neighbourhood, alongside two co-defendants. He is 19 years old, unemployed, and his case is being heard at the Crown Court. He was picked up by Sara, a nurse with the liaison and diversion team at the magistrates court at his first hearing, as his mother mentioned to his solicitor that he has a diagnosis of moderate ID and ASD. His family were present and discussed him with Sara, who was able to advocate on Daniel's behalf, furnishing the court with information about his ID, ASD, general vulnerability and risks of harm he posed to himself, should he be sent to custody. As a result, he was bailed to stay with his family instead of being remanded into custody. When his case was committed to the Crown Court, psychiatric reports considering Daniel's fitness to plead were instructed. Although this was positive, Daniel was likely to be tried alongside his co-defendants. This could have been problematic as there was the fear that his case would have been considered in the same way as his neurotypical co-defendants.

Daniel was given a community link worker, named Tim, who was part of the wider liaison and diversion service. Tim supported Daniel and his family through the process. During the bail period, Tim was able to access a psychological report of Daniel's cognitive functioning through the liaison and diversion service. This psychological report became pivotal in the proceedings. One psychiatric report concluded that Daniel was not fit to plead and suggested an additional diagnosis of ADHD. The other report found him fit according to the Pritchard criteria. The psychological report was able to provide contextual information about Daniel's cognitive functioning, and establish that he was suffering from a mild–moderate ID, which was likely complicated by his ASD and possible ADHD. The psychologist conducting the report was of the opinion that Daniel would be fit to enter a plea provided he was supported by an intermediary and reasonable adjustments were made to his case.

On the available evidence, the judge concluded Daniel was fit to plead and agreed to a series of adjustments to his proceedings in order to ensure a fair trial. This included having his case heard separately to his co-defendants, him being seated in the well of his court next to the intermediary and solicitor, and a ground rules hearing in which it was agreed how questions should be put to Daniel and how the intermediary would alert the court if he was struggling to understand or needed additional breaks.

Daniel was found guilty of possession of a bladed article but was acquitted of the other charges. He received a community order with a mental health treatment requirement [97] to ensure he received support and treatment in the community, and was provided with a social worker specialising in care for autism.

Conclusion

Many criminal defendants have underlying neurodevelopmental disorders, and high levels of morbidity go undetected [98, 99]. Identifying those who require assessment and support remains problematic [100]. There has been an international drive to identify mental disorder through liaison and diversion services, but these have tended to prioritise serious mental illness. Significant progress is needed to better identify and meet the needs of individuals with ADHD, ASD and ID [38, 63]. Once identified, defendants require expert assessment of their abilities to participate in trial and fitness to plead but, even amongst psychiatric assessors, understanding of neurodevelopmental disorders and utilisation of cognitive measures can be limited.

Furthermore, educating the judge, jury and court staff about how neurodevelopmental disorders manifest themselves in defendants may prevent wrongful assumptions to be made regarding behaviour presentations in court or omissions made [84]. Procedural adjustments such as familiarising the defendant with the courtroom, simplifying language, allowing frequent breaks, shorter sitting sessions, sensory adjustments such as limiting distractions and lowering lighting can all be implemented to assist vulnerable individuals at court. Specialist intermediaries are increasingly available to assess and support with communication difficulties [101]. While it is inevitable that some individuals with severe impairments will never be fit to plead, identifying needs and providing support where possible will ensure that the removal of a defendant from criminal justice processes will be the last resort.

References

1. Rossner M, Tait D, McKimmie B, Sarre R. The dock on trial: courtroom design and the presumption of innocence. *Journal of Law and Society* 2017; 44(3): 317–44.

2. Young S, Moss D, Sedgwick O, Fridman M, Hodgkins P. A meta-analysis of the prevalence of attention deficit hyperactivity disorder in incarcerated populations. *Psychological Medicine* 2015; 45(2): 247–58.

3. Hellenbach M, Karatzias T, Brown M. Intellectual disabilities among prisoners: prevalence and mental and physical health comorbidities. *Journal of Applied Research in Intellectual Disabilities* 2017; 30(2): 230–41.

4. Allely CS, Cooper P. Jurors' and judges' evaluation of defendants with autism and the impact on sentencing: a systematic Preferred Reporting Items for Systematic Reviews and Meta-analyses (PRISMA) review of autism spectrum disorder in the courtroom. *Journal of Law and Medicine* 2017; 25(1): 105–23.

5. Chaplin E, McCarthy J, Forrester A. Defendants with autism spectrum disorders: what is the role of court liaison and diversion? *Advances in Autism* 2017; 3 (4): 220–8.

6. Gudjonsson G, Joyce T. Interviewing adults with intellectual disabilities. *Advances in Mental Health and Intellectual Disabilities* 2011; 5(2): 16–21.

7. Søndenaa E, Palmstierna T, Iversen VC. A stepwise approach to identify intellectual disabilities in the criminal justice system. *European Journal of Psychology Applied to Legal Context* 2010; 2: 183–98.

8. Talbot J, Jacobson J. Adult defendants with learning disabilities and the criminal courts. *Journal of Learning Disabilities and Offending Behaviour* 2010; 1(2): 16–26.

9. Council of Europe. European Convention for the Protection of Human Rights and Fundamental Freedoms. Council of Europe Treaty Series 005. Council of Europe, 1950.

10. Duff RA. *Trials and Punishments*. Cambridge University Press, 1991.

11. *R* v. *Pritchard* (1836) 7 C&P 303.

12. Brown P. Unfitness to plead in England and Wales: historical development and contemporary dilemmas. *Medicine, Science and the Law* 2019; 59(3): 187–96.

13. *R* v. *Davies* (1853) 3 C&K 328.

14. *R* v. *M(John)* [2003] EWCA Crim 3452.

15. *R* v. *Marcantonio* [2016] EWCA Crim 14.

16. Exworthy T. Commentary: UK perspective on competency to stand trial. *Journal of the American Academy of Psychiatry and the Law* 2006; 34(4): 466–71.

17. Rogers TP, Blackwood NJ, Farnham F, Pickup GJ, Watts MJ. Fitness to plead and competence to stand trial: a systematic review of the constructs and their application. *Journal of Forensic Psychiatry and Psychology* 2008; 19 (4): 576–96.

18. Owusu-Bempah A. The interpretation and application of the right to effective participation. *International Journal of Evidence and Proof* 2018; 22(4): 321–41.

19. *Stanford* v. *UK* [1994] ECHR 6.

20. *T and V* v. *UK* [2000] 30 EHRR 121.

21. Law Commission of England and Wales. *Unfitness to Plead – Volume 2: Draft Legislation*. The Stationary Office, 2016.

22. Vassall-Adams G, Scott-Moncrieff L. Capacity and fitness to plead: the yawning gap. *Counsel* 2006; 3: 2–3.

23. *R* v. *Presser* [1958] VR 45.

24. Freckleton I. *Fitness to stand trial under Australian law*. In Mackay R, Brookbanks W, eds., *Fitness to Plead: International and Comparative Perspectives*. Oxford University Press, 2018: 153–174.

25. *Dusky* v. *United States*, 362 US 402 (1960); 80 S Ct 788.

26. Bonnie RJ. Fitness for criminal adjudication: the emerging significance of decisional competence in the United States. In Mackay R, Brookbanks W, eds., *Fitness to Plead: International and Comparative Perspectives*. Oxford University Press, 2018; 175–206.

27. Morse SJ. Involuntary competence in united states criminal law. In Mackay R, Brookbanks W, eds., *Fitness to Plead: International and Comparative Perspectives*. Oxford University Press, 2018; 207–30.

28. Shah A. Making fitness to plead fit for purpose. *International Journal of Criminology and Sociology* 2012; 1: 176–97.

29. Brown P. Modernising fitness to plead. *Medicine, Sciences and the Law* 2019; 59(3): 131–4.

30. Victorian Law Reform Commission. *Review of the Crimes (Mental Impairment and Unfitness to be Tried) Act 1997*. Victorian Law Reform Commission, 2014.

31. Law Commission of England and Wales. *Unfitness to Plead (Consultation Paper No.197)*. The Stationery Office, 2010.

32. Mental Capacity Act 2005. Available at: www.legislation.gov.uk/ukpga/2005/9/contents.

33. Brown P. Unfitness to plead in England and Wales: historical development and contemporary dilemmas. *Medicine, Science and the Law* 2019; 59(3): 187–96.

34. Peay J. Fitness to plead and core competencies: problems and possibilities. LSE Legal Studies Working Paper No 2/2012. 2012. Available at: https://eprints.lse.ac.uk/44734/1/Fitness_plead_author.pdf.

35. *R v. Murray (Aisling)* [2008] EWCA Crim 1792.

36. Maher G. Unfitness *for trial in Scots law*. In Mackay R, Brookbanks W, eds., *Fitness to Plead: International and Comparative Perspectives*. Oxford University Press, 2018; 81–104.

37. Mackay R. On being insane in Jersey: Part 3 – the case of *Attorney General v. O'Driscoll*. *Criminal Law Reports* 2004; April: 291–6.

38. McCarthy J, Chaplin E, Hayes S, Søndenaa E, Chester V, Morrissey C, et al. Defendants with intellectual disability and autism spectrum conditions: the perspective of clinicians working across three jurisdictions. *Psychiatry, Psychology and Law.* 2021: 29(5): 698–717.

39. Mackay R, Kearns G. An upturn in unfitness to plead? Disability in relation to the trial under the 1991 Act. *Criminal Law Review* 2000; July: 532–46.

40. Mudathikundan F, Chao O, Forrester A. Mental health and fitness to plead proposals in England and Wales. *International Journal of Law and Psychiatry* 2014; 37(2): 135–41.

41. Rogers TP, Blackwood N, Farnham F, Pickup G, Watts M. Reformulating fitness to plead: a qualitative study. *Journal of Forensic Psychiatry and Psychology* 2009; 20 (6): 815–34.

42. Gudjonsson GH, Sigurdsson J, Bragason O, Newton A, Einarsson E. Interrogative suggestibility, compliance and false confessions among prisoners and their relationship with attention deficit hyperactivity disorder (ADHD) symptoms. *Psychological Medicine* 2008; 38(7): 1037–44.

43. Law Commission of England and Wales. *Unfitness to Plead – Volume 1: Report (Law Com. No 364).* The Stationery Office, 2016.

44. NHS England. Liaison and diversion standard service specification 2019. Available at: www.england.nhs.uk/wp-content/uploads/2019/12/national-liaison-and-diversion-service-specification-2019.pdf.

45. Lally SJ. What tests are acceptable for use in forensic evaluations? A survey of experts. *Professional Psychology: Research and Practice* 2003; 34(5): 491.

46. Warren JI, Chauhan P, Kois L, Dibble A, Knighton J. Factors influencing 2,260 opinions of defendants' restorability to adjudicative competency. *Psychology, Public Policy, and Law* 2013; 19(4): 498–508.

47. Fogel MH, Schiffman W, Mumley D, Tillbrook C, Grisso T. Ten year research update (2001–2010): evaluations for competence to stand trial (adjudicative competence). *Behavioral Sciences and the Law* 2013; 31(2): 165–91.

48. Brown P, Stahl D, Appiah-Kusi E, Brewer R, Watts M, Peay J, et al. Fitness to plead: development and validation of a standardised assessment instrument. *PLOS One.* 2018; 13(4): e0194332.

49. Brewer RJ, Davies GM, Blackwood NJ. Fitness to plead: the impact of autism spectrum disorder. *Journal of Forensic Psychology Practice* 2016; 16(3): 182–97.

50. Committee on the Rights of Persons with Disabilities. Convention on the Rights of Persons with Disabilities: general comment No. 1 (2014) Article 12: equal recognition before the law. UNCRPD, 2014.

51. Committee on the Rights of Persons with Disabilities. Concluding observations on the initial report of Republic of Korea, 29 October 2014, CRPD/C/KOR/CO/1. UNCRPD, 2014.

52. Committee on the Rights of Persons with Disabilities. Concluding observations on the initial report of Ecuador, 27 October 2014, CRPD/C/ECU/CO/1. UNCRPD, 2014.

53. Committee on the Rights of Persons with Disabilities. Views adopted by the Committee under article 5 of the Optional Protocol, concerning communication No. 7/2012 (Noble vs Australia). UNCRPD, 2016.

54. Minkowitz T. Rethinking criminal responsibility from a critical disability perspective: the abolition of insanity/ incapacity acquittals and unfitness to plead, and beyond. *Griffith Law Review* 2014; 23 (3): 434–66.

55. Freckelton I, Keyzer P. Fitness to stand trial and disability discrimination: an international critique of Australia. *Psychiatry, Psychology and Law.* 2017; 24(5): 770–83.

56. Faraone SV, Sergeant J, Gillberg C, Biederman J. The worldwide prevalence of ADHD: is it an American condition? *World Psychiatry* 2003; 2(2): 104.

57. Kirley A. Diagnosis and classification of ADHD in adulthood. In Fitzgerald M, Bellgrove M, Michael Gill M, eds.,*Handbook of Attention Deficit Hyperactivity Disorder.* John Wiley & Sons, 2007: 37–52.

58. McCarthy S, Wilton L, Murray ML, Hodgkins P, Asherson P, Wong IC. The epidemiology of pharmacologically treated attention deficit hyperactivity disorder (ADHD) in children, adolescents and adults in UK primary care. *BMC Pediatrics* 2012; 12(1): 1–11.

59. Mohr-Jensen C, Steinhausen H-C. A meta-analysis and systematic review of the risks associated with childhood attention-deficit hyperactivity disorder on long-term outcome of arrests, convictions, and incarcerations. *Clinical Psychology Review.* 2016; 48: 32–42.

60. Satterfield JH, Faller KJ, Crinella FM, Schell AM, Swanson JM, Homer LD. A 30-year prospective follow-up study of hyperactive boys with conduct problems: adult criminality. *Journal of the American Academy of Child and Adolescent Psychiatry* 2007; 46(5): 601–10.

61. Savolainen J, Mason WA, Bolen JD, Chmelka MB, Hurtig T, Ebeling H, et al.

The path from childhood behavioural disorders to felony offending: investigating the role of adolescent drinking, peer marginalisation and school failure. *Criminal Behaviour and Mental Health* 2015; 25(5): 375–88.

62. Young S, Goodwin EJ, Sedgwick O, Gudjonsson GH. The effectiveness of police custody assessments in identifying suspects with intellectual disabilities and attention deficit hyperactivity disorder. *BMC Medicine* 2013; 11(1): 1–11.

63. Brown P, Bakolis I, Appiah-Kusi E, Hallett N, Hotopf M, Blackwood N. Prevalence of mental disorder in defendants at criminal court in submission. *BJPsych Open.* 2022; 8(3): E92.

64. Young SJ, Adamou M, Bolea B, Gudjonsson G, Müller U, Pitts M, et al. The identification and management of ADHD offenders within the criminal justice system: a consensus statement from the UK Adult ADHD Network and criminal justice agencies. *BMC Psychiatry* 2011; 11 (1): 1–14.

65. Buitelaar NJ, Ferdinand RF. ADHD undetected in criminal adults. *Journal of Attention Disorders* 2016; 20(3): 270–8.

66. Gudjonsson GH, Young S. An overlooked vulnerability in a defendant: attention deficit hyperactivity disorder and a miscarriage of justice. *Legal and Criminological Psychology* 2006; 11(2): 211–18.

67. Gudjonsson GH, Young S, Bramham J. Interrogative suggestibility in adults diagnosed with attention-deficit hyperactivity disorder (ADHD). A potential vulnerability during police questioning. *Personality and Individual Differences* 2007; 43(4): 737–45.

68. Kassin SM, Gudjonsson GH. The psychology of confessions: a review of the literature and issues. *Psychological Science in the Public Interest* 2004; 5(2): 33–67.

69. Gudjonsson GH. *The Psychology of Interrogations and Confessions: A Handbook* John Wiley & Sons, 2003.

70. Young S. Coping strategies used by adults with ADHD. *Personality and Individual Differences* 2005; 38(4): 809–16.

71. Young S, Thome J. ADHD and offenders. *World Journal of Biological Psychiatry* 2011; 12(sup1): 124–8.

72. Mackay R, Mitchell B, Howe L. A continued upturn in unfitness to plead: more disability in relation to the trial under the 1991 Act. *Criminal Law Review* 2007; July: 530–45.

73. *Crown Prosecution Service* v. *P* [2007] EWHC 946 (Admin), [2008] 1 WLR 1005 at [10].

74. Attwood B. *Make Your Own Picture Stories for Kids with ASD (Autism Spectrum Disorder): A DIY Guide for Parents and Carers*: Jessica Kingsley Publishers, 2015.

75. Baron-Cohen S. *Autism and Asperger Syndrome*. Oxford University Press, 2008.

76. Korkmaz B. Theory of mind and neurodevelopmental disorders of childhood. *Pediatric Research* 2011; 69(8): 101–8.

77. Ali S. Autistic spectrum disorder and offending behaviour: a brief review of the literature. *Advances in Autism* 2018; 4(3): 109–21.

78. Lerner MD, Haque OS, Northrup EC, Lawer L, Bursztajn HJ. Emerging perspectives on adolescents and young adults with high-functioning autism spectrum disorders, violence, and criminal law. *Journal of the American Academy of Psychiatry and the Law Online* 2012; 40(2): 177–90.

79. Murphy D. Understanding offenders with autism-spectrum disorders: what can forensic services do?: commentary on … Asperger syndrome and criminal behaviour. *Advances in Psychiatric Treatment* 2010; 16(1): 44–6.

80. Murphy D. Extreme violence in a man with an autistic spectrum disorder: assessment and treatment within high-security psychiatric care. *Journal of Forensic Psychiatry and Psychology* 2010; 21(3): 462–77.

81. Woodbury-Smith M, Clare I, Holland AJ, Watson PC, Bambrick M, Kearns A, et al. Circumscribed interests and 'offenders' with autism spectrum disorders: a case-control study. *Journal of Forensic Psychiatry and Psychology* 2010; 21(3): 366–77.

82. Sabet J, Underwood L, Chaplin E, Hayward H, McCarthy J. Autism spectrum disorder, attention-deficit hyperactivity disorder and offending. *Advances in Autism* 2015; 1(2): 98–107.

83. Maras KL, Bowler DM. Eyewitness testimony in autism spectrum disorder: a review. *Journal of Autism and Developmental Disorders* 2014; 44(11): 2682–97.

84. Berryessa C. Defendants with autism spectrum disorder in criminal court: a judges' toolkit. *SSRN Electronic Journal* 2021; June.

85. Taylor K, Mesibov G, Debbaudt D. Autism in the criminal justice system. *North Carolina Bar Journal* 2009; 14(4): 32–6.

86. Cooper P, Backen P, Marchant R. Getting to grips with ground rules hearings: a checklist for judges, advocates and intermediaries to promote the fair treatment of vulnerable people in court. *Criminal Law Review* 2015; 6: 417–32.

87. Barry-Walsh JB, Mullen PE. Forensic aspects of Asperger's syndrome. *Journal of Forensic Psychiatry and Psychology* 2004; 15 (1): 96–107.

88. Freckelton I. Autism spectrum disorder: forensic issues and challenges for mental health professionals and courts. *Journal of Applied Research in Intellectual Disabilities* 2013; 26(5): 420–34.

89. Haskins BG, Silva JA. Asperger's disorder and criminal behavior: forensic-psychiatric considerations. *Journal of the American Academy of Psychiatry and the Law* 2006; 34(3): 374–84.

90. Katz N, Zemishlany Z. Criminal responsibility in Asperger's syndrome. *Israel Journal of Psychiatry* 2006; 43(3): 166.

91. McKinnon I, Thorp J, Grubin D. Improving the detection of detainees with suspected intellectual disability in police

custody. *Advances in Mental Health and Intellectual Disabilities* 2015; 9(4): 174–85.

92. White AJ, Batchelor J, Pulman S, Howard D. The role of cognitive assessment in determining fitness to stand trial. *International Journal of Forensic Mental Health* 2012; 11(2): 102–9.

93. Brewster E, Willox EG, Haut F. Assessing fitness to plead in Scotland's learning disabled. *Journal of Forensic Psychiatry and Psychology* 2008; 19(4): 597–602.

94. Murphy GH, Clare IC. Adults' capacity to make decisions affecting the person: psychologists' contribution. In Bull, R, Carson D, eds., *Handbook of Psychology in Legal Contexts*. Wiley, 1995: 97–128.

95. Talbot J. Prisoners' voices: experiences of the criminal justice system by prisoners with learning disabilities. *Tizard Learning Disability Review* 2010; 15(3): 33–41.

96. Howard K, McCann C, Dudley M. 'I was flying blind a wee bit': professionals' perspectives on challenges facing communication assistance in the New Zealand youth justice system. *International Journal of Evidence and Proof* 2019; 24(2): 104–20.

97. Molyneaux E, Vera San Juan N, Brown P, Lloyd-Evans B, Oram S. A pilot programme to facilitate the use of mental health treatment requirements: professional stakeholders' experiences. *The British Journal of Social Work* 2021; 51 (3): 1041–59.

98. Forrester A, Till A, Simpson A, Shaw J. Mental illness and the provision of mental health services in prisons. *British Medical Bulletin* 2018; 127(1): 101–9.

99. Ali A, Ghosh S, Strydom A, Hassiotis A. Prisoners with intellectual disabilities and detention status. Findings from a UK cross sectional study of prisons. *Research in Developmental Disabilities* 2016; 53–54: 189–97.

100. Hensel JM, Casiano H, Chartier MJ, Ekuma O, MacWilliam L, Mota N, et al. Prevalence of mental disorders among all justice-involved: a population-level study in Canada. *International Journal of Law and Psychiatry* 2020; 68: 101523.

101. Henderson E. 'A very valuable tool': judges, advocates and intermediaries discuss the intermediary system in England and Wales. *International Journal of Evidence and Proof* 2015; 19(3): 154–71.

Chapter 19

Fitness to Plead Procedures in Relation to Mental Health and Capacity Legislation

Harinder Bains and Jane M. McCarthy

Introduction

People with intellectual disability (ID), which is also referred to as learning disability in the UK, may be subject to unfitness to plead proceedings in court due to the nature of their disability. ID is defined by onset in the developmental period, with deficits in intellectual functions and adaptive functioning. When people have conditions that affect their cognitive ability such as ID or autism spectrum disorder, and are subject to criminal proceedings, their disability may affect their fitness to plead in court. There is no current statutory test to assess a person's fitness (or unfitness) to plead and this is determined by a common law test called the Pritchard test [1]. The Pritchard test has evolved over the years but is still seen to be inconsistent with modern trial processes and current psychiatric thinking. There are also inconsistencies in the application of the test.

People with ID in England and Wales are also subject to legislation such as the Mental Capacity Act 2005 (MCA 2005) [2] and in Section 1 of the Mental Health Act 1983 (as amended in 2007) (MHA 2007) [3], although for ID to be considered a mental disorder for the purpose of detention under the MHA 2007, they should display abnormally aggressive or seriously irresponsible behaviour. This chapter explores issues with current fitness to practice proceedings for people with ID with a specific focus in relation to the Mental Health Act and Mental Capacity Act and the recommendations of the Law Commission report of 2016 [4]. Chapter 17 provides a detailed overview of mental health legislation in the UK. Chapter 18 covers the defence of fitness to plead in detail, including recommendations of the 2016 Law Commission report and the right to a fair trial.

A significant challenge for unfitness to plead procedures is the accurate and timely identification of those accused who are unfit to plead and those who may require adjustments to the trial process to effectively participate in the trial. This is particularly relevant when people have disabilities and vulnerabilities. Also, legal professionals may not have sufficient awareness and understanding of how to address this issue, which may give rise to difficulties in participating for people with ID [4]. There is currently no statutory entitlement to assistance from an intermediary who may be able to help vulnerable defendants (an intermediary is a communication expert whose role is to facilitate a witness's or defendant's understanding of, and communication with, the court). This is further complicated by the fact that there is no registration scheme for intermediaries assisting defendants. There is also no qualification requirement, no professional conduct regulation or any continuing professional development or supervision arrangements. This is likely to affect their ability and effectiveness in assisting people with neurodevelopmental conditions and particularly ID [4].

The Law Commission considered that some of the terminology currently used such as a finding of 'disability' such that the defendant is deemed 'unfit to plead' is out-dated and risks labelling a defendant in a way that may be objectionable to him or her and to others affected. For lay people, the term 'unfitness to plead' provides no clear understanding or description of what the court has considered or concluded and hence is even more challenging for people who have cognitive issues to understand. The test, as it is currently formulated, looks not only at the ability to enter a plea, but also at other abilities required for a defendant to engage meaningfully in trial. The Law Commission focused on reformulating the test into one that assesses the defendant's capacity to participate effectively in his or her trial, as discussed in Chapter 18, which lays out the test in a more understandable way.

Discrepancy between Unfitness to Plead and Capacity as Defined in the MCA 2005

People who suffer neurodevelopmental disabilities are also more likely to be subject to provisions of the MCA 2005 [2]. Under this Act, a person lacks capacity in relation to a civil matter if at the material time he or she is unable to make a decision for himself or herself in relation to that matter because of an impairment of, or a disturbance in, the functioning of the mind or brain. Also, being able to make a decision requires being able to understand the information relevant to the decision, retain that information, use or weigh it in the decision-making process and communicate the decision.

As seen in the case of Moyle [5], in criminal proceedings a defendant will be found fit to plead even where his or her ability correctly to appraise, believe, weigh up and validly use information regarding legal proceedings is impaired. This gives rise to significant discrepancy between the test for fitness in criminal proceedings and the test for capacity in civil proceedings [6]. This discrepancy seemingly creates the potential for a conflicting assessment where the same individual could be found fit to plead in relation to a murder indictment, but lacking in capacity if there are any civil proceedings.

At the moment, there is no statutory presumption of capacity but criminal courts proceed on an assumption that people are fit to plead unless established otherwise. This was confirmed to be the correct approach by the Court of Appeal in the case of Ghulam [7]. Lord Justice Stanley Burnton held that the requirement from two registered medical practitioners in the Criminal Procedure (Insanity) Act 1964 [8] is the determination of whether the defendant is unfit to plead. In contrast, there is a statutory presumption of capacity for civil proceedings and Section 1 of the MCA 2005 requires that a person 'must be assumed to have capacity' unless it is established otherwise.

The Law Commission recommended that if a decision to adopt alternative procedures is taken, it should be done with caution and only done where it is in the best interest of the defendant. This recommendation does parallel the approach in civil proceedings under the MCA 2005, where there is statutory obligation to act in the person's best interest if they are found to lack capacity in relation to a decision.

Then there is also the issue of expert evidence for a finding of lack of capacity. Currently, a finding of unfitness to plead is based on the evidence of two or more registered medical practitioners [8] and at least one of them has to be approved under Section 12 of the MHA 2007, which designates a registered medical practitioner as having special experience in the diagnosis and treatment of mental disorder. In practice, a consensus of psychiatric medical opinion is needed. The issue for people who have ID is that the experts may not have expertise or experience of working with people with such disabilities. It is recommended that professionals who are routinely involved in assessing capacity, such as psychologists, should be involved in the process as a second expert [9]. This would allow the opportunity for experts with experience of working with capacity issues in people with ID to be involved in the assessment of unfitness to plead.

Specific Issues with Section 35 and Section 36 of the MHA 2007

The Law Commission considered Sections 35 and 36 of the MHA 2007, used by the courts for the assessment and treatment of defendants awaiting trial, as being adequate in the light of the 12-month period proposed by the Law Commission report [4] for assessing unfitness to plead.

Section 35 of the MHA 2007 provides for remand of a defendant to hospital for a report on his or her mental condition to be prepared. It is applicable to any defendant arraigned before the Crown Court for an offence punishable with imprisonment, including murder, prior to conviction. It is not available in the summary courts prior to conviction or a finding that the defendant did the act, unless the defendant consents. Remand is limited to 28 days, with the right of extension for periods of 28 days up to 12 weeks in total. Section 36 of the MHA 2007 provides for the remand of an accused to hospital for treatment. It is applicable to any individual in the Crown Court in custody awaiting trial for an offence which is imprisonable, other than an offence the sentence for which is fixed by law, such as murder. It is therefore not applicable to a defendant awaiting trial or determination of facts in relation to a murder charge. It is not available in the magistrates' court and Section 36 has the same time limitation as Section 35 above.

Considerable difficulty is therefore encountered in cases of murder before trial of determination of facts, if the person needs treatment in hospital. Courts tend to rely on Section 35 of the MHA 2007 for remand in hospital and then, because Section 35 does not confer power to treat, the responsible clinician may have to use Section 3 of the MHA 2007 to add a treatment component. According to Section 35 of the MHA 2007, remand reaches its maximum extension at 12 weeks. If the defendant still requires treatment, the court has to rely on agreeing with the Ministry of Justice for a transfer under Section 48 of MHA 2007, on the basis that the defendant needs urgent treatment, to avoid the defendant inevitably being remanded in custody. The only alternative that currently exists is to grant the defendant bail and rely on their continued detention in hospital under a civil sectioning order. It has been recommended by the Law Commission [4] report that Section 36 of the MHA 2007 be extended to apply to defendants remanded in custody for offences where the penalty is fixed by law, such as murder. It also recommends extension of duration of remand under Section 36 to a maximum of 12 months, with the Crown Court reviewing every 12 weeks.

The Law Commission also made recommendations for reform of the procedures in the magistrates' courts for dealing with defendants who have participation difficulties. If these were enacted, a similar extension of Section 36 of the MHA 2007 to be applicable in the magistrates' court was recommended, albeit with some adjustment, where the defendant faces trial on imprisonable matters. The Law Commission also recommended the application of Section 35 of the MHA 2007 in the magistrates' court be extended to cover all defendants who are awaiting trial or determination of the facts on imprisonable matters [4].

This will entail simplification of the process and will hence assist people with neurodevelopmental conditions, including those with ID, to understand the process. People with such disabilities may be also at risk due to their vulnerabilities and hence are better looked after in a hospital rather than a prison environment.

Representation for the Defendant

The court has the duty to appoint a representative to put forward the case for defence at a Section 4A hearing under the Criminal Procedure (Insanity) Act 1964. This can be someone who is different from the person who has represented the defendant until this point in the proceedings. The duty of the court here is to appoint someone who is the right person for the task. The responsibility placed on the person so appointed is quite different to the responsibility placed on an advocate, where he or she can take instructions from a client. Criminal procedure rules set out factors for the court to take into account in exercising its power to appoint a representative [10]. The representative is not bound to follow the defendant's instructions if they do not agree that the instructions are in their best interest.

The appointment of a representative parallels the function of an independent mental capacity advocate (IMCA) under the MCA 2005. The function of the IMCA is also to act in the best interest of the patient when they do not have capacity to make a decision. This will no doubt assist people who are unfit to plead due to a lack of capacity associated with ID. Some of the trial procedures that are recommended, such as a two-stage process, are likely to be difficult to understand for people with cognitive disability, and to have a representative acting in their best interest is likely to assist them in participating in the trial process.

Removal of the Mandatory Restriction Order

The Law Commission considered the requirement that a defendant be suitable for a hospital order before a mandatory restriction order under Criminal Procedure (Insanity) Act 1964 can be made. This was brought in following the amendment of the 1964 Act by the Domestic, Violence, Crime and Victims Act 2004 [11].The concern is that this may lead to 'arbitrary outcomes' and this is discriminatory against defendants who have a treatable 'mental disorder' under the meaning of the MHA 2007. Such a defendant, following a finding that he or she had committed the offence of murder, would be subject to an indefinite mandatory restriction order without any limit of time, regardless of whether or not he or she represented a risk of serious harm to the public. Another defendant in an identical position, but who does not suffer a treatable mental disorder, would receive, at most, a supervision order for a maximum of two years, however significant the risk he or she presented of serious harm to the public.

This means that people with ID who have a mental disorder by virtue of having abnormally aggressive or seriously irresponsible behaviour could similarly be subject to an indefinite restriction order. This approach is out of step with the Equality Act 2010 [12] and Article 14 of the United Nations Convention on the Rights of People with Disabilities [13], which places an absolute prohibition on people being deprived of liberty on the basis of disability alone.

Involving Liaison and Diversion Services in Courts

The Law Commission recommended that the Criminal Practice Directions [14] be amended to require the court or the parties to make use of liaison and diversion services at court, when these are available, so that the defendant can have an initial assessment where there are doubts as to his or her capacity but it is unclear whether a full expert assessment is required [14].

The UK's Department of Health [15] pointed out that effective liaison and diversion services are essential in providing early assessment on the offender's pathway through the criminal justice system. This report recommend that such services should work in courts and in police stations where they will liaise with all agencies involved in the criminal justice/health interface, providing advice and information as necessary. They would be open to all offenders whether they have ID, a personality disorder or mental health issues. It was recommended they provide a series of assessments which are able to meet the needs of the person in the criminal justice system. The liaison and diversion services would be involved in helping courts and police make informed decisions about charging and sentencing, meet healthcare needs of offenders and focus in reducing the number of people with ID and mental health problems who are in prison unnecessarily.

In 2009, only around one-third of magistrates' courts had liaison and diversion services and they varied significantly in coverage, size, composition, governance, funding arrangements and quality. The report promoted the development of such services over the next five years [15]. The roll-out of NHS England-commissioned liaison and diversion services achieved 100% coverage across England in March 2020 [16]. This scheme is seen to have the potential to revolutionise the identification and screening of defendants with unfitness to plead or capacity issues. The development of such liaison service is likely to help vulnerable people with neurodevelopmental disabilities to seek access to appropriate services at an early stage in the offender pathway and, where appropriate, could help avoid them being subjected to unnecessary and stressful proceedings in courts, which in such cases would have eventually led to disposal to hospital care in any case.

Supervision Orders in the Community

The Law Commission reviewed the option of supervision orders as a disposal option, following unfitness to plead procedures. There is concern about whether probation services would have the expertise to monitor supervision orders for vulnerable individuals such as those with ID. Probation services tend to operate on a coercive basis and it is appreciated that this may not be the best approach [4]. There would also be concern about vulnerable individuals attending probation services alongside convicted offenders, an issue that is likely to become more prominent, as national probation services take on only high-risk and high-profile offenders, which is a recommendation from Ministry of Justice in their consultation 'Transforming rehabilitation: a strategy for reform-response to consultation' [17].

The Law Commission recommended that supervision orders as a disposal option be amended so that the local authority in which the person is resident has sole responsibility for supervising the defendant. A significant proportion of supervised individuals will have ID. They may not need the treatment under a supervision order and hence need no clinical involvement in their supervision. In such circumstances, they would not need a medical supervising officer. The local authority may therefore be in a better position to fulfil this role. Their involvement in safeguarding procedures would also assist them in this role. Many of these individuals with ID will already have involvement with the local authority. It has, however, been noted that further training may be required to assist officers in this role and focused training on the needs of people with ID is likely to assist the effective fulfilment of this role

Conclusion

The Law Commission has recommended a capacity-based approach to assessing fitness to plead. There are considerable challenges with how this will be implemented for people with mental health needs and cognitive disabilities, and discrepancies have been discussed with how this would work for criminal and civil procedures. The Law Commission proposed changes to current mental health legislation; for example, that Section 36 of the MHA 2007 be extended to apply to defendants remanded in custody for offences where the penalty is fixed by law, such as murder. There is also appreciation for the need for representation and support when people with mental health needs interact with legal systems, and how some of the existing statutory arrangements can adversely affect people with mental health needs and neurodevelopmental disabilities. It is not surprising that there are identified gaps in training for professionals working in the legal system. There is a recognised need for diversion of people with such conditions into more appropriate healthcare systems and supervising them with suitable arrangements in the community.

References

1. *R* v. *Pritchard* (1836) 7 C&P 303.

2. Mental Capacity Act 2005. Available at: www.legislation.gov.uk/ukpga/2005/9/contents

3. Mental Health Act 1983 (as amended 2007). Available at: www.legislation.gov.uk/ukpga/1983/20/contents.

4. Law Commission of England and Wales. *Unfitness to Plead – Volume 1: Report (Law Com. No 364)*. The Stationery Office, 2016.

5. *R* v.*Moyle* [2008] EWCA Crim 3059.

6. Vassall-Adams G, Scott-Moncrieff L. Capacity and fitness to plead: the yawning gap. *Counsel* 2006; 3: 2–3.

7. *R* v.*Ghulam* [2009] EWCA Crim 2285.

8. Criminal Procedure (Insanity) Act 1964. Available at: https://www.legislation.gov.uk/ukpga/1964/84

9. Mackay R, Kearns G. An upturn in unfitness to plead? Disability in relation to the trial under the 1991 Act. *Criminal Law Review* 2000; July: 532–46.

10. Gov.UK. Criminal procedure rules and practice: directions 2020. Available at: www.gov.uk/guidance/rules-and-practice-directions-2020.

11. Domestic Violence, Crime and Victims Act 2004. Available at: www.gov.uk/government/publications/the-domestic-violence-crime-and-victims-act-2004.

12. Equality Act 2010. Available at: www.legislation.gov.uk/ukpga/2010/15.

13. United Nations. Convention on the Rights of Persons with Disabilities (CRPD). Available at: www.un.org/development/desa/disabilities/convention-on-the-rights-of-persons-with-disabilities.html.

14. Criminal Practice Directions [2015] EWCA Crim 1567.

15. Department of Health. Improving health, supporting justice. 2009. Available at: www.choiceforum.org/docs/justicebd.pdf.

16. NHS England. About liaison and diversion. 2020. Available at: www.england.nhs.uk/commissioning/health-just/liaison-and-diversion/about/ -accessed 11th December 2022

17. Ministry of Justice. Transforming rehabilitation: a strategy for reform. 2013. Available at: https://consult.justice.gov.uk/digital-communications/transformingrehabilitation/results/transforming-rehabilitation-response.pdf.

Chapter 20

Forensic Services for Neurodevelopmental Disorders: An English Perspective

John Devapriam and Harinder Bains

Introduction

In England and the wider UK, policy and service development for people with neurodevelopmental disorders with forensic needs have evolved over the years with a complex dynamic between care in the community, hospital inpatient care, criminal justice system pathways and changes in mental health/capacity legislation. Most policy and practice have been based on people with intellectual disability (ID) (with or without autism), but the needs of those with autism spectrum disorder (ASD) (without ID) and attention deficit hyperactivity disorder (ADHD) with forensic needs are becoming more recognised, leading to specialist services and adaptations to existing services being developed to address the needs of this population. As criminal justice pathways and mental health/ capacity legislation is being discussed in other chapters, this chapter focuses on community and inpatient hospital services for people with neurodevelopmental disorders within England.

Historically, most people with ID were cared for in long-stay institutions, which ranged from workhouses and prisons during the industrial revolution to local-authority-built special asylums in the late nineteenth century. The first private school dedicated for the training of people with ID was set up in Paris [1], influenced by the work of Édouard Séguin and Jean Mark Gaspard Itard. This led to an interest in people with ID as a separate entity, which led to Seguin continuing the same work in the USA and founding, in 1876, what is known today as the American Association of Intellectual and Developmental Disabilities.

In the early twentieth century, legislation in England and Wales led to care of people with ID being in special asylums, which focused on training and rehabilitation and on lifelong containment and isolation from society. In the 1920s and 1930s, medical interest in the research into the biological basis of 'mental deficiency', and the involvement of prominent people of the medical profession such as Professor Lionel Penrose, led to these asylums becoming designated as hospitals when the National Health Service (NHS) was introduced in 1948. With the Mental Health Act 1959, compulsory admission to hospital was possible on the basis of mental sub-normality and care became polarised between hospital and community, with numbers in hospital increasing until the 1970s [2]. When people with ID were cared for in hospitals, it was assumed that all the healthcare needs could be met in that setting. However, the segregated nature of the hospitals made access to mainstream health services difficult and inequitable. Two large-scale hospital inquiries by the Department of Health and Social Security of Ely hospital in 1969 [3] and Farleigh hospital in 1971 [4] revealed overcrowding, understaffing and serious ill-treatment.

Influential publications by Goffman [5] and Morris [6], describing the dehumanising effects of institutions, coupled with changing attitudes throughout the Western world, led to closure of large-scale asylums and shift of care to the community [7].

Following the de-institutionalisation movement of the 1980s, patients moved into the community. By the 1990s there was greater acknowledgement of both the basic and special healthcare needs of people with ID, and that people with ID have the same rights of access to NHS services as everyone else, but that they may require assistance to use these services. This was accompanied by an increasing focus on community ID teams providing a range of services including those for mental health and behavioural difficulties [8]. The community ID teams were multidisciplinary, offering advice and support to families and carers as well as direct work with individuals with ID. These teams varied in composition but usually included social workers, nurses, speech and language therapists, occupational therapists, physiotherapists, clinical psychologists, psychiatrists and other therapists. By 1993, following the publication of the Mansell report [9], there continued to be significant focus on 'de-institutionalisation' and moving people out of big hospital settings into communities. The Disability Discrimination Act 1995 and the 'Valuing people' white paper [10] further propelled the movement of people from institutional type settings into community settings. By the time of the second Mansell report [11] there were less than 5,000 people in institutional settings. As a result of all the above policy interventions over the years, the number of people with ID living in hospital accommodation in England and Wales fell dramatically from 64,173 in 1970, to 6,404 in 1998 [12], and was just over 2,000 in May 2020 [13].

More recently, following institutional abuse uncovered in Sutton and Merton Trust, Cornwall ID services, Winterbourne View hospital and Whorlton Hall hospital, NHS-commissioned services for people with ID, both in the NHS and the independent sector, have come under the spotlight. A general theme that has emerged from abuse scandals and inquiries is that there is a widespread failure to design, commission and provide services locally and a failure to assess the quality and outcomes being delivered in hospitals for adults with ID [14].

In response to the Winterbourne View hospital scandal, the Transforming Care programme was launched in England and a national service model, 'Building the right support', was developed for the provision of better services for people with ID and ASD, focused around nine key principles [15]. The first focused upon helping people with ID and ASD to live good and meaningful lives in their communities, something which is exceptionally important for those who may be at risk of engaging in offending behaviours. The further principles focused upon ensuring that: family and paid care staff are appropriately supported; individuals have choice as to where they live and who they live with; individuals have access to mainstream and specialist health and social care support within community settings, inclusive of specialist forensic support; and, when hospital is needed, there are clear safeguards in place to help ensure the provision of high-quality care and a short length of stay.

Unfortunately, 'Building the right support' did not achieve all of its objectives, with around the same number of people with ID (i.e., just under 2,500) remaining in hospital in March 2019 at the end of the programme as there were when the plan was implemented in 2015 [13]. The NHS long-term plan [16] places emphasis on quicker ASD assessments and improving quality of services and this is likely to lead to the need for more services focusing on needs of people with ASD and is backed by £2.3 billion investment in improved mental health services. The NHS long-term plan also committed to a reduction of inpatient provision by a further 50% in England by 2024.

Table 20.1 Tiered mode of care for ID services [18]

Tier 1 encompasses primary care and other mainstream services	It is the tier of service provision that serves the general health, social care and educational needs of people with ID and their families. The community ID team and the psychiatrist have limited direct clinical contact in this tier. Nevertheless, they are involved in activities which may influence patients' care, and interacting with this tier is essential to the training of ID psychiatrists.
Tier 2 is general community ID services	At this level the person with ID starts to use specialist ID services. Most specialist services are provided jointly between health and social services or are moving towards such a model.
Tier 3 is a highly specialised element of community ID service	This includes areas of specialised needs such as epilepsy, dementia, challenging behaviour, pervasive developmental disorders and out-patient forensic services.
Tier 4 is specialist inpatient services	This includes all specialist inpatient services for people with ID, ranging from local assessment and treatment services to high secure forensic services.

Tiered Model of Service Provision

The service model in the UK is a combination of generic and specialist services spanning across hospital and community services. Currently in England, most people with ID live fairly independent lives in the community. Of the 900,000 adults with the condition, at any point in time, 191,000 (21%) have contact with specialist ID services and 3,035 (0.3%) receive treatment in psychiatric inpatient settings, including specialist ID hospitals [17]. It is also estimated that that 6,000 people with ID are in UK prisons at any point in time.

Acknowledging nuances in the structural set-up of commissioning and provision of services in the four countries of the UK, the service provision for people with neurodevelopmental disorders can best be described as a tiered model [18] – tiers 1 to 3 constitute the community element of care provision and Tier 4 constitutes the hospital-based element of care provision. The tiered care model and care pathway strives to enable the right care to be delivered by the right people and at the right time and place (see Table 20.1).

The tiered model of service provision from a forensic perspective for people with neurodevelopmental disorders can be described as in Table 20.2 [19]. This model involves multiple agencies across health, social care, education, employment, criminal justice and community/home support agencies [13]. As Figure 20.1 illustrates, an extensive workforce is required, with all agencies delivering support to people with neurodevelopmental disorders who engage in offending behaviours.

The tiered model is described in more detail in the next section, starting with Tier 4.

Tier 4: Specialist Inpatient Services

Tier 4 is further categorised into six types of inpatient beds, as described in Table 20.3, ranging from secure beds (high medium and low secure), acute admission beds in specialist

Table 20.2 Tiered model of care for forensic services for people with ID (reproduced from Devapriam and Alexander [19])

Tier 1	Enabling other agencies (primary care and other mainstream services including criminal justice system) to support offenders with ID: provision of training, supervision and raising awareness of issues in relation to offenders with ID
Tier 2	Supporting community ID teams and other agencies to assess and manage offenders with ID: signposting and providing advice
Tier 3	Hands-on assessment and management of offenders with ID: providing the specialist component of risk assessment and management of offenders with ID using structured professional judgement
Tier 4	Care and treatment of offenders with ID within inpatient facilities (categories 1–6, as described in Table 20.3)

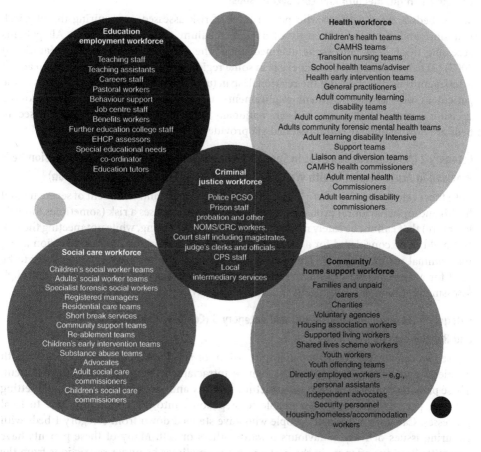

Figure 20.1 Multiple agencies are involved in helping to deliver high quality support to people with ID and ASD who are at risk of engaging in offending behaviours (reproduced from [13, p. 9]). CAMHS: child and adolescent mental health services; CRC: community rehabilitation companies; EHCP: education, health, and care plan; NMSO: National Offender Management Service; PCSO: police community support officer.

Table 20.3 [20] Categories of inpatient beds within Tier 4 for people with ID and mental health and/or severe behavioural problems

Category 1	High, medium and low secure (forensic) beds
Category 2	Acute admission beds within specialist ID units
Category 3	Acute admission beds within generic mental health settings
Categories 4 and 5	Forensic rehabilitation and continuing care beds
Category 6	Other beds including those for health, respite and specialist neuropsychiatric conditions

and mainstream mental health settings and forensic and complex care rehabilitation beds. The different categories are described in more detail below.

Category 1 (High, Medium and Low Secure Beds)

Secure beds are for patients who pose a level of risk assessed as requiring the physical, relational and procedural security of a high, medium or low secure unit. All patients accessing these beds tend to be detained under the Mental Health Act 1983 (amended 2007) [21]. A streamlined process exists in some regions for access to these units – an access assessment is undertaken and the relational, structural and procedural security needs of the patient as well as the treatment requirements are established before a commissioning decision is made. High secure beds are nationally commissioned, medium and low secure beds are now regionally commissioned via provider collaboratives.

Category 2 (Acute Admission Beds in Specialist ID units) and Category 3 (Acute Admission Beds Provided in Acute Mental Health Wards or Such Wards with a Specialist ID Function)

Both these categories of beds are intended for the assessment and treatment of severe mental health and/or behavioural problems, of an intensity which poses a risk (sometimes forensic in nature) that cannot be safely managed in a community setting, while not meeting the risk threshold to be considered for a secure bed and depending on the stage of diversion along the criminal justice pathway. These units complement community services and are to be used for a short period of time to mitigate risk therapeutically and to enable a thorough assessment of mental health needs in a controlled environment by specialist staff.

Category 4 (Forensic Rehabilitation) and Category 5 (Complex Continuing Care and Rehabilitation)

These two categories refer to inpatient provision for several patients whose mental health problems and behavioural difficulties remain intractable in spite of optimum treatment. These patients continue to need the structure, security and care offered by a hospital setting for long periods of time or are unable to step down into the community due to legal processes. Category 4 is mostly people who have stepped down from category 1 beds with enduring issues of risky behaviours towards others or self. Many of these patients have committed serious offences in the past and may sometimes be under restrictions from the Ministry of Justice. Although they have gone through offence-specific and other treatment programmes, their current risk assessments still emphasise the need for robust external supervision and ongoing therapeutic input. However, because of the long length of stays and out of area nature of these provisions, they have come under criticism from regulators [22].

Category 6 (Other Types of Beds)

This includes specialist beds for some neuropsychiatric conditions such as epilepsy and movement disorders. At present, this service provision is limited to a few specialised national units, including those with ASD.

It is recognised that for years there has been lack of information in relation to service models for people with ASD [23]. Hence, there is no benchmark or service specification, but good practice recommends a therapy-based approach to managing treatment pathways [24]. Patients with ASD admitted to forensic services are a heterogeneous group. They usually have other comorbidities including mental illness such as schizophrenia, mood disorders, personality disorders and sometimes other neurodevelopmental conditions such as ADHD and ID. This presents the challenge of managing a group of individuals, all of whom have social communication difficulties but different needs in a group therapeutic setting.

It is recognised that people with neurodevelopmental conditions are more likely to experience mental health issues [25]. Those using forensic neurodevelopmental services tend to have more complex needs and services therefore need to be able to meet these needs. The principle of management remains based on understanding psychological, social and health needs [24] and multidisciplinary teams in such services need to be structured to meet these needs. Services therefore need specialist experience with input from psychologists, occupational therapist, nurses, psychiatrists, speech and language therapists and social workers.

In forensic services there are also security needs and the need to manage the physical, procedural and relational security of the environment. Relational security may pose unique risks in an environment shared by several people with neurodevelopmental disabilities [26]. Security needs of individuals can conflict with the rehabilitation and therapeutic focus in such an environment.

Tiers 1 to 3: Community Services

Several NHS trusts have moved resources from closure of inpatient services and redirected these into intensive community support teams (ICSTs). In regions where ICSTs have been established, there has been reduction in admissions to inpatient care. However, this is primarily in the community pathway described above, as the patients needing a secure pathway need admission to an inpatient facility, which is usually secure and under provisions of the Mental Health Act. Similarly, ICSTs have not been involved in case management of out-of-area patients in secure services either because of the design of the service or because they do not have the time and resources to do this in addition to their community-based role. The effect of ICSTs has therefore been primarily the reduction in use of assessment and treatment, and locked rehabilitation beds.

Specialist forensic community teams have developed in certain regions of the country. These services and care pathways have been set up through local initiatives [19]. A national model for outreach forensic services for people with neurodevelopmental disabilities has been proposed [13]. There are considerable resources for therapeutic management of high-risk patients in inpatient settings. Provision of such services in the community has been dependent on local innovation and limited by resources and clinical expertise in the community. It has been argued that the lack of investment in community services has had a disproportionate effect on the care and rehabilitation of offenders with ID [27]. There needs to be a focus on 'bridging the gap' between therapeutic risk management in inpatient and community setting with a focus on joint working, information and resource sharing and a more supportive approach to the transition from secure to community care. This usually involves working across different organisations, which are sometimes geographically separate. Hence there is need for formal management of such care pathways with oversight from commissioning bodies.

Developing Services for People with Neurodevelopmental Disorders with Forensic Needs

This can be approached in several ways. Where there is no pre-existing written model of care, a starting point is to identify the existing tacit or implicit model of care by mapping existing services, their estate, human resources and levels of activity, pathways and processes. The model needs to be underpinned by a vision, and a commonly used approach is to engage stakeholders in a process involving planning, action, and evaluation. This model therefore needs involvement of all relevant stakeholders [28].

A model of care should be derived from clinical science that is consistent, methodical, cumulative and capable of being evaluated objectively. Human rights, medical ethics, legal structures and processes are integral to this. Then there are legal structures and processes that shape service demands and processes. A final design needs to be accepted by the clinical experts who have clinical responsibility [29]. This can usually be achieved by using the commissioning cycle framework and the five-stage model of care pathway development [28], as outlined below.

The commissioning cycle consists of the following:

(1) assessing the needs of the local population, engaging stakeholders (including patients and their families) and clinical leaders/champions
(2) reviewing services and undertaking a gap in service analysis
(3) understanding key health and care risks and developing a strategy to mitigate risk
(4) deciding on commissioning priorities by using evidence-based and cost-effectiveness analysis
(5) strategic planning using local and national drivers
(6) contract implementation with providers of services, with clear objectives and outcomes
(7) provider development through identifying workforce and resource needs to deliver services
(8) managing provider performance from a quality and financial perspective.

A care-pathway-based approach to service development addresses the variation in practice and ensures standardisation and personalisation (using personalised care plans) of services. Care pathways can be both operational and clinical in nature and developed usually in five stages:

(1) stage 1: map the patient's journey through the care system
(2) stage 2: embedding standards across both mental health and physical health; the standards could include regulatory, contractual, clinical, continuous learning from incidents and values-based standards

(3) stage 3: develop the service structure around the patient's journey

(4) stage 4: develop the workforce – identifying the tasks and level of skills required to undertake the tasks (e.g., functional mapping by Skills for Health (www .skillsforhealth.org.uk))

(5) stage 5: operationalise, evaluate, improvise.

The key elements of a model of care include clear and defined goals for admission. These include generic goals in a forensic service of reducing violence, recovery, providing effective treatment options, managing length of stay and providing a population-based service that is sustainable. This needs to be done with an emphasis on quality, particularly as these are specialist high-cost and low-volume services. The service should have defined care pathways, and these include admission and discharge pathways. There needs to be collaborative approach involving clinical teams in the service, commissioning bodies and community care provision. Treatment modalities need to be defined and this should be evidenced based and in line with what is accepted good practice. Finally, any service should have a process of evaluation to support good quality care and a model that is able to imbibe learning and improve.

The aim of any service should be to provide a high-quality specialist service focusing on engagement in an individualised and outcome-focused treatment and rehabilitation programme in a suitable environment. The environment should address the needs of patients (e.g., be 'autism friendly' for people with ASD) in a physical sense and the therapeutic input focuses on creating a therapeutic milieu conducive to addressing specific needs, risk management and enable patients to move to live safely, with appropriate support in the community.

Each patient admitted or transferred into such a service should have the following standards to meet the person's health and care needs:

(1) *A structured transition into service.* This includes working with the service where the patient is admitted from by introducing structured care plans that can then be followed into the service. This assists with some of the difficulties with transition, as for example this can be a particularly difficult phase for people with ASD, as most patients will struggle with change. A relatively smoother transition also means that patients can facilitate early engagement with the multidisciplinary team in the service. Some of the patients admitted to specialist services will have previously been placed in services that are not 'specialist' services and hence it is helpful for them, and for staff who will be working with them, to have such a period of transition.

(2) *Providing a safe, robust, and individually tailored environment.* The ward environment is a crucial element in providing a suitable and therapeutic service for patients with neurodevelopmental conditions. For an autism specialist service, the physical environment should be designed as per guidance outlined by the National Autistic Society (www.autism.org.uk). Staff should have experience and training of working with people with ASD and work with patients to design individualised care plans regarding their individual environment. The aim is to provide an environment which provides regular positive feedback for appropriate behaviour, gives positive role models, supports patients to take an increased responsibility in their day-to-day living and empowers them in skills of decision making and exercising positive choices. It is important that such an environment is underpinned by positive behaviour support (PBS) with all patients having a PBS plan in place.

(3) *Multidisciplinary therapeutic treatment plan.* The multidisciplinary care plans should be implemented prior to admission. These care plans should be outcome based and individually based on the treatment needs of the patent. Patients may have comorbid mental and physical health conditions, which along with other psychosocial considerations will form the framework for expected care-plan outcomes. Care plans will be based on needs formulations that are based on assessed needs at the time of assessment. There should be the opportunity to review these with NHS England case managers, commissioners and care coordinators through the pre-admission (or post-admission in some cases) care and treatment reviews. The care plans should include interventions and projected time frames, with expected outcomes. The multidisciplinary team should ideally be able to provide the liaison and transition support necessary for safe and smooth movement in and out of the service to improve transition and continuity of care.

(4) *Access to therapy and range of activities.* The approach to multidisciplinary treatment and rehabilitation plan should focus on opportunities to promote a lifestyle with dignity and have access to a range of educational, leisure, vocational, sporting and community skills sessions that are focused on rehabilitation. There should be opportunities to access therapeutic, individual and group sessions specifically designed to meet the individual needs of the patient. This includes adapted offence-related work and adapted sex-offender treatment. Patients should be encouraged wherever possible to engage in ward-based mindfulness practice. Indirect therapies such as drama and art therapy are helpful in engaging patients who may otherwise struggle to engage in psychological work.

(5) *Risk management.* Each patient should have an individualised risk management plan that includes a positive risk-taking approach wherever this is possible. The service should have the necessary physical and procedural elements, but particularly focus on therapeutic relational security, as this is essential for people with ASD. Individualised PBS plans help define and drive this element of therapeutic work.

(6) *Communication and sensory needs.* The treatment plan must include communication, functional and sensory assessments, and amalgamate this into multidisciplinary team care plans and risk management. Communication passports should be used where necessary.

(7) *Pathway approach to discharge.* A multi-agency care pathway approach is required, with involvement from community teams through care coordination, to facilitate seamless delivery of care pathways stepping down from higher levels of security. Where patients don't have local community care coordination, this needs to be established as soon as possible after admission through commissioners and community teams. Close working with community and commissioning teams is essential for successful and timely discharge into community placements. Joint working with community teams and providers is essential for translating hospital-based care plans into community-based ones.

(8) *Interface with external agencies.* The teams should also maintain interface with other external agencies (such as social services, Ministry of Justice, police, Court of Protection) involved in the patient's treatment plan, as this is essential in the delivery of a transparent and dynamic risk-management approach. There is always scope for improving communication with the Ministry of Justice to facilitate movement of

patients through the care pathway (for restricted patients). An example of this would be to inform the Ministry of Justice of discharge plans at an early stage and informing them of likely time frames to discharge.

(9) *Health action plans.* All patients must have health action plans based upon individual healthcare issues and needs. There are increased healthcare vulnerabilities in this patient group and hence the emphasis on health action plans and reducing inequalities. This has recently been brought into sharper focus by the coronavirus (COVID-19) pandemic.

(10) *Person-centred care.* Person-centred care is one of the fundamental standards of care. People should be involved as 'a partner' in a collaborative approach to their care. People who receive personalised care plans are more responsive to their needs. The regulator Care Quality Commission has identified lack of person-centred care as a significant issue for ID services. Accessible information about health and care options help involve people in their care. This should be supported by involvement of carers and families and, where needed, a flexible advocacy provision [31]. Rehabilitation into community settings requires effective and appropriate family and carer support.

Conclusion

On its 70th anniversary, the NHS in England published its 10-year long-term plan with the triple aim of providing integrated care, reducing health inequalities and focusing on prevention. In the context of service models for people with neurodevelopmental disorders, especially ID and ASD, the steer is on drawing from learning from the new care models in tertiary mental health services, where local providers will be able to take control of budgets to reduce avoidable admissions, enable shorter lengths of stay and end out-of-area placements [16]. There will be increased investment in intensive, crisis and forensic community support and there will be a focus on improving the quality of inpatient care across the NHS and independent sector.

Further bed closure initiatives need to be supported by effective discharge planning by tackling not only financial-resource barriers but also commissioning clinical, therapeutic and risk-management resources. While there may be a minority of people who need longer-term inpatient care, either due to the nature of risk or offending, it should be possible that most people in inpatient facilities can be discharged and rehabilitated if there are suitable facilities and resources available in the community to meet their needs. One of the challenges for patients with neurodevelopmental disorders is that, at the time of discharge, there are several factors which can delay discharge. The specialist forensic expertise needed for the safe management of patients in the community is variable. There is anecdotal evidence that where there are well-resourced and effective forensic teams such as community-based forensic intellectual and neurodevelopmental (FIND) teams, it is easier to discharge patients. This is partly linked to a degree of 'nervousness' in community settings about meeting the complex needs of this patient group. FIND teams are also able to provide other support such as training staff and helping them understand the patient's needs.

There is also a lack of specialist providers in the community, and placements are therefore difficult to find. Future emphasis needs to be on developing specialist pathways spanning across inpatient and community services and planning this pathway as a continuum. This needs to be supported by better communication and shared resource management. An emphasis on early involvement of community services and with a similar emphasis on inpatient services supporting community services in designing care plans for this complex group of patients.

There is likely to be a shift in needs of patients being looked after in forensic neurodevelopmental services. This is understandable as the need for inpatient care is affected by resources in the community. For example, better resourced community care is known to reduce reliance on inpatient care

In future, inpatient services are therefore likely to encounter a dynamic environment, with the challenge of meeting changing demands along with the challenge of working collaboratively with stakeholders in community, who until now have been limited by resources to meet the needs of this complex group. This will involve clinical provisions being flexible and adapting to these changing needs. Such changes also mean that clinical expertise will also need to be developed in line with changing service demands.

References

1. Maulik P, Harbour CK, McCarthy J. Epidemiology. In Tsakanikos E, McCarthy J, eds., *Handbook of Psychopathology in Adults with Developmental and Intellectual Disability: Research, Policy and Practice.* Springer Science, 2014.

2. Lindsey M (2003). New patterns of service. In *Seminars in the psychiatry of learning disabilities.* Editors: Fraser W, Kerr M. Royal College of Psychiatrists.

3. Department of Health and Social Security (1969). *Report of the Committee of Inquiry into Allegations of Ill Treatment and Other Irregularities at Ely Hospital, Cardiff (Cmnd 3975).* London: HMSO.

4. Department of Health and Social Security (1971). *Report of the Farleigh Hospital Committee of Inquiry (Cmnd 4557).* London: HMSO.

5. Goffman E. *Asylums: Essays on the Social Situation of Mental Patients and Other Inmates.* Doubleday Anchor, New York 1961.

6. Morris P (1969). *Put Away: A Sociological Study of Institutions for the Mentally Retarded.* London: Routledge and Kegan Paul.

7. Department of Health (1971) *Better services for the mentally handicapped (white paper).* London.

8. Lindsey M (2000) Services for people with learning disability and mental health problems. *Mental Health Review,* 5, 5–18.

9. Department of Health (1993) *Services for People with Learning Disabilities and Challenging Behaviour or Mental Health Needs (Chairman: Prof. J L Mansell).* London: HMSO

10. Department of Health *Valuing people: a new strategy for learning disability for the 21st century.* 2001. Available at: https://assets.publishing.service.gov.uk/government/uploads/system/uploads/attachment_data/file/250877/5086.pdf.

11. Department of Health (2007) *Services for People with Learning Disabilities and Challenging Behaviour or Mental Health Needs: Revised edition (Chairman: Prof. J L Mansell).* London: HMSO.

12. Braddock D, Emerson E, Felce D, et al (2001). Living circumstances of children and adults with mental retardation or developmental disabilities in the United States, Canada, England and Wales and Australia. *Mental Retardation and Developmental Disabilities,* 7, 115–21.

13. Health Education England. *Working in Community Settings with People with Learning Disabilities and Autistic People Who Are at Risk of Coming into Contact with the Criminal Justice System.* Health Education England, 2021.

14. Department of Health. Transforming care: a national response to Winterbourne View hospital Department of Health Review: final report. 2012. Available at: https://asse

ts.publishing.service.gov.uk/government/uploads/system/uploads/attachment_data/file/213215/final-report.pdf.

15. Department of Health. Building the right support: a national plan to develop community services and close inpatient facilities for people with a learning disability and/or autism who display behaviour that challenges, including those with a mental health condition. 2015. Available at: www.england.nhs.uk/wp-content/uploads/2015/10/ld-nat-imp-plan-oct15.pdf.

16. Department of Health and Social Care. NHS long term plan. Available at www.longtermplan.nhs.uk.

17. Devapriam J, Rosenbach A, Alexander R. In-patient services for people with intellectual disability and mental health or behavioural difficulties. *BJPsych Advances* 2015; 21(2): 116–23.

18. Royal College of Psychiatrists. Future role of psychiatrists working with people with learning disabilities. Faculty of psychiatry of learning disability, Faculty report FR/LD/1. 2011. Available at: www.rcpsych.ac.uk/docs/default-source/members/faculties/intellectual-disability/id-futureroleofpsychiatristsinld-services.pdf?sfvrsn=33500689_4.

19. Devapriam J, Alexander R. Tiered model of learning disability forensic service provision. *Journal of Learning Disabilities and Offending Behaviour* 2012; 3(4): 175–85.

20. Royal College of Psychiatrists. People with learning disability and mental health, behavioural or forensic problems: the role of in-patient services Royal College of Psychiatrists' Faculty of Psychiatry of Intellectual Disability Faculty Report FR/ID/03. Available at: www.rcpsych.ac.uk/docs/default-source/members/faculties/intellectual-disability/id-fr-id-03.pdf?sfvrsn=cbbf8b72_2.

21. Mental Health Act 1983 (as amended 2007). Available at: www.legislation.gov.uk/ukpga/1983/20/contents.

22. Care Quality Commission. Mental health rehabilitation inpatient services. Results from the 2019 information request. Available at: www.cqc.org.uk/sites/default/files/20201016_MH-rehab_report.pdf.

23. Alexander R, Langdon P, O'Hara J, Howell A, Lane T, Tharian R, et al. Psychiatry and neurodevelopmental disorders: Experts by experience, clinical care and research. *British Journal of Psychiatry* 2021; 218(1): 1–3.

24. National Institute of Health and Care Excellence. Autism spectrum disorder in adults: diagnosis and management. Clinical Guideline [CG142]. Available at: www.nice.org.uk/guidance/cg142.

25. Langdon P, Alexander R, O'Hara J. Highlights of this issue. *British Journal of Psychiatry* 2021; 218(1): A3.

26. National Health Service. See, think, act. Available at: https://assets.publishing.service.gov.uk/government/uploads/system/uploads/attachment_data/file/320249/See_Think_Act_2010.pdf.

27. Taylor JL, McKinnon I, Thorpe I, Gillmer BT. The impact of transforming care on the care and safety of patients with learning disabilities and forensic needs. *British Journal of Psychiatry Bulletin* 2017; 41: 205–8.

28. Jaydeokar S, Devapriam J, McCarthy J, Kapugama C, Bhaumik S. Models of service development and delivery for people with intellectual disability. In Bhaumik S, Alexander R, eds., *Oxford Textbook of Psychiatry of Intellectual Disability*. Oxford University Press, 2020: 289–96.

29. Kennedy HG. Models of care in forensic psychiatry. *BJPsych Advances*.; 2022; 28 (1): 46–59.

30. Care Quality Commission. Better care in my hands: a review of how people are involved in their care. 2016. Available at: www.cqc.org.uk/sites/default/files/20160519_Better_care_in_my_hands_FINAL.pdf.

Offenders with Neurodevelopmental Disorders in Four Nordic Countries

Erik Søndenaa and Søren Holst

Introduction

The Nordic countries share a social democratic, universal and humanistic view that offenders should not be punished or sentenced to prison if they are considered not accountable for their offending behaviour. However, the countries differ in a variety of legal and clinical frameworks. This chapter presents both the status and differences in Sweden, Finland, Denmark and Norway concerning offenders with neurodevelopmental disorders.

The Nordic welfare model describes how the Nordic countries (Denmark, Sweden, Norway, Finland and Iceland) have organised their social security systems, health services and education. The uniqueness of this model is in the sense that basic welfare arrangements are a citizen's rights. The basic welfare arrangements are also defined for the individual and the financing is collective via taxation. An important aspect of this basic principle is that there is no direct relationship between entitlements and financing for the individual. Although this principle is not applied without exceptions, there are strong universal elements in basic arrangements, such as education, hospital care, social benefits, care of elderly people and basic pensions for all people, including those with intellectual disability (ID) [1]. This welfare model aims to offer services at an early stage and to treat more harmful behaviour as regular care instead of criminalisation of people with ID. One problem arises when an offender is a person with borderline or mild ID; she or he has significant intellectual problems without being administratively diagnosed as a person with ID. The more recent knowledge of the vulnerabilities among some people with neurodevelopmental disorders, especially concerning violent offending, has also called for new integrations to the Nordic welfare model of social and criminal caring. These groups are not included in the local ID services and they are not within the scope of social caring and preventive programmes.

The Nordic welfare model has often been associated with a high degree of solidarity, national cohesion and egalitarianism [2]. There has been a tradition of comprehensive welfare services and programmes, ensuring social and health services, social security, education, employment and housing for all. One particular aim has been to stabilise the economy to ensure that the basic needs of the population are met. The relatively mild penal policy has been explained as rooted in high levels of social trust and political legitimacy, as well as consensual and negotiating political cultures [3].

The Nordic countries have different traditions and histories concerning the treatment of offenders with ID. Denmark (in 1911) and Sweden (in 1928) established forensic institutions for offenders with ID [4]. Norway and Finland did not establish a segregated forensic system for offenders with ID during this period, but included offenders with ID in general institutions for people with ID or into forensic mental health services [5, 6]. These national differences have two possible explanations. First, the economy and welfare systems are different, and hence such services have been prioritised differently. Second, the highly influential enthusiasts who raised the issue of such special care as a priority were Danish. In Denmark, Christian Keller dedicated his working life to forensic ID services [4]. The 'Kellerske Anstalter' (institutions) and the island-based institutions Livø and Sprogø in Denmark have housed several hundred offenders with ID during the first part of the twentieth century [4]. Promoted by numerous professionals who were dedicated proponents of eugenics, similar institutions became common in industrialised Europe and the USA [7].

Population Studies in the Nordic Countries Concerning Neurodevelopmental Disorders

A Swedish birth cohort ($n = 15,117$) from 1953 was studied over 30 years [8]. After 30 years, a small group of people who had attended special ID classes ($n = 192$) was retrieved from the health and criminal registers and compared with non-ID people. The odds of people with ID being convicted of a crime were higher compared with people without ID. Specifically, males with ID were about three times as likely (odds ratio [OR] = 3.12, 95% confidence interval [CI] 2.17–4.49) and females with ID were nearly four times as likely (OR = 3.73, 95% CI 2.00–6.94) to be convicted. In violent convictions, the odds were even higher (males: OR = 5.45, 95% CI 3.38–8.80; females: OR = 24.77, 95% CI 8.86–69.2) [8]. The study, however, has been criticised in recent years for biased sampling [9].

Schwartz and colleagues studied a birth cohort of 21,513 men born in Finland in 1987, with intelligence quotient (IQ) measured by the Finnish Defense Forces Education Development Center, combined with information from the Central Register for Criminal Records, covering crimes committed between the ages of 15 and 21 years [10]. The results showed a consistent linear negative correlation between IQ and criminal offending. They also found curvilinear tendencies for the highest and lowest IQ scores. One explanation for the curvilinearity is that offending behaviours are not considered offending because the adaptive or intellectual functioning is below a certain level. Another explanation is simply that people with less adaptive and intellectual functioning are more law-abiding individuals. These studies have been influential by both addressing the issue of ID and crime [8] and by supporting essential knowledge about the association between ID and crime [10].

Large studies of birth cohorts have also been conducted in Sweden [11, 12]. Moberg et al. followed up 49,000 men after assessment by the Swedish Armed Forces in 1970 and found a strong connection between IQ and violent crime on record, 35 years after this assessment [11]. Heeramun et al. [12] followed up 295,000 children in the Stockholm region, of which 5,700 met the criteria for autism spectrum disorder (ASD) at the age of 15 years. With follow-up until the age of 27, they found that ASD correlated with violent crime, assuming a comorbid attention deficit hyperactivity disorder (ADHD)/conduct disorder. Cases of ASD and ID without ADHD did not show such a correlation with violent crime. A previous population-based register study of child and adolescent mental health services in Stockholm, including 3,391 people, found associations between ADHD and tic disorders with violent crimes, but no such association in people with ASD or obsessive–compulsive disorder.

Nordic Research on Issues Concerning Offenders with Neurodevelopmental Disorders

In recent years, Swedish researchers have published important contributions to the field on neurodevelopmental disorders related to offending behaviour [13–15]. It is interesting that Moberg et al. [11] found a clear connection between IQ and later violent convictions, Billstedt et al. [13] found an increased proportion of young convicted men (violent crimes) with ASD and Heeramun et al. [12] found in particular the combination of ASD and ADHD as a risk factor for violent crime. Thus, in cases of low IQ and symptoms of ASD and ADHD, there may be a particular risk of violent crime.

In 1990, the Danish psychiatrist Lund published an article that focused on ID offenders in Denmark. There was a significant decrease in the number of 'mentally retarded offenders', from 290 in 1973 to 91 in 1984 [16]. Lund explained this reduction in the number of convicted people with ID by a shorter sentence and a 'dramatic' fall in the number of borderline ID offenders, who in the research exhibited more recidivism. On the other hand, the decrease in total sentences was opposed by the fact that the types of crime were altered from less crime against property to more violence, arson and sexual offences. The figures for violence, arson and sexual offences have increased from 110 in 1984 to 151 in 2019 (+37%; [17]). Every year, the Danish Ministry of Justice publishes a report of how many ID offenders have been sentenced, the type of sentence and the type of crime for ID offenders, among other factors.

The life and treatment of ID offenders has been rarely studied in Denmark, but in the last decades there has been an increase in research in the field. An example is a two-volume research report on this topic, by workers at Aalborg University, which describes ID offenders (the target group), provides some of their narratives and examines the legal framework and the social pedagogic practice and treatment [18, 19]. A thesis has looked at the impact, advantages and disadvantages of the social pedagogic treatment [20, 21]. In 2013, Holst and Lystrup undertook a project in which they focused on ID offenders who were sentenced for arson [22, 23].

During the last decade, the study of neurodevelopmental disorders including ID in Norway has focused on epidemiological, service and legal issues. The prevalence of inmates with potential ID was as high as 10.8% [24], and later studies have been conducted to examine whether a potential ID diagnosis was known during the criminal justice proceedings in such cases. Studies have explored different legal applications [25, 26], the awareness of ID in courts and by the police [27] and correctional service adjustments in cases involving prisoners with ID [28].

A nationwide Norwegian study focusing on ASD in 48 forensic examinations resulted in a series of papers [29–31]. The study identified that most ASD diagnoses occurred when these individuals were adults, the diagnostic validity was weak, the background characteristics of these people was similar to other offenders and some had experienced criminal justice as problematic based on their neurodevelopmental difference.

There has been a prominent increase in the proportion of Norwegian prisoners who are sexual offenders. This growth follows increased penalties for such crimes. Many studies have emphasised that offenders with neurodevelopmental disorders are more frequent among sex offenders than among other subgroups of offenders (Simpson & Hogg [32]). Søndenaa and Spro [26] found that sex offenders with ID were mostly given a reduced sentence.

Legislation and Offenders with Neurodevelopmental Disorders

All the Nordic countries have a forensic mental health service commissioned by the courts for the purpose of declaring whether the alleged offender was suffering from a mental disorder or ID at the time of the offence [33]. The forensic examination provides a basis for determining whether the person's mental state at the time of the offence may have influenced the capacity to understand and control her or his behaviour. There are varying practices concerning the assessment and identification of charged individuals with neurodevelopmental disorders in the Nordic countries.

The Nordic countries have been very early compared to other countries worldwide in establishing conditional and suspended sentences. This was initially reserved for first-time offenders or for short sentences. These alternatives have subsequently been used in the combination between social care and criminal suspension, with shared responsibilities between community services and criminal justice services. The basic principles and priorities of the sentencing systems of the Nordic countries have much in common, but there are some differences. Political tendencies in the last two decades have been somewhat contradictory but at the same time have succeeded in controlling the use of imprisonment and expanding the use of community penalties. Imprisonment rates increased until 2005 and have been stable or declining since then [34].

A Nordic community of forensic mental health research and practice has been active in the last three decades, and their interests beyond traditional mental health conditions have been growing.

Sweden

The Swedish criminal code, Section 3, states that a connection between the conduct of the accused and their diminished development, experiences or ability to judge is a mitigating circumstance for the penalty [35]. Swedish legislation does not include the concept of criminal responsibility. According to Swedish law, in principle all adults are accountable but, if you suffer from a serious mental disorder, you can be sentenced to care instead of imprisonment. A disorder due to lack of development such as ID can, if the conditions are sufficiently pronounced and disabling, constitute a so-called 'serious mental disorder', which is the basis for the court to sentence to care instead of imprisonment. The Swedish court stated in 2010 that young people with neurodevelopmental disabilities cannot comply with the requirement of 'socially degrading behaviour' in Section 3 of the Swedish code (1990:52) if their behaviour is a direct symptom of their disability. A white paper (SOU 2015:71) proposed that there should no longer be obstacles to provide compulsory care to young people with neurodevelopmental disabilities who need care because of their own behaviour [36]. Those authors noted that a lack of implementation of the white paper recommendations means that many young people with neurodevelopmental disorders and delinquent behaviour receive unsatisfactory treatment.

Denmark

It is a fundamental principle in the Danish Penal Code that all offenders who by law are assessed to be intellectually disabled or have a severe psychiatric disorder are not punishable by law [37]. The underlying principle is that criminal intent requires the offender to have committed the offence intentionally and that she or he is able to understand the implications of her or his crime when committing it. A person with ID does not have the capacity to comprehend fully the consequences of a particular situation or her or his actions. Penal sentencing is therefore deemed

Table 21.1 Number of people with ID sentenced by the Danish Penal Code since 2001, odd years [17])

2003	2005	2007	2011	2013	2015	2017	2019
52	84	72	140	111	148	120	167

Note: No data from 2009 because of a lack of registration from the Ministry of Justice.

to be meaningless in most cases. Danish criminal law determines that offenders with ID need social pedagogic help and support to ensure that they do not engage in further criminal activity.

The Danish Penal Code stipulates:

Section 16. Persons who, at the time of the act, were irresponsible on account of mental illness, or a state of affairs comparable to mental illness, or who are severely mentally defective are not punishable.

Persons who, at the time of the act were slightly mentally defective are not punishable.

In Denmark, you are considered to have ID if your IQ is less than 70, according to the WHO's International Classification of Diseases 10th Revision (ICD-10), which is equivalent to the definition in ICD-11 in which the terminology is 'Disorders of intellectual development' [38]. If the IQ is slightly higher than 70 and if the convicted has significant social problems, drug abuse or sexual problems that reduce their level of functional capacity, a psychiatrist can assess that the person should be judged as if she or he has ID.

There are three laws in Denmark pertaining to adult criminals: the Danish Penal Code [39], the Danish Psychiatric Act [40] and the Danish Consolidation Act [41]. An individual who is convicted of a criminal offence under the Danish Penal Code receives her or his sentence and is then transferred to the Danish prison and probation service, the authority that administers the Danish prison system. If a mentally ill person commits a crime, she or he is not punishable (Section 16 of the Danish Penal Code), but is referred for treatment in one form or another under the provisions of the Danish Psychiatric Act. When a person with ID commits a crime, she or he is not punishable (Section 16 of the Code), but is placed in a residential unit according to the provisions of the Danish Consolidation Act on Social Services.

There are five types of sentences that apply to individuals who are mentally disabled and have committed a crime in Denmark [42]. They lie on a continuum from the mildest measure: supervision by the municipality, an arrangement according to which the offender with ID shall comply with the supervisory authority's provisions on matters relating to residence and work, to the most intrusive: placement in a secure unit for people with ID.

An issue that is unique to Denmark is the distinction between people with ID and those with other psychiatric or neurodevelopmental disorders. In the latter cases, the convicted person will be transferred to a psychiatric ward for treatment, or a special prison.

There has been an increase in sentences by the Danish Penal Code for people with ID in recent decades (Table 21.1). The reason for this is not completely clear, but a probable hypothesis is that there is now better screening of the accused in the initial legal, social and psychiatric examinations.

Norway

According to Section 20 of the Norwegian Penal Code people above the age of 15 who commit crimes and are found to be 'mentally retarded to a high degree' (*psykisk utviklingshemmet i høy grad*) are not criminally responsible and cannot be punished [43]. The legal term 'mental retardation to a high degree' is not defined in the Norwegian Penal Code but has been elaborated through relevant legal sources and covers people with an intellectual functioning level corresponding to an IQ of less than 55. People with ID who commit crimes and do not meet the criteria of being 'mentally retarded to a high degree' – that is, those who have an IQ above 55 – are viewed as criminally responsible and are thus given a regular sentence, to be served either in prison or in society (e.g., community service). When the person has mild ID, defined as having an IQ of 55–75 – which is considered mentally disabled to a lesser degree according to Penal Code Sections 78(d) and 80(g) – there is the possibility for the court to reduce the sentence.

Recent changes in the punitive legislation have made adjustments to include offenders with neurodevelopmental disorders and other functional deficits (i.e., dementia) as not criminally responsible. The government (Prop. 154L [2016–2017]) has proposed including more offenders by both elevating the functional threshold of the offender and prosecuting less serious offences when not-responsible offenders have been convicted. The term 'serious mental health disorder' has been replaced with a more inclusive term, namely 'strongly deviant mental condition'. The latter term includes neurological disorders, infections, delirium or neurodevelopmental disorders (Prop. 154L p. 76). The number of forensic psychiatric examinations has increased during the past decade, from 335 in 2010 to 547 in 2019 [44]. Between 5% and 10% of all examinations have concluded with the observed individual having ID.

There has been controversy in Norway surrounding the case of Anders Breivik when it comes to considering ASD and offending behaviour, as the forensic experts were of the opinion that the diagnosis was personality disorder [45].

Finland

According to Section 4 of the Finnish Penal Code, the perpetrator is not criminally responsible if at the time of the act she or he has a mental illness, severe mental deficiency or a serious mental disturbance. In terms of forensic psychiatric assessments, Finnish law permits a forensic psychiatric examination if the offence is punishable, an evaluation can be justified and the accused gives consent to be examined [6]. As in the other Nordic countries the forensic psychiatric assessment must consider the question of criminal responsibility due to mental illness, severe mental deficiency, mental disturbance or serious cognitive disturbances. Interestingly, the number of full forensic psychiatric examinations has decreased in the last decade, from 300 to 80–100 [6]. Out of these examinations, less than 5% of people have ID [6, 45]. Männynsalo et al. studied all the forensic psychiatric examination reports of people with ID over a decade [46]. They found that the single most common crime was arson, often related to substance use.

Housing and Placements for Offenders with Neurodevelopmental Disorders

Sweden

The Swedish legislation says that all defendants found guilty are convicted and held responsible for the crime regardless of their mental state at the time of their crime. If they are considered to have acted under a severe mental disorder, they will not be sentenced to prison, but to mental healthcare (Chapter 30, Section 6) [35]). The so-called 'prison ban' prevents offenders with severe conditions (including neurodevelopmental disorders) from being sentenced to prison. Swedish courts impose imprisonment to a convicted person with a neurodevelopmental disorder only if there are exceptional grounds to do so (Section 6 of the Swedish code). The court considers whether (a) the offence has a high penalty value, (b) there is less need for psychiatric care or (c) the crime was caused by a self-inflicted condition. Probation is the alternative (Section 9 of the Swedish code) to imprisonment if the court finds that a probation sentence will prevent reoffending. Probation is also considered in combination with a provision of community services, and such a provision is appropriate in view of the character of the individual and other circumstances.

Denmark

In Denmark, ID offenders are treated in residential units. The staff are mainly social pedagogues and there are usually very few healthcare professionals assigned. A social pedagogue is a professional with three and a half years of training in social education with focus on social training and development. They mainly work with marginalised and vulnerable people, for example young people with social problems, drug users, people with ID and psychiatric patients. If the ID offender has other or multiple psychiatric disorders, she or he will be referred to a psychiatrist, and medication is often prescribed. The majority of ID offenders are placed in residual units all over the country, except those who are sentenced to secure wards and are admitted to the national institution called Kofoedsminde. As of 2021, about 70 people have such a sentence in Denmark. This country also has one secure institution for juvenile ID offenders (mostly 15–18 years old). In 2013, 12 juveniles were among the 111 offenders sentenced as described in Table 20.1.

People who have a neurodevelopmental diagnosis such as ADHD or ASD would normally be transferred to prisons or psychiatric hospitals. They are assessed by psychiatric and psychological specialists working in psychiatric wards in the Danish healthcare system or at the institution of Herstedvester near Copenhagen, managed by the Danish prison and probation service. This facility specialises in a variety of offenders with different disorders including ASD, ADHD and other neurodevelopmental diagnoses. The treatment available includes medical and psychotherapeutic interventions and social and relational training.

Norway

Most offenders with neurodevelopmental disorders are considered responsible subjects by Norwegian courts. The accused person will be considered not responsible if she or he is defined as having a 'strongly deviant mental condition', which most often includes both a neurodevelopmental disorder and ID or ID with IQ of less than 55. If not responsible because of ID, the offender can be sentenced to mandatory care and will be secured in highly professional local community-based habilitation services for three years at a time. Very few offenders are sentenced within this system (1–2 per year, 10–12 at any one time), but the incidence has increased in recent years, with a total number of people receiving such a sentence of about 20, in 2021.

Offenders with neurodevelopmental disorders (mostly ASD) can be sentenced to forensic mental healthcare if it is comorbid to conditions that classify the person within the category 'strongly deviant mental condition'. This incarceration is institutional and based on the principles of secure mental health services. Norwegian criminal law can also give reduced sentences to convicted people who are declared not criminally responsible. This then includes both people with a mild degree of ID and more high-functioning autism.

Norway introduced a new service for rehabilitation and the return back to home for vulnerable long-term prisoners in 2013. People with a neurodevelopmental disorder often need a strong and prepared service in the local community to succeed in the transfer from imprisonment to independent living. The coordinators of this service have described their work as a patient, slow and labour-intensive effort. They have to time the process at an early stage and the results are very encouraging, with good housing and day-time activity along with adapted social and health services [28].

Finland

Finland has two large forensic state hospitals (Niuvanniemi and Vahna Vasa) with a total of approximately 300 beds. There are also forensic mental health beds in general psychiatric hospitals (100 beds) and in prison wards (50 beds). The state forensic hospitals have facilities to treat mentally ill and dangerous offenders, while the general psychiatric hospitals and prison wards serve offenders who lack criminal responsibility or prisoners who are suspected of being mentally ill [47, 48]. Männynsalo et al. showed that a large proportion of offenders with ID are known to the services based on triple diagnosis – substance abuse, mental illness and ID [46]. Thus, there is the need for close, long-term cooperation among specialists in the field of ID, substance abuse services and mental health services. The most challenging part of this cooperation, however, seems to be providing good-quality treatment programmes and support systems for people with ID with such complex needs.

Treatment and Care of Offenders with Neurodevelopmental Disorders

Sweden

The Swedish courts have stated that young people with neurodevelopmental disabilities cannot be compelled to comply with the requirement of 'socially degrading behaviour' if their behaviour is a direct symptom of their disability. Criminal justice services usually do not have the competency required to assess or understand such disabilities and many of these young offenders do not obtain the care they need [36].

Denmark

There is no systematised and standardised way of handling ID offenders in Denmark. Each residential facility plans treatment based on individual needs. This work is planned, described and evaluated in the resident offender's individual work plan. The individual work plan is a statutory instrument. The social pedagogic staff working with the offender prepares the work plan. External experts may be involved if there is a need for this, usually being psychologists and psychiatrists. The offender's home municipality approves the action plan.

The basic thinking behind the treatment with ID offenders in Denmark is that the offender should develop and improve her or his or social skills. This is achieved, for example, through contact and interaction with staff and fellow residents, schooling, employment and activities of daily living. Social pedagogic interaction and treatment are primarily based on a model focused on learning theory, an approach of recognition and on an understanding that ID offenders often commit crimes as a result of their disabilities. Medical treatment is administered if the psychiatrist deems it to be appropriate. Unless a particular condition is attached to the sentence, the offender may in principle desist from complying with staff recommendations. Treating ID offenders is therefore based largely on a voluntary approach, cooperation and trust.

Norway

A prison cohort study [24] concluded that 10.8% of the randomly selected prisoners had an IQ less than 70. These prisoners were not eligible from most prison rehabilitation efforts like work-directed education and crime-prevention programmes. This improved knowledge about the significant proportion of people with ID in this prison study [24] has resulted in several initiatives, both within research and in practical changes. In 2013, all prisons hired release coordinators to follow vulnerable people from imprisonment to release. By adjusting this process with better adaptation to the life circumstances in freedom with housing, work, family, network and social activities, these coordinators have contributed to improved welfare for many former prisoners with ID or other neurodevelopmental conditions [28]. Identification within the prison health services and education about ID or ASD to prison staff are offered in several prisons. Since Norway ratified the United Nations Convention of the Rights of Persons with Disabilities in 2013, there has been a request for educational support to courts and police on how to identify and communicate to fulfil the requirements of a more equal treatment.

Norwegian offenders with ASD have been found to experience several conflicting issues at the early stage of the criminal proceedings [30]. One of the interviewed individuals said that he was 'interrupted when I was supposed to give testimony in court', and most have described the trial as very challenging and stressful. One said, 'I was afraid all the time, sweated heavily and just wanted to finish as fast as possible', and, 'It was terrible in court with a lot of people present'. By contrast, the interviewed people who were or had been in prison answered that they coped well in these circumstances. Most of them reported that they enjoyed the firm structure and the routines, and one said, 'I enjoyed myself in prison, and that is in contrast to what the forensic experts said, who claimed that prison would be bad for me'.

Finland

Männynsalo found that 25% of the offenders with ID also had substance dependency [46]. Other mental health conditions in this sample were rare. About 50% of the offenders with ID were placed in special care residences for people with ID, with national guidelines for the principles of nursing care. These guidelines were, according to Männynsalo, not sufficiently followed because of an insufficient structure in the majority of cases [45] . A more integrative and consistent service provision model is required with the use of multi-skilled key workers. Better cooperation among caregivers is a definite problem in Finland concerning offenders with ID and their long-term needs for treatment and care.

Table 21.2 A summary of how offenders with ID or severe mental health problems are considered in the Nordic countries

	Criminal non-responsibility	Placements	Treatment
Denmark	IQ < 70, severe mental health problems	Social service facilities	Social pedagogic
Finland	IQ < 70, severe mental health problems	Mental health facilities or correctional services	Mental healthcare
Norway	IQ < 55, severe mental health problems	Mental health facilities or correctional services	Mental healthcare
Sweden	No concept of criminal non-responsibility	Mental health facilities or correctional services	Mental healthcare

Conclusion

The Nordic countries are often described within the frame of a common Nordic welfare model; however, there are marked differences in criminal cases involving offenders with neurodevelopmental disorders (Table 21.2). The Swedes have recognised the presence of this group of offenders, but they consider that all adults are accountable for their actions. The other Nordic countries have differing thresholds for considering a person criminally irresponsible. These limits are set at IQ < 70 in Denmark and Finland and at IQ < 55 in Norway. The treatment of offenders with ID and other neurodevelopmental disorders within the criminal law is unclear. The treatment facilities reflect the legal rules, and an inclusive perspective as in Sweden provides no separate treatment facilities for offenders with neurodevelopmental disorders. While the Swedes have recognised the presence of these offenders, who are served within an integrated criminal care system, Norway and Denmark have special units, with Denmark based on social pedagogic treatment and Norway on mental health services. The care and welfare for non-offending people with ID and other neurodevelopmental disorders are much more similar in the Nordic countries, with community-based integrated services and group homes. As Männynsalo et al. noted [46], there is a gap between offenders with neurodevelopmental disorders receiving integrative and consistent services, with the use of multi-skilled key workers based on cooperation among caregivers, and the reality of what occurs in practice within criminal care settings.

References

1. Andersen TM. Challenges to the Scandinavian welfare model. *European Journal of Political Economy* 2004; 20(3): 743–54.

2. Christiansen NF. *The Nordic Model of Welfare: A Historical Reappraisal.* Museum Tusculanum Press, 2006.

3. Lappi-Seppälä T. Trust, welfare, and political culture: explaining differences in national penal policies. *Crime and Justice* 2008; 37(1): 313–87.

4. Kirkebæk B. Da de aandssvage blev farlige [When the mentally deficient became dangerous]. Forlaget SocPol. 1995.

5. Søndenaa E, Gudde C, Thomassen Ø. Patients with intellectual disabilities in the forensic asylums 1915–1982: before admission. *Scandinavian Journal of Disability Research* 2015; 17(1): 14–25.

6. Seppänen A, Joelsson P, Ahlgren-Rimpiläinen A, Repo-Tiihonen E. Forensic psychiatry in Finland: an overview of past,

present and future. *International Journal of Mental Health Systems* 2020; 14: 1–8.

7. Rafter NH. *Creating Born Criminals.* University of Illinois Press, 1997.

8. Hodgins S. Mental disorder, intellectual deficiency, and crime: evidence from a birth cohort. *Archives of General Psychiatry* 1992; 49(6): 476–83.

9. Lindsay WR, Dernevik M. Risk and offenders with intellectual disabilities: reappraising Hodgins (1992) classic study. *Criminal Behaviour and Mental Health* 2013; 23: 151–7.

10. Schwartz JA, Savolainen J, Aaltonen M, Merikukka M, Paananen R, Gissler M. Intelligence and criminal behavior in a total birth cohort: an examination of functional form, dimensions of intelligence, and the nature of offending. *Intelligence* 2015; 51: 109–18.

11. Moberg T, Stenbacka M, Tengstrom A, Jonsson EG, Nordstrom P, Jokinen J. Psychiatric and neurological disorders in late adolescence and risk of convictions for violent crime in men. *BMC Psychiatry* 2015; 15: 299.

12. Heeramun R, Magnusson C, Gumpert CH, Granath S, Lundberg M, Dalman C, et al. Autism and convictions for violent crimes: population-based cohort study in Sweden. *Journal of the American Academy of Child and Adolescent Psychiatry.* 2017; 56(6): 491–7.

13 Billstedt E, Anckarsater H, Wallinius M, Hofvander B. Neurodevelopmental disorders in young violent offenders: overlap and background characteristics. *Psychiatry Research* 2017; 252: 234–41.

14. Krona H. On lifetime violent criminality in a Swedish forensic psychiatric cohort. 2020. Available at: www.lunduniversity.lu .se/lup/publication/0e2a599f-e361-4826- a4ff-35afff4767f4.

15. Lundström S, Forsman M, Larsson H, Kerekes N, Serlachius E, Långström N, et al. Childhood neurodevelopmental disorders and violent criminality: a sibling control study. *Journal of Autism and Developmental Disorders* 2014; 44(11): 2707–16.

16. Lund J. Mentally retarded criminal offenders in Denmark. *British Journal of Psychiatry* 1990; 156(5): 726–31.

17. Justitsministeriet. Nye foranstaltningsdomme i 2019. Forskningskontoret, Copenhagen. 2020.

18. Breumlund A, Hansen IB. Domsanbragte udviklingshæmmede. Hvorfra-Hvorhen? II: Beboerperspektiver på forandringer [Sentenced people with developmentally disabillity. From where to where? User perspectives on change]. Aalborg Universitet, 2014. Available at: https://vbn .aau.dk/ws/portalfiles/portal/201355186/f_ rdig_Domsanbragte_2_NETTET.pdf.

19. Ringø P. Domsanbragte udviklingshæmmede Hvorfra-Hvorhen? I: Den socialpædagogiske indsats på et botilbud for voksne udviklingshæmmede med dom [Sentenced people with developmentally disability. The social peadagogic efforts at a residential unit for adults with developmental disabilities who are convicted]. Aalborg Universitet, 2014. Available at: https://viden.sl.dk/media/728 9/domsanbragte_web.pdf.

20. Rømer M. *Det socialpædagogiske arbejde på botilbud med domfældte udviklingshæmmede: rammebetingelser og dilemmaer* [The socio-educational work in residential facilities with convicted mentally disabled people: framework conditions and dilemmas]. Social-og specialpædagogik: Akademisk Forlag, 2015: 255–68.

21. Rømer M. Dømt til socialpædagogik: Et studie af dilemmaer i den socialpædagogiske indsats på et botilbud for domfældte voksne med udviklingshæmning. Aalborg University. 2016. DOI: https://doi.org/10.5278/vbn .phd.socsci.00061.

22. Holst S, Lystrup D. *Brandstiftelse. Hærværk, Kommunikation eller Fascination. En Undersøgelse af Udviklingshæmmede Brandstiftere* [Fire Setting. Vandalism, communication or fascination? A study of developmentally disabled fire setters]. Kofoedsminde, 2013.

23. Holst S, Lystrup D, Taylor JL. Firesetters with intellectual disabilities in Denmark.

Journal of Intellectual Disabilities and Offending Behaviour 2019; 10(4): 72–81.

24. Søndenaa E, Rasmussen K, Palmstierna T, Nøttestad J. The prevalence and nature of intellectual disability in Norwegian prisons. *Journal of Intellectual Disability Research* 2008; 52(12): 1129–37.

25. Søndenaa E, Olsen T, Kermit PS, Dahl NC, Envik R. Intellectual disabilities and offending behaviour: the awareness and concerns of the police, district attorneys and judges. *Journal of Intellectual Disabilities and Offending Behaviour* 2019; 10(2): 34–42.

26. Søndenaa E, Spro M. Lettere psykisk utviklingshemmede i strafferettslig forstand: en gjennomgang av alle registrerte saker fra Lovdata 2002–2014. *Lov og rett* 2016; 55(08): 504–16.

27. Søndenaa E, Friestad C, Storvik BL, Johnsen B. Criminal responsibility and challenges in the criminal justice system for people with intellectual disability in Norway. *Bergen Journal of Criminal Law and Criminal Justice* 2019; 7(1): 97–109.

28. Friestad C, Johnsen B, Storvik BL, Søndenaa E. Innsatte med utviklingshemming: en deskriptiv undersøkelse av ulike etaters arbeid med identifikasjon og tilrettelegging. 2020. Available at: https://sifer.no/wp-content/uploads/2020/06/Rapport-innsatte-utviklingshemming_PDF.pdf.

29. Helverschou SB, Rasmussen K, Steindal K, Søndanaa E, Nilsson B, Nøttestad JA. Offending profiles of individuals with autism spectrum disorder: a study of all individuals with autism spectrum disorder examined by the forensic psychiatric service in Norway between 2000 and 2010. *Autism* 2015; 19(7): 850–8.

30. Helverschou SB, Steindal K, Nøttestad JA, Howlin P. Personal experiences of the criminal justice system by individuals with autism spectrum disorders. *Autism* 2018; 22(4): 460–8.

31. Søndenaa E, Helverschou SB, Steindal K, Rasmussen K, Nilson B, Nøttestad JA. Violence and sexual offending behavior in people with autism spectrum disorder who

have undergone a psychiatric forensic examination. *Psychological Reports* 2014; 115(1): 32–43.

32. Simpson MK, Hogg J. Patterns of offending among people with intellectual disability: a systematic review. Part 1: methodology and prevalence data. *Journal of Intellectual Disability Research* 2001; 45(5): 384–96.

33. Holmberg G. Forensic psychiatric practice in the Nordic countries. *Nordic Journal of Psychiatry* 1998; 51(S39): 7–14.

34. Lappi-Seppälä T. Nordic sentencing. *Crime and Justice* 2016; 45(1): 17–82.

35. Swedish Government. The Swedish criminal code. Available at: www.government.se/498db0/contentassets/7a2dcae0787e465e9a2431554b5eab03/the-swedish-criminal-code.pdf.

36. Justermark J, Lagneteg M. Tvångsvård av unga med neuropsykiatriska funktionsnedsättningar: Tillämpning av rekvisitet 'socialt nedbrytande beteende' [Compulsory care of young people with neuropsychiatric disabilities: Application of the requirement 'socially degrading behavior']. PhD Thesis. Ørebro University, 2019.

37. FreseJensen M, Greve V, Høyer G, Spencer M. *The Principal Danish Criminal Acts, The Danish Criminal Code, The Danish Correction Act, The Administration of Justice Act.* DJØF Publishing Association of Danish Lawyers and Economists, Copenhagen, 2006.

38. World Health Organization. International Classification of Diseases 11th revision. 2022. Available at: www.who.int/standards/classifications/classification-of-diseases.

39. Danish Criminal Code. Available at: www.ojp.gov/ncjrs/virtual-library/abstracts/danish-criminal-code-english-version.

40. Retsinformation. Psykiatriloven. Available at: www.retsinformation.dk/eli/lta/2019/936.

41. Retsinformation. Serviceloven. Available at: www.retsinformation.dk/eli/lta/2020/1287.

42. Rigsadvokaten [Director of Public Prosecutions]. Meddelelse nr. 5/2007, Behandling af straffesager vedrørende psykisk afvigende kriminelle og personer omfattet af straffelovens § 70. 2007 [A governmental document published by the Director of Public Prosecutions and the Ministry of Justice as a guide to interpret the current law.]

43. The Norwegian Penal Code, Available at: https://lovdata.no/dokument/NLE/lov/200 5-05-20-28.

44. Statens sivilrettsforvaltning, 2020. Available at: https://img4.custompublish.com/getfile .php/4838511.2254.lz7wjtnwu7lkqw/A%CC %8Arsrapport+2020.pdf?return=www .sivilrett.no.

45. Faccini L, Allel CS. Mass violence in individuals with autism spectrum disorder and narcissistic personality disorder: a case analysis of Anders Breivik using the 'path to intended and terroristic violence' model. *Aggression and Violent Behavior* 2016; 31: 229–36.

46. Männynsalo L, Putkonen H, Lindberg N, Kotilainen I. Forensic psychiatric perspective on criminality associated with intellectual disability: a nationwide register-based study. *Journal of Intellectual Disability Research* 2009; 53(3): 279–88.

47. Salize HJ, Dressing H. *Placement and Treatment of Mentally Disordered Offenders: Legislation and Practice in the European Union*. Pabst Science Publishers, 2005.

48. Kaltiala-Heino R. Involuntary commitment and detainment in adolescent psychiatric inpatient care. *Social Psychiatry and Psychiatric Epidemiology* 2010; 45(8): 785–93.

Chapter 22

Forensic Neurodevelopmental Disabilities: A Perspective from Ontario, Canada on Pathways and Services

Voula Marinos, Lisa Whittingham, Jessica Jones
and Richard D. Schneider

Introduction

It has been over a decade since the last institution dedicated to individuals with developmental disabilities closed in Ontario, Canada. While efforts have been made to recognise the breadth of neurodevelopmental disorders, government policies and provision of services continue to focus on individuals labelled as having developmental disabilities. In the most recent legislation [1], the term 'developmental disabilities' is used synonymously with the DSM-5 [2] clinical definition of intellectual disability (ID) – or learning disability in the UK – to describe who is eligible to receive government-funded services. This has resulted in providing supports and services for only a small fragment of the population with neurodevelopmental disorders (e.g., persons with fetal alcohol spectrum disorders (FASD) or autism spectrum disorder (ASD) that also have significant cognitive impairments).

Like many other Western countries, large institutions were the dominant form of residential care for individuals with developmental disabilities in Ontario for the first part of the twentieth century. Initially promoted as safe environments away from society where individuals could receive specialised healthcare and education, these institutions were gradually closed due to their overcrowding, lack of demonstrated success, cost and decreased ability to meet demand [3]. Changes in legislation and government-funded services in the community developed in tandem with the closing of institutions, resulting in a wide range of housing options, community programming and staffing support models to promote positive well-being and foster independent functioning [4].

Also identified in Ontario's legislation [1] is the central structure for the provision of 'developmental services' for adults with developmental disabilities, known provincially as Developmental Services Ontario (DSO). Providing a single point of access for all government-funded services, these agencies are charged with administering resources necessary for optimal community inclusion and equitable access to community services as non-disabled citizens.

While the most recent changes to Ontario's legislation addressing the supports and services for individuals with developmental disabilities may have focused on increasing the opportunities for personal choice, independence and community inclusion [1], proper implementation and evaluation has been hindered by long waitlists, uneven access to supports and services and lack of innovative cross-sector collaboration and interministerial solutions [5]. This lack of adequate resources, as outlined in a recent

Ombudsman report [5] and a governmental select committee [6], has also resulted in many individuals with developmental disabilities and their care providers experiencing crises, and subsequently being left without appropriate community supports or being housed inappropriately in a variety of institutional settings (e.g., hospitals, long-term care homes, detention centres) [5]. Consequently, increased community care and participation has also meant increased exposure to environmental risks. Individuals with developmental disabilities are more likely to experience problematic interpersonal situations, high-risk behaviours and maladaptive responses, which can lead to their engagement with the law and the criminal justice system [7, 8].

Aligned with international [9], federal [10] and provincial [11] legislation, the Canadian federal and provincial governments and the legal system have diligently and respectively attempted to ensure that individuals with developmental disabilities are afforded the opportunity to access justice in the criminal justice system. This has included building a number of supports and legal services around alleged offenders with developmental disabilities to ensure a fair and equitable process through the criminal justice system, from the point of arrest to final sentencing or disposition.

Using two composite case studies, this chapter outlines legal pathways consistent with the Criminal Code of Canada [12] and the scaffolding of services and supports for this population in Ontario, Canada. We elaborate on the advantages and challenges of ensuring both equitable justice and therapeutic jurisprudence, recognising that this population still remains one of the most marginalised and vulnerable in our society today.

As individuals with developmental disabilities proceed through the criminal justice system they interface with a number of services and programs from the social care sector. Their pathways include a number of junctures where decision making by different stakeholders across sectors is required pertaining to legal determinations of either criminal fitness (to stand trial) and culpability as well as the healthcare presence of a contributory mental illness or disorder. This chapter illustrates that, despite having similar profiles, people with developmental disabilities can have vastly different access, processes and outcomes depending upon a number of variables including legal factors (i.e., severity of the offence, offence history) and extra-legal factors (i.e., support network, discretion of multiple decision makers, legal resources, jurisdiction). For example, court diversion, established in Ontario as an alternative to prosecution while addressing an accused's underlying needs, can be non-existent or weakly endorsed by one jurisdiction, while in others it may be well supported with early identification, diversionary court support workers and/or robust mental health courts with enhanced links to community resources and a multidisciplinary team for planning support [13].

Decision-Making Junctures

Figure 22.1 illustrates the points of time or junctures while navigating both the adult criminal justice and mental health system in Canada. From this figure, it can be seen that having information about developmental disabilities and its use in decision making by justice professionals at various points can influence the outcomes for persons with developmental disabilities. For the purposes of this chapter, we follow two cases through their respective junctures and outline the various roles and responsibilities of stakeholders and options.

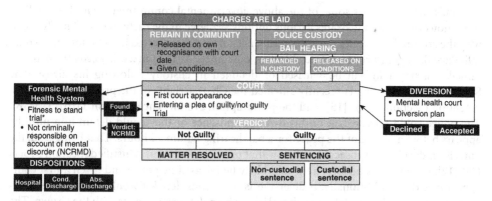

Figure 22.1 The criminal justice and forensic system processes [14]

Case Study 22.1 Tim: legal pathways and diversion

Tim is a 19-year-old man with mild ID and a history of attention deficit hyperactivity disorder (ADHD) living in Toronto, an urban city. He lives in a group home after being apprehended by children's services at a young age due to familial neglect. Tim attends a high-school life skills program and participates in a cooperative placement at a garage with the goal of making it paid employment. Tim has been in and out of trouble during high school with his impulsivity and aggression. He has had difficulties in the home with staff conflict, he has been suspended from school a number of times and has had a number of police warnings for making threats towards teachers and peers. More recently, he threatened the principal and was charged with uttering threats. He was subsequently expelled from the rest of his school year and possibly his final year.

Justice Involvement and Legal Pathways

In Tim's case, upon being charged, he would likely experience a trajectory through the criminal justice system. Recognising the impact that justice involvement can have and the over-representation of specific marginalised groups, diversionary options are increasingly considered to facilitate community rehabilitation. Diversion courts, based on the principles of therapeutic jurisprudence [16], are increasingly being used to address the needs of persons with mental health, addictions and/or cognitive disabilities who come into contact with the legal system, in order to assess and treat identified 'root causes' and other contributory or mitigating factors. In Ontario, the Ministry of the Attorney General's policy on diversion excludes eligible offences that are relatively serious (e.g., firearms offences, robbery, sexual assault, murder) and considers other, less serious, offences appropriate (e.g., theft, mischief) for those accused who have little to no previous record and are considered low risk [17]. The existence of a criminal record or previous participation in diversion does not cause an individual to be excluded.

Tim's case highlights some of the above governmental commitments and legal obligations; however, it also illustrates various options available in the early stages of involvement with the criminal justice system and the diversity of responses across jurisdictions that could influence divergent processes and different outcomes. At the outset, it needs to be determined whether Tim will be released or detained in custody following his arrest. The Supreme Court of Canada recently affirmed the Charter rights of the presumption against detention (Section 11(e)) [15], and the presumption of innocence (Section 11(b)) [15, 18]. The police could release Tim on his own recognisance or they could detain him until he appears before a justice of the peace for a bail hearing within 24 hours. That being said, the onus is on the Crown prosecutor to show that pre-trial detention is justified (Section 515(1) (2)) [12]. Given Tim's history, he would likely be released by police and given a first court appearance date. Additionally, if diversion is to be considered it would typically be advocated as an option by the defence counsel, though final discretion rests with the Crown. The defence counsel or the Crown would also ascertain whether fitness is a question for Tim. If there are concerns for fitness of the accused at any stage of the proceedings, the defence or Crown, whoever makes an application to the court, has the burden of proof, then the judge can make a fitness assessment order (Section 672.11 (a)) [12]. Although Tim has mild ID without other known comorbidities or concerning presentation, it does not appear as if fitness is an issue. Tim is presumed to be fit so long as counsel is of the view that he maintains a rudimentary factual understanding of his legal predicament and can instruct counsel.

If Tim is identified as a person with developmental disabilities, he will be referred to a diversion court worker and/or a dual diagnosis justice case manager (DDJCM). Recognising the challenges faced by persons with neurodevelopmental disorders and mental health issues involved in the criminal justice system, external agencies provide support to courts in all regions of Ontario through specialised case managers who assist these individuals and their caregivers in navigating the court processes and legal logistics. It is interesting to note within the available developmental services in Ontario, the DDJCM can assist even if the diagnosis is suspected but not yet confirmed or the individual has not yet been deemed administratively eligible for developmental services, recognising the gaps in service mandates between sectors [19]. Their role within the system is to advocate on behalf of the individual for accommodations in the justice process and to advocate to justice professionals on both sides of the court [17, 19]. Since there are limits in the law on whether diversion is possible, the DDJCM may advocate for acknowledging the presence of a developmental disability at the time of diversion or sentencing, depending on the offence. In cases eligible for diversion, the DDJCM will help to develop a diversion treatment plan. There are often wide variations in the plans that are crafted by the DDJCMs due to inconsistencies in service mandates and infrastructure across the regions (e.g., access to forensic mental health services, appropriate residential programs, specialty clinical services).

Given the nature of Tim's offence and the presence of his mild ID and ADHD, he would likely be eligible for diversion. He would then be given the option of participating or remaining in the regular prosecutorial stream. If accepted by the Crown attorney and admitted, the DDJCM would work with Tim and his care providers to develop a 'diversion plan', involving rehabilitation and the establishment of supports in the community. This may be through formal referral to a diversion court or it may be through the generic court, depending on what specialty courts are available in the region (e.g., diversion and/or mental health courts).

As Tim's developmental disability is known, he would likely not need to be referred for a psychodiagnostic assessment. Instead, the DDJCM would focus on connecting Tim to adult developmental services, which are not currently involved. This would include connecting him with a DSO case manager to complete the required assessment for confirming eligibility and access to developmental services. This assessment involves a structured interview incorporating the Application for Developmental Services and Supports (ADSS) and the Support Intensity Scale (SIS) [20]. The ADSS and SIS are standardised measures developed to assess what an individual's goals are and the associated supports and services required to participate in various activities of daily living (e.g., employment, home management) [20].

Following this assessment, Tim would be referred to the various developmental services which reflect the person-centred goals that make up his diversion plan. This may include healthcare needs including psychiatric, psychological, rehabilitation or behavioural supports. Services may also address any offence-contributing factors such as underlying mental health issues, psychosocial, functional or behavioural factors contributing to or associated with his offending behaviour. However, as noted above, waitlists in Ontario remain long despite qualification for supports and services. In addition, many clinical services are accessible by referring to either generic hospital or healthcare teams, or, if in his jurisdiction, a dual diagnosis team that provides consultation to primary care and developmental agencies. In Ontario, there are no inter-ministerial regional 'learning disability' teams as in the UK; services are siloed within either social services or health.

For Tim specifically, based on available services in the region, his diversion plan may include assessments from psychiatry to consult on possible pharmacological interventions to reduce his anger; from psychology to recommend possible psychotherapeutic or diagnostic interventions to mediate his aggression; or from occupational therapy to improve his functional independence in the community; or behavioural supports to provide positive programming. In addition, his social support needs may entitle him to funding for employment supports if he is not to return to school – an entitlement for individuals with developmental disabilities up to the age of 21 in Ontario through post high-school life-skills training [21]. If housing is an issue for his transition into adulthood and away from family care, his lead agency may facilitate appropriate residential options, for example congregate care or supported independent living. Further, he may also be referred to a case manager or adult protective support worker to assist in service navigation in the future and reduce risk of recidivism by successful community integration and access to supports.

If available in his jurisdiction, an alternative pathway for Tim is diversion to a specialised mental health court. Availability of formal diversion to mental health courts, in addition to the services provided, vary by jurisdiction – typically by size of jurisdiction and population base [21]. Larger urban centres are more likely to have more robust, regular, dedicated courts with a designated judge and affiliated multidisciplinary teams and programs, and greater resources. Subject to the resources available in Tim's jurisdiction, he would certainly be a candidate to diversion to a mental health court if available. While mental health courts vary across the province, there are some key similarities in process: the Crown and mental health court support worker (or the DDJCM) are most likely to process the individual for eligibility; there is an established link between the alleged offence and the mental health diagnosis or cognitive disability; the accused is willing to participate in treatment or rehabilitation; there is an exclusion of serious offences; there is a plan developed in consultation with the Crown, the accused and/or their care providers and defence counsel; and the plan created addresses the individual's mental health needs by making connections to relevant community services [22].

In Tim's case, similar to working with the DDJCM to develop a diversion plan, the mental health court diversion would open the door to developmental services and supports within the community and liaise with the school for supported placement if deemed appropriate. Regardless of whether Tim gets a diversion plan via a mental health court or a traditional generic court, upon completion of the court requirements, he would then return to court where the charges would be either stayed or withdrawn by the Crown.

If Tim is not viewed as eligible for any of the forms of diversion (e.g., he threatened the principal by bringing a weapon to school in an attempt to resolve the conflict), and assuming on the facts that fitness is not an issue, he would then have the option of pleading guilty or proceeding to trial and pleading not guilty. This tactic would ideally be discussed with the defence counsel. If found guilty, a pre-sentence report could be ordered by the court to assist in sentencing (Section 721(1)) [12]. Sentencing options include non-custodial and custodial sentences (Part XXIII, Section 716) [12]. Tim's sentence would likely range from an absolute discharge or conditional discharge (no record of conviction) to a conviction with a suspended sentence. A conditional discharge or a suspended sentence may both include a probation order with particular requirements/obligations designed to ensure Tim's success.

Diversion to the Forensic Mental Health System

The second case of John (Case Study 22.2) illustrates diversion to the forensic mental health system. In John's case, upon being charged and appearing in court, John would likely be diverted away from the criminal justice system to the forensic mental health system. Given his significant cognitive deficits, which have played a considerable role in his previous lack of success in intervention, it should be accounted for in his potential legal response and rehabilitative options. Given the aggravating facts of the case, his history of sexualised behaviours, the alleged victim being a minor and offence of a sexual nature, decisions around release or detention will be determined before a justice of peace within 24 hours for a bail hearing.

Case Study 22.2 John: a tale of forensic mental health diversion

John is a 25-year-old man with a fetal alcohol spectrum disorder. He lived at home in a rural community with his mother and younger siblings until the age of 20. John is supported by a developmental service agency which provides a respite worker on weekends. However, during the week he has no planned activities. John has a childhood history of sexually inappropriate behaviour including sexualised language and inappropriate touching. He has attended a social-sexual education group but his success was hindered by his comprehension difficulties. Recently, he was charged with sexual assault upon a minor after an incident which was alleged to have involved 'groping' with a neighbourhood child. He was admitted to hospital where an assessment diagnosed a moderate level of ID and extremely low adaptive behaviour or independent functioning. He was transferred to the local forensic mental health program for psychiatric assessment including a fitness evaluation.

Additionally, or even prior to a bail hearing, given his background and recent assessment of having a moderate level of ID, there may be questions about John's ability to participate in his trial in a meaningful way or his legal 'fitness to stand trial'. Section 2 of the Criminal Code of Canada [12] defines 'unfit to stand trial' as:

> unable on account of mental disorder to conduct a defence at any stage of the proceedings before verdict is rendered or to instruct counsel to do so, and, in particular, unable on account of mental disorder to
> a. understand the nature or object of the proceedings,
> b. understand the possible consequences of the proceedings, or
> c. communicate with counsel.

If fitness to stand trial is a concern raised by either the defence or the Crown, John can be ordered by a judge for a fitness assessment (Section 672.11) [12]; further fitness assessments can be ordered at any stage throughout the proceedings (Section 672.12) [12]. Assessments are typically undertaken by a psychiatrist interview within 5 days although it should not exceed 30 days, with extensions not exceeding 60 days. These fitness assessments are either completed following admission to a forensic mental health hospital ward or, in some jurisdictions, while being held in a detention centre. At some mental health courts, assessments may be conducted on a 'stand down' basis by a psychiatrist who attends the court on a daily basis.

As set out in Section 672.38(1) of the Criminal Code of Canada [12], each province is responsible for setting up review boards that are responsible for the oversight of individuals who have been found unfit to stand trial or received a verdict of not criminally responsible on account of mental disorder (NCRMD). In Ontario, the tribunal sits in panels of at least five members consisting of a judge, psychiatrist, lawyer, another mental health professional licensed to practice medicine or psychology and a public member (Bill C-30). The Taylor case sets out the test of 'limited cognitive capacity' in determining fitness [23]. The application of such case law and its implementation has a low threshold in Ontario, requiring that the accused merely understand the proceedings against him and can communicate with counsel without necessarily having the capacity to make decisions within their best interests [24]. Some argue that this test falls short of providing adequate protections for mentally disordered accused and that meaningful participation requires at least a modicum of rationality [25].

Accordingly, if found fit, John may be detained in jail, in hospital (Section 672.46(2)) [12] or released until trial. If found unfit, the Crown may apply to the court for a treatment order. At this hearing the judge hears testimony from a psychiatrist regarding John's likelihood of becoming fit without treatment within a 60-day period. If granted, the order provides for involuntary treatment for up to 60 days. Hence, his 'treatability' comes into question. For individuals with developmental disabilities, this is an equivocal question given the organic and chronic nature of their cognitive impairments.

If John remains unfit at the conclusion of the 60-day treatment order then he is remanded to the Ontario Review Board (ORB) [26], which monitors his progress until it is of the view that John is 'fit', at which point he would be returned to court so that the issue may be re-tried.

If John is found unfit following a judge-ordered assessment and likely treatment (e.g., pharmacological intervention is deemed ineffective), an alternative pathway is explored. An accused who is repeatedly and permanently found unfit and who does not pose a significant threat to public safety should be handed a stay of proceedings within 30 days [27]. For individuals who are found unfit, there are two dispositions available – a detention disposition, by which the individual is detained in hospital, or a conditional discharge (allowed to live in community with conditions similar to a probation order). The individual's disposition is reviewed not less than yearly by the ORB [26]. In John's case, the least restrictive and preferred disposition would likely be a conditional discharge given the potential for a supervised community placement with the oversight of a probation order and regular monitoring to mitigate risk and recidivism.

Alternatively, if John is found fit, he may plead guilty or proceed to trial; if found not guilty, he will be released. But, if it is determined at trial that John has committed the act, the question of culpability or criminal responsibility may arise. If criminal responsibility is not an issue, then John's developmental disorder will be considered at sentencing, possibly as a mitigating factor similar to Tim (see Section 718.2(a)(i)) [12]. A pre-sentence report completed by a probation officer could be ordered pursuant to Section 721.1 of the Criminal Code [12] to determine the risk and treatment needs of John, particularly if the judge is considering time served in pre-trial detention or a reduced sentence.

If John returns to the community, an additional risk assessment may be completed by a psychiatrist or psychologist to determine the level of community risk and recommended risk-mitigating supports to be implemented and monitored. For individuals with developmental disabilities, this may be extremely relevant. They are likely to return to a community residential setting with different staffing models and thus the threshold for risk tolerance by such agencies needs to be accounted for in determining individuals' overall level of risk in returning to the community; for example, the presence of staff supervision and unsupervised community access [28].

If John is found to have committed the otherwise criminal act he may, nevertheless, be found NCRMD pursuant to the provisions of Section 16 of the Criminal Code of Canada [12]:

(1) No person is criminally responsible for an act committed or an omission made while suffering from a mental disorder that rendered the person incapable of appreciating the nature and quality of the act or omission or of knowing that it was wrong.

If John is found NCRMD then the ORB will make one of three dispositions (Section 672.54) determined to be the least onerous and least restrictive. The ORB will take into consideration: the safety of the public, which is the paramount consideration; the mental condition of John; the reintegration of John into society; and the other needs of John. The dispositions may be: (a) absolute discharge; (b) conditional discharge; or (c) detained in custody in a hospital.

Given John's profile, which includes a moderate level of ID, low adaptive functioning and a history of significant developmental service supports, it is likely that he will be detained in hospital while a viable and sustainable community plan is developed. It is possible that, with additional services ensuring safety for the public, a reduced probability of reoffending and ongoing supervision, John could be placed into the community in a supervised living arrangement. Upon review, which must occur not less than annually, John would be given an absolute discharge should the evidence not support a finding that he constitutes a 'significant threat to the safety of the public'. The ORB states: 'An accused may be connected to a variety of community agencies and services which, together with family support, may attenuate any threat to such an extent that an absolute discharge may be appropriate' [26].

If John is discharged conditionally, he is allowed to live in the community but may be required to abide by strict oversight conditions such as requiring him to report to a hospital, refrain from the use of drugs or alcohol, not associate with particular individuals and report changes of address [26]. Each annual review would address the need for a gradual and scaffolded transition plan of faded supervision and recommended privileges within the community and an adequate oversight and monitoring plan by responsible community stakeholders. Once released into the community, he would most likely be required to also abide by conditions that would mitigate any ongoing risk of recidivism.

Any limitation placed upon John's liberty must have a logical nexus to a risk posed. Gratuitous limitations are unlawful. If the hospital is of the view that psychiatric 'treatment' is required, that can be included in a disposition with John's consent (Section 672.55 (1)) [12]. Otherwise, the hospital would have to pursue treatment possibilities pursuant to the provisions of the provincial mental health legislation. Dispositions are orders pursuant to the Criminal Code of Canada [12] and not provincial civil mental health legislation. We are not aware of any specialist developmental disability units anywhere in Canada within the forensic hospital system.

In addition to the services and lead agency involved in John's return to the community, the DDJCM may work with the forensic case manager to develop a sequential plan for conditional discharge and absolute discharge. It is likely that a conditional discharge will be implemented first, to 'prove' that the plan works, with community commitments to service provision that mitigates John's risk to the community. If there is evidence that the plan is sustainable and working and there is 'buy-in' from the individual and their support network, the ORB must issue an absolute discharge should John, with these supports, not be seen as constituting a significant threat to the safety of the public.

In John's case, and in many cases with developmental disabilities, the success of either conditional or absolute discharges depend not only on the immediate services or treatment supports provided following the court's verdict but more so on the long-term planning and commitment to mitigating risk and reducing recidivism while residing in the community. This goal can be, at times, in conflict with overarching policies and care philosophies of developmental agencies, which facilitate increasing community independence and a stepped approach to self-reliance. In John's case, given his poor adaptive functioning, the need for some model of permanent residential supervision is clear; however, continued structured supports is also equally important to ensure full community participation while minimising risk. This balance of risk management versus optimal community participation illustrates a fragile phenomenon known in community care for individuals with developmental disabilities as 'dignity of risk' or one's right to self-determination and the right to take reasonable risks essential for self-dignity; however, this can be offset by either paternalistic approaches about duty of care or, in contrast, overly optimistic perspectives of one's needs. Indeed, this is the balancing of factors that the Canadian parliament has articulated, as set out in Section 672.54 of the Criminal Code [12], as discussed above.

John may, therefore, need a community risk-management plan developed with the DDJCM and their services, to ensure adequate, appropriate and ongoing supports to ensure a smooth transition into community care and also confirmation for the criminal justice system that his risk of recidivism remains low. This may include a period in a specialised treatment home for offenders with developmental disorders or residential supervision that provides 24-hour monitoring – few and hard to access across Ontario. Both services are at a premium and likely require an inter-ministerial arrangement for funding and follow-up responsibility. Also of importance is the ability of John's lead developmental agency upon discharge to accept his level of risk and their ability to manage the respective responsibility.

Given his profile, John will likely be found NCRMD and be discharged conditionally. It will be up to the case manager assigned to him in the hospital and the DDJCM to assist John in navigating the DSO process (similar to what was described for Tim). The risk assessment completed for the ORB will be used to help determine the type of setting that John should live in; however, it is likely that he will remain in hospital beyond what is clinically needed given the long waitlists for services, particularly for residential care (i.e., group homes) [5]. Further, there may be differences between what forensic professionals and community agencies feel is appropriate and reasonable for mitigating risk given differences in mandates and resources [5]. For example, while forensic professionals may feel that a group home with other adults is a suitable placement, agencies may not be willing to place an individual with a history of sexual offending in a home with individuals they perceive to be vulnerable or that cannot provide 24-hour eyes-on supervision.

John will also be eligible for the same services (e.g., recreational/housing, employment supports) as Tim through the DSO; however, due to the lack of specialised services (e.g., forensic disability services), he may be restricted to rely on generic forensic or justice services that have limited familiarity with developmental disabilities or developmental services that have limited experiences and capacity for supporting people with criminogenic needs.

Common Challenges between Cases

Although their cases are similar in that both Tim and John were identified as having developmental disabilities either early on or at the point of contact, they have experienced very different trajectories through the criminal justice system, including regionalised differences due to the availability of resources and dedicated services to offenders with developmental disabilities across Ontario. As demonstrated by John's case, a division continues to exist between the criminal justice system and community services. This has created gaps for ORB patients, which has meant extended stays in hospitals and short-term service plans that are cobbled together with generic services [5]. In addition, the long waitlists and regionalised differences in available services have also meant that there is limited capacity in the community to prevent both Tim and John from initially becoming involved in the criminal justice system or preventing further involvement once they have entered [29].

Early identification meant that both individuals were afforded the opportunity to be supported by the DDJCM, and for diversions that prevented miscarriages of justice; however, individual differences, excluding offence-specific factors, meant that different legal options were exercised. In both cases, the DDJCM would have played an important role communicating with justice professionals about what having a developmental disability meant to each individual and helping to facilitate accommodations [19]. Despite efforts to increase the accessibility of the justice system for individuals with disabilities [10, 11], there remains a lack of awareness and adequate knowledge within the criminal justice system about the unique situation and possible mitigating factors to offenders with developmental disabilities. Despite the predominant philosophy of both the criminal justice system and developmental services in supporting inclusion and equitable justice for all individuals with developmental disabilities, there are significant divisions of accountability between the criminal justice system, the mental health sector and the developmental services sector. It is important to ensure that there is therapeutic justice and a shared collaborative responsibility for both the community at large and for the individual.

Conclusion

In Ontario, supports and services have focused on individuals diagnosed with ID (labelled as developmental disabilities), meaning that a large number of individuals with neurodevelopmental disabilities are not eligible for government-funded services. Tim and John are not unique but represent a wide range of individuals with developmental disabilities who come into contact with the Canadian criminal justice system; and most likely not dissimilar to other countries' experiences.

This discussion has attempted to provide both clinicians within the field of developmental disabilities, and mental health workers and legal practitioners who want exposure to relevant forensic issues, a window into possible pathways for such individuals as they journey across junctures from arrest to final disposal or sentencing. As you can see from the discussion of the above case studies, the outcomes of individuals with developmental disabilities vary greatly in Ontario, Canada; however, all result from coexistent legislative and policy viewpoints that recognise the importance and need for ensuring equitable and therapeutic justice for such individuals. Further, the differences in implementation and success across jurisdictions inevitably depend upon the provision of adequate and appropriate local resources. These differences depend less so on intersectoral commitment to protecting the public, reducing risk and facilitating rehabilitation for individuals with developmental disabilities through safe community management.

References

1. Services and Supports to Promote the Social Inclusion of Persons with Developmental Disabilities Act, 2008, S.O. 2008, c. 14. Available from: www.ontario.ca/laws/statute/08s14.

2. American Psychiatric Association. *Diagnostic and Statistical Manual of Mental Disorders, 5th edition: DSM-5*. American Psychiatric Association, 2013.

3. Brown I, Radford JP. The growth and decline of institutions for people with developmental disabilities in Ontario: 1876–2009. *Journal of Developmental Disabilities* 2015; 21(2): 7–27.

4. Griffiths D, Owen F, Condillac R, eds. *A Difficult Dream: Ending, Institutionalization for Persons with Intellectual Disabilities with Complex Needs*. NADD Press, 2016.

5. Dubé, P. Nowhere to turn: investigation into the Ministry of Community and Social Services' responses to situations of crisis involving adults with developmental disabilities. 2016. Available at: www.ombudsman.on.ca/resources/reports-and-case-summaries/reports-on-investigations/2016/nowhere-to-turn.

6. Legislative Assembly of Ontario. Inclusion and opportunity: a new plan for developmental services in Ontario. 2014. Available at: https://connectability.ca/wp-content/uploads/2014/06/5.2-GO-Select-Committee-Development-Services-Final-Report-2014.pdf.

7. Jones J. Persons with intellectual disabilities in the criminal justice system: review of issues. *International Journal of Offender Therapy and Comparative Criminology* 2007; 51(6): 723–33.

8. Lunsky Y, Raina P, Jones J. Relationship between prior legal involvement and current crisis for adults with intellectual disability. *Journal of Intellectual and Developmental Disability* 2012; 37(2): 163–8.

9. UN General Assembly. Convention on the Rights of Persons with Disabilities: resolution adopted by the General Assembly, 24 January 2007, A/RES/61/106. Available at: www.refworld.org/docid/45f973632.html.

10. Accessible Canada Act(S.C. 2019, c. 10). Available at: https://laws-lois.justice.gc.ca/PDF/A-0.6.pdf.

11. Accessibility for Ontarians with Disabilities Act, 2005, S.O. 2005, c. 11. Available at: www.ontario.ca/laws/statute/05a11.

12. Criminal Code(R.S.C., 1985, c. C-46) (Can). Available at: https://laws-lois.justice.gc.ca/PDF/C-46.pdf.

13. Human Services and Justice Coordinating Committee. Mental health courts in Ontario: a review of the initiation and operation of mental health courts across the province. Available at: https://ontario.cmha.ca/wp-content/uploads/2017/11/Mental-Health-Courts-in-Ontario-1.pdf.

14. Prokop J, Huisman T, Marr, G. Understanding the offender with a dual diagnosis. Available at: www.community-networks.ca/wp-content/uploads/2015/11/understanding_the_offender_w_dd-jan.2010.pdf.

15. Canadian Charter of Rights and Freedoms, Part I of the Constitution Act, 1982, being Schedule B to the Canada Act 1982 (UK), 1982, c 11, s 91(24). Available at: https://laws-lois.justice.gc.ca/eng/const/page-15.html.

16. Wexler DB, Winick, BJ. Therapeutic jurisprudence as a new approach to mental health law policy analysis and research. *University of Miami Law Review* 1991; 45: 981–1004.

17. Ministry of the Attorney General. Crown Prosecution manual. Available at: www.ontario.ca/document/crown-prosecution-manual.

18. *R. v. Antic* [2017] 1 SCR 509. Available at: https://scc-csc.lexum.com/scc-csc/scc-csc/en/item/16649/index.do.

19. Southern Network of Specialized Care. Understanding special needs offenders who have dual diagnosis. Available at: www.community-networks.ca/wp-content/uploads/2015/11/understanding_the_offender_w_dd-jan.2010.pdf.

20. Ministry of Children, Community and Social Services. Policy directives for application entities. 2013. Available at: www.ontario.ca/page/ministry-children-community-and-social-services.

21. Ministry of Education. Special education in Ontario: Kindergarten to grade 12. Available at: www.ontario.ca/edu.

22. Human Services and Justice Coordinating Committee. Mental health courts in Ontario: a review of the initiation and operation of mental health courts across the province. 2017. Available at: https://ontario.cmha.ca/wp-content/uploads/2017/11/Mental-Health-Courts-in-Ontario-1.pdf.

23. *R v. Taylor* 1992 CanLII 7412 (ON CA), [1992] OJ 2394 (ON CA). Available at: https://scc-csc.lexum.com/scc-csc/scc-csc/en/item/14276/index.do.

24. *R v. Whittle* [1994] 2 SCR 914. Available at: https://scc-csc.lexum.com/scc-csc/scc-csc/en/item/1165/index.do.

25. Schneider RD. Fitness to be sentenced. *Criminal Law Quarterly* 1998–1999; 261: 261–3.

26. Ontario Review Board. About us. Available at: www.orb.on.ca/scripts/en/about.asp#history.

27. R v. Demers [2004] 2 SCR 489. Available at: https://scc-csc.lexum.com/scc-csc/scc-csc/en/item/2160/index.do?site_preference=normal.

28. Marinos V, Stromski S, Whittingham L, Griffiths D. *Intellectual and Developmental Disabilities and the Criminal Justice System.* NADD Press, 2020.

29. Whittingham L, Durbin A, Lin E, Matheson FI, Volpe T, Dastoori P, et al. The prevalence and health status of people with developmental disabilities in provincial prisons in Ontario, Canada: a prospective cohort study. *Journal of Applied Research in Intellectual Disabilities* 2020; 33(6): 1368–79.

Forensic Aspects of Neurodevelopmental Disorders: An Australasian Perspective

Catherine Franklin

Introduction

Australasia is a broad term, used to refer to the countries of Australia, Aotearoa New Zealand, Papua New Guinea and the neighbouring islands of the Pacific. These countries range from the developed (Australia and Aotearoa New Zealand) to the least developed (some of the Pacific Islands); the remainder, including Papua New Guinea, are considered developing countries (see Figure 23.1). As services, frameworks and approaches are so rudimentary in the developing nations and non-existent in the least developed, this chapter briefly describes the situation in the developing nations before describing services and frameworks in Australia and Aotearoa New Zealand in greater detail.

Papua New Guinea and Pacific Island Nations

Papua New Guinea has a population of 7.6 million people and is the largest Pacific Island nation. Papua New Guinea and some of the other Pacific Islands were under colonial administration by Britain and Germany in the late 1800s and later occupied by Japan during World War II. Independence was only gained for Papua New Guinea from Australia in 1975, and for Samoa from New Zealand in 1962. Until recently, nearly 90% of the population of these nations lived in rural and often very remote communities, but rapid urbanisation is occurring and this percentage is decreasing with time. While Papua New Guinea is a signatory to the United Nations Convention on the Rights of People with Disabilities, and has begun to develop policy on disability in recent years, this has not yet translated to changes in legislation or practice.

For most Papua New Guineans and Pacific Islanders, accessing basics including employment, education and healthcare locally is challenging. While some of these countries have begun to develop policy on disability in recent years, they have not yet included consideration of disability into their legislation, health or education systems. Attitudes to disability reflect the medical model and a charity model, where people with a disability are viewed as disordered and/or defective. They are often kept away from the community and suffer multiple disadvantages. Australian and New Zealand government and non-government aid organisations continue to work with Papua New Guinea and Pacific Island nations to improve conditions for their population, including for people with disability, and progress is being made.

Australia and Aotearoa New Zealand

While both Australia and Aotearoa New Zealand have long histories that pre-date British colonisation in the late eighteenth century, it is this latter part of their history that has shaped their current legal and healthcare systems. British colonisation also had lasting

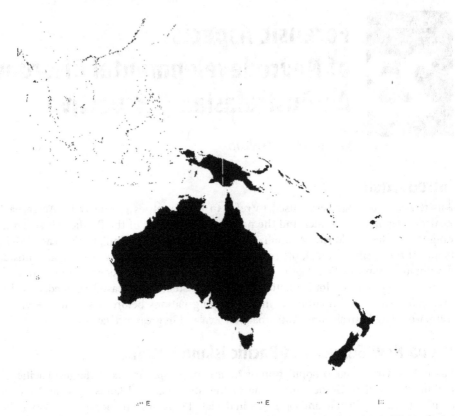

Figure 23.1 Map of Australasian region. Source: https://en.wikipedia.org/wiki/Australasia#/media/File:Location_A ustralasia_cylindrical.png.

effects on the Indigenous people of both countries, who continue to suffer inequity and stigma, resulting in a number of difficulties including poorer health outcomes and over-representation in forensic settings.

Improvements in the social care and support of people with neurodevelopmental disorders are in process in both countries. Australia has recently seen the introduction and implementation of the National Disability Insurance Scheme (NDIS), providing indi-vidualised access and funding to a variety of services and supports, including supported independent living, allied health services and specialised behaviour supports. Each individ-ual is provided with a specific budget and can choose where their funding is spent. This model relies on the private sector to deliver the services which individuals are funded to access. It is currently significantly more challenging under this system for people with neurodevelopmental disorders, and a history of having committed an offence, to identify and access services. It is of course hoped that the private sector will grow to meet demand, but this process is hampered by the lack of capacity in education, training and provision of mainstream services.

The government of Aotearoa New Zealand has very recently announced it is transform-ing the disability support system, promising increased inclusion and choice for people with disability. This process of change has been very slow and undergone several different iterations in recent years, without significant change occurring to date.

Healthcare in Australia and Aotearoa New Zealand

Australia and Aotearoa New Zealand both have universal free healthcare provided federally and administered regionally, although this is changing to federal administration in Aotearoa New Zealand. They also both have additional private (i.e., non-government funded) healthcare choices through optional private health insurance schemes for those who can afford it.

De-institutionalisation occurred in both countries at similar times and, like some other countries, this seems to have been associated with a de-coupling of health services from the social care and support of people with neurodevelopmental disorders. This has been identified as one of the aetiological factors for the well-established lack of capacity in neurodevelopmental disorder healthcare in in Australia and Aotearoa New Zealand. This lack of capacity to support individuals with neurodevelopmental disorders is evident at systemic, organisational and individual levels and is a major and recurring theme when considering forensic aspects of such disorders in Australia and Aotearoa New Zealand.

People with neurodevelopmental disorders in Australia and Aotearoa New Zealand rely on mainstream healthcare services for provision of their physical and mental healthcare. While there are often small, specialised physical and/or mental healthcare teams in capital cities, these are often staffed with part-time staff and have limited capacity, with very few able to provide ongoing follow-up. This leaves many mainstream health services with no access to additional support or advice from specialised neurodevelopmental disorder health services. A related issue is the lack of capacity in mainstream healthcare services to work with people with neurodevelopmental disorders: reviews of undergraduate and postgraduate healthcare worker education indicate very limited exposure to these disabilities, which is reflected in the mainstream health workforce, and the structure and accessibility of mainstream healthcare services [1, 2]. This lack of capacity has practical effects: there is under-detection of neurodevelopmental disorders in healthcare settings and diagnostic overshadowing contributes to misdiagnosis and inadequate care.

For people with neurodevelopmental disorders who have committed, or are at increased risk of committing offences, this lack of capacity has significant, yet perhaps predictable, impacts including the longer length of stay and greater length of admissions known for people with a neurodevelopmental disorder in Australia [3] and difficulties in coming off forensic orders [4]. The lack of capacity in neurodevelopmental disorder healthcare has been raised by the Royal Australian and New Zealand College of Psychiatrists (RANZCP) [5] and underlined again in the hearings of the Australian Disability Royal Commission [6]. While this Royal Commission's primary intent was to focus on the abuse and neglect of people with intellectual and developmental disabilities, it has deemed it necessary to include a focus on neglect in the healthcare system, with specific hearings on the use of psychotropic medications in people with intellectual and developmental disabilities and on provision of health professional education in this area [6].

Cultural and Historical Considerations

The Indigenous people of Australia and Aotearoa New Zealand are distinct and very different groups of people. However, there are some themes common to both countries. Working with the Indigenous people of Australia and Aotearoa New Zealand requires an understanding of their cultural context, background and history, as this directly affects interviewing and the assessment and evaluation of mental illness. The practice of engaging the individual in interview and discussing personal issues is challenging across different cultures and working with Indigenous clients is no different in this respect. Further, the reasons behind an offence may seem illogical, even beyond comprehension, if viewed through the lens of a person of European descent, but may make perfect sense when understood in the context of an Indigenous person's culture and historical background.

Cultural security refers to the practice of recognising the language, customs, attitudes and beliefs of cultural groups within the health system and throughout the provision of services. Addressing the inequities experienced by Indigenous people of both countries has been established as a priority for some time, but effecting change has been more difficult. There is now increasing emphasis on the requirement for culturally safe approaches for the Indigenous people of Australia and Aotearoa New Zealand, and approaches specific to each country are further described later in this chapter.

Legislative Frameworks in Australia and Aotearoa New Zealand

The specifics of legislative frameworks applicable to people with neurodevelopmental disorders who commit offences vary across both countries, and also across each different state and territory of Australia. There has been recent progress and overall significant improvements in legislation. These changes have attempted to identify and provide discrete and different pathways for people with neurodevelopmental disorders, compared to those who have committed offences while suffering mental illness. Some different examples are outlined below. Unfortunately, these changes in legislation alone have not been sufficient to lead to improved outcomes as, in most cases, people with neurodevelopmental disorders are still managed by the mainstream mental health services who lack capacity in this area as described above.

The criminal justice systems of both countries reflect the English common law, which provides, in some way, for a defence of 'mental illness' to be raised against the prosecution of a crime. This defence is derived from common-law rules based on the nineteenth-century case of M'Naghten and has two aspects relevant to the future of the defendant. First, the defendant is not considered guilty of the crime for which they have been charged, and a verdict of not guilty by reason of mental illness applies. Second, the defendant can still be subject to an ongoing order by the court, which may include detention and care for their mental illness in an appropriate environment. In most areas, this is a treatment facility run by health professionals in a non-correctional setting. The rationale for this is that the individual is not guilty of a crime and that their primary need is for medical care and rehabilitation. The purpose of the ongoing order is either to ensure the individual receives the necessary medical care and rehabilitation to assist in recovery from the effects of mental illness and allow the individual to resume their place in the community or to ensure that an individual with cognitive impairment receives appropriate support to manage their disability. It is fundamentally not meant to be a punitive order.

However, the RANZCP has issued a position statement in relation to people who are found unfit to stand trial, expressing concern that these people (including those with neurodevelopmental disorders who commit offences) are subject to laws and detention conditions that may violate their human rights and cause long-term harm [7]. In particular, there is concern that 'people in Australia and New Zealand are being held in jails or corrective services custody, despite having never been convicted of a crime or placed on remand, and that the conditions of release are becoming increasingly severe and punitive.' The position statement identifies key principles endorsed by the RANZCP to be applied to the treatment and detention of forensic patients. The RANZCP advocates the adoption of these principles in all Australian and New Zealand jurisdictions and continues to advocate that all forensic patients receive treatment in accordance with these principles.

A Focus on Australia

Australia is a vast country, approximately 32 times the land size of the UK and 80 percent the size of the USA, but has a population of only 24 million people, which equates to about one-third of the population of the UK and one-thirteenth of the population of the USA (see Figure 23.2). The population is 3.3% Indigenous First Nations Australians. In 2016, 26% of Australia's population was born overseas and this figure continues to increase, with most of these people born in England, followed by New Zealand, then China and then India.

Healthcare System in Australia

Medicare, the national scheme to provide basic healthcare to all Australians, was introduced in 1984. It is funded by the federal government, in part through a 2% levy on Australians' income. There is also an incentive for Australians to have private health insurance, through an additional 1–1.5% levy on those with higher income who do not have private health insurance. General practice and outpatient private specialist medical services are funded federally directly through Medicare, whereas inpatient and community health services are

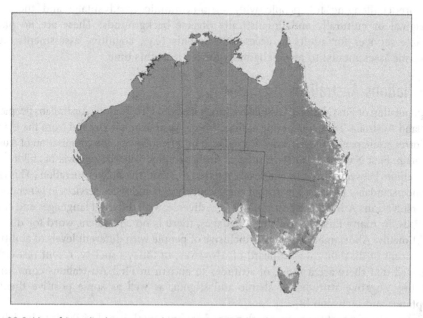

Figure 23.2 Map of Australia showing population density (2016). Lighter areas show the greatest density. Source: https://commons.wikimedia.org/wiki/File:Australian_population_density_2016.png.

administered by the state and territory governments, through partial federal funding. This means that each state and territory can (and does) spend different proportions of their budget on healthcare. As such, the quality and availability of healthcare differs significantly across states and territories of Australia. Australia's significant land area also means that there are challenges in providing services to those living in rural and remote areas, and services here can be rudimentary or non-existent, requiring some people to travel large distances to access healthcare.

Mental Healthcare for People with Neurodevelopmental Disorders in Australia

The variety (and paucity in relation to population size) of Australian neurodevelopmental disorder mental healthcare services is shown in Table 23.1. This illustrates that there are no specialised acute inpatient units for people with neurodevelopmental disorders in Australia and that community health services are variable and very small in relation to the population they serve. A number of services cater to both physical and mental health problems in the one service. Provision of services for autistic people who do not have intellectual disability (ID) is very scarce and not currently an area of focus for the government, who have only recently begun to focus on ID as an area of need.

Individuals who are participants in the NDIS can now also access funding for allied health services in relation to their disability. This includes funding to access psychological services, occupational therapists, nurses, speech pathologists, dieticians and exercise physiologists. The NDIS attempts to differentiate between treatment for healthcare and disability and will only fund treatment for disability-related conditions, but this does include, for example, challenging behaviour or assistance with communication. Access to the NDIS can be more challenging for people with socio-economic disadvantage and those from Aboriginal or culturally and linguistically diverse backgrounds. There are no publicly available services for adults to access assessments (e.g., cognitive assessments, autism diagnostic assessments) to prove eligibility for NDIS at this time.

First Nations Australians

The population of First Nations Australians, which includes First Nations Australians people from mainland Australia, Tasmania or one of the offshore Australian islands) and from the islands of the Torres Strait, part of Queensland, was reduced by 90% following the colonisation of Australia by Britain. First Nations Australians suffered further trauma with the removal of children from their families between the 1860s and 1960s, referred to as the 'the stolen generation'. This history has understandably fuelled a mistrust of community health and social services in general.

First Nations Australians communities are diverse, with different languages and cultural practices. In many First Australians languages, there is no equivalent word for disability. Traditionally, Aboriginal culture was inclusive of people with different levels of ability, and the concept of disability was unheard of. However, in today's society, recent research has suggested that there are a range of attitudes to autism in First Australians communities, including negative attitudes of shame and stigma, as well as some positive themes of acceptance and inclusion [8].

Culturally, support for people with neurodevelopmental disorders tends to be delivered within the extended family rather than by professional service providers, in both

Table 23.1 Specialist neurodevelopmental disorder adult mental health services in Australia[a]

State	Total Population (million)	Aboriginal population (million)	Torres Strait Islander (%)	Name of community service[b]	Staff full-time equivalent[c]	Mental health services	Autistic clients without ID	Physical health	Inpatient services
Queensland	4.8	3.7	0.4	MIDAS SMHIDS	5 8	Clinics Home visits	Clinics -	Clinics	- -
New South Wales	7.7	3.3	0.1	3DN DDHU SIDMHOS	-	Clinic Clinic Clinical assessments	- Clinic	- Clinic -	- -
Victoria	6.7	0.9	0	CDDH VDDS MHIDI-Adult Casey Transition Support Unit	5.7	Clinic Clinic Home visit Clinic Home visit -	- Clinic Home visit Clinic Home visit -	Clinic	21 step-downbeds[d]
South Australia	1.7	2.4	0.1	CDH	5.4	Clinic	Clinic	Clinic	-
Western Australia	2.7	3.8	0.1	-	-	-	-	-	-
Tasmania	0.5	5.1	0.3	Mental health and ID service	3	Clinic	-	-	-
Northern Territory	0.3	29.0	0.4	-	-	-	-	-	-

Table 23.1 (cont.)

State	Total Population (million)	Aboriginal population (million)	Torres Strait Islander (%)	Name of community service[b]	Staff full-time equivalent[c]	Mental health services	Autistic clients without ID	Physical health	Inpatient services
Australian Capital Territory	0.4	1.8	0	Mental health service for people who inject drugs	4.8	Clinic	–	–	–

[a] Subject to change, as a number of states are undergoing major changes in services at the time of writing. [b] Abbreviations: 3DN, Department of Developmental Disability Neuropsychiatry; CDDH, Centre for Developmental Disability Health; CDH, Centre for Disability Health; DDHU, Developmental Disability Health Unit; MHIDI, Monash Health Mental Health and Intellectual. Disability Initiative; MIDAS, Mater Intellectual Disability and Autism Service; SMHIDS, Specialist Mental Health in Intellectual Disability Service; SIDMHOS, Specialist Intellectual Disability Mental Health Outreach Service. VDDS, Victoria Developmental Disability Service [c] Staff numbers are indicative only and not available for all services. [d] Slow-stream 2–5-year transition inpatient to community.

metropolitan and remote settings. Some of the cultural beliefs relevant in this setting are around time, confidentiality and cultural practices when conducting interviews. Beliefs relating to time concern the circular rather than linear concept of time, where past, present and future exist together in the same space and time and there are no fixed start and end points. People's right to keep secret and sacred their cultural knowledge (information that is restricted under customary law) is important. There may be several sensitive or taboo subjects that present problems in interviews. Even if these are acknowledged as such, they may not be able to be discussed due to fear about 'payback', which can prevent the person returning home. Averting eye contact can be a sign of respect; to make direct eye contact can be considered rude, especially if it is cross-gender. The terms 'aunty' and uncle' are used to show respect for someone older; this does not necessarily mean that someone is a blood relative.

Rates and Diagnosis of Neurodevelopmental Disorders in First Nations Australians

Current estimates are that ID is nearly four times as prevalent in First Australians than in the general population. This is thought to be multifactorial and possible causes include socio-economic disadvantage, maternal alcohol or drug use and poor physical conditions and health [9]. Prevalence rates for autism appear to be similar in First Australians and the general population, although they may be less likely to be accurately diagnosed [10]. Current evidence suggests that the diagnosis of neurodevelopmental disorders may be missed in First Australians, where there are cultural and language barriers to assessment, as well as greater difficulty in obtaining developmental history [11]. At the same time, the lack of culturally safe and valid screening and diagnostic tools may also mean that First Australians score artificially lower on intelligence tests and obtain false positives on autism screening. The use of First Australian liaison officers and interpreters to assist in conducting assessments is recommended [12]. The Kimberley Indigenous Cognitive Assessment (KICA) [13] has been designed and validated with Aboriginal people, but it is designed as a dementia screen and is not inclusive of all domains usually assessed for a diagnosis of ID. The Guddi protocol is a culturally safe tool developed to assess neurocognitive disability and mental health issues affecting First Australians. It incorporates a 'yarning' method, which is built on principles from the Aboriginal cultural form of conversation of the same name [14].

Forensic Issues and A First Nations Australian with Neurodevelopmental Disorders

Research in this area is less well developed than in the general population, but tends to suggest that there are higher levels of cognitive impairment (due to neurodevelopmental disorders or acquired brain injury) in First Australians who commit offences than non-First Australians offenders [15]. First Australians with cognitive disability are also associated with greater risk of entering the criminal justice system, with higher incidence of police contact, particularly at a younger age [15].

Principles to Consider When Interviewing a First Nations Australian

First Nations cultures values the connection to country and community, reflected in the importance of engagement and rapport when interviewing a First Nations Australian Practical tips include taking extra time to talk about where the person is from, and where the interviewer is from. Allowing extra time, approaching issues more gently, for example asking about general matters first and illness-related issues later, are all practical suggestions that have been identified by First Australians to assist in this process. Engagement is broader than with the person alone and should extend to the person's family and community. At the same time, confidentiality is very important, and this can be difficult if different family members are providing care and support. Check with the person as to what they are comfortable with people knowing. This is balanced with the need for the community to understand what is happening for the person. Shame can be felt if confidentiality is breached. An interpreter may be required. Wherever possible, it is recommended to involve a First Australian worker.

Support for First Nations Australian with Neurodevelopmental Disorders

First Australians with neurodevelopmental disorders are equally eligible to access the NDIS but they encounter barriers to accessing services. These include geographical barriers (most services are provided in urban centres), language and cultural barriers and lack of culturally safe services. Individuals and families may need to move from their remote communities to urban centres in order to access support. Within Aboriginal communities, individuals and families have also reported lack of awareness and understanding. Community support has been identified as a key protective factor [10]. For First Australians with neurodevelopmental disorders and complex support needs, including those who have committed an offence, it can be extremely difficult to find suitable service providers. Those in prisons or mental health units suffer double disadvantage, in settings that lack capacity to support First Australians and also people with neurodevelopmental disorders.

Australian Legislative Frameworks for People with Neurodevelopmental Disorders Who Commit Offences

Australia was originally colonised by the British in 1788 and its Westminster system of government and law is inherited from Britain. In Australia, individual states have legislative jurisdiction over the criminal justice and mental health systems [16]. Australia has recently developed the 'National Statement of Principles Relating to Persons Unfit to Plead or Found Not Guilty by Reason of Cognitive or Mental Health Impairment' (the National Principles) [17]. These are best-practice principles, which recognise the rights of individuals with impairment due to cognitive or mental health reasons. They seek to identify safeguards throughout legal processes and beyond, during the period in which a person is subject to orders. The National Principles have been endorsed by all states and territories of Australia with the exception of South Australia, which advised that the principles are inconsistent with their current legislative provisions, policies and procedures. In South Australia, these are weighted more heavily towards the protection of the community, reflected in their sentencing laws. The states and territories which have endorsed the National Principles will implement these in the context of their own legislation, policy and procedures.

The approach to people with neurodevelopmental disorders who offend is also variable across different states and territories of Australia (see Table 23.2). Most states and territories do not have a specialised service response, and management of people with neurodevelopmental disorders who have committed a serious offence is undertaken by general forensic or generic mental health services, where staff often have little or no specialised skills or knowledge of neurodevelopmental disorders. The one exception is the Mental Health Court in Queensland, as described below.

Table 23.2 Forensic disability services in Australia (from the Australian Bureau of Statistics [18])

Australian state	Total population (million	Aboriginal population (%)	Torres Strait Islander (%)	Separate forensic disability service	Specialised facility disability administered	Specialised facility health administered	Specialist unit in prison
Queensland	4.8	3.7	0.4	–	10 beds	–	–
New South Wales	7.7	3.3	0.1	Custody and community	–	–	8 additional support units
Victoria	6.7	0.9	0	Yes	14 beds 5 step-down beds	–	35 + 25 (male)
South Australia	1.7	2.4	0.1	–	–	10-bed unit in forensic mental health unit	–
Western Australia	2.7	3.8	0.1	–	10 beds	–	–
Tasmania	0.5	5.1	0.3	–	–	–	–
Northern Territory	0.3	29.0	0.4	–	8 beds + step-down beds	–	–
Australian Capital Territory	0.4	1.8	0	–	–	–	–

Services for People with Neurodevelopmental Disorders Who Are Subject to Legislation within Different States

Queensland

Queensland's Forensic Disability Service (FDS) facility commenced in 2011 as part of the Queensland government's reforms in response to the Carter Inquiry [19]. It is a purpose-built medium-secure 10-bed facility designed for the involuntary detention and care of people who have been found unfit to stand trial as a result of neurodevelopmental disorders or cognitive disability. It is provided by the Department of Communities (not Health) and has been at the centre of recent reviews and concerns around the length of detention and quality of care, including use of restrictive practices. In practice, people subject to a forensic order (disability) may be managed under the Department of Communities in the FDS or under the Department of Health in the mental health system.

Queensland's Mental Health Court is unique. It is designed to provide a separate pathway for cases where an individual has been charged with a serious offence and is thought to have been of unsound mind at the time and/or is temporarily or permanently unfit to stand trial [16]. A serious offence is considered one that cannot be heard and determined by a magistrate [20]. The Mental Health Court operates at Supreme Court level and consists of two Supreme Court judges and, for people with neurodevelopmental disorders, two independent psychiatrists or clinicians with experience working with people with neurodevelopmental disorders. In cases where the finding is that the individual is of unsound mind and/or permanently unfit to plead, the possible outcomes are provision of a forensic order (disability), forensic order (mental health) or no order.

In Queensland, a forensic order (disability) can specify various conditions, including that the individual be housed at a stand-alone forensic disability facility [7]. Other conditions can be similar to a forensic order (mental health), including that the person reside at an approved address, abstain from alcohol and illicit substances, is complaint with prescribed medication and attends psychiatric follow-up at his or her local government-funded mental health service (where he or she is monitored by a general adult psychiatrist without training in neurodevelopmental disorders psychiatry). This has been raised as an issue of concern by various stakeholders and in formal reviews of the forensic disability system [4]. Additional concerns relate to the trend for forensic disability orders to continue indefinitely, given the permanent nature of disability and the lack of access to specialised behaviour support and intervention for this group with complex needs.

New South Wales

New South Wales has a state-wide community forensic disability service that operates separately to forensic mental health services. It consists of a multidisciplinary team, which assists with assessments and addresses disability support needs of people with neurodevelopmental disorders who have committed offences. New South Wales also has the Community Justice Program, which provides services to people with neurodevelopmental disorders exiting the criminal justice system [4].

Victoria

Victoria has a specialised forensic disability service and two facilities for those on custodial supervision orders. These specialist forensic disability facilities are funded and administered by the Department of Disability Services and function as residential treatment programs. Victoria's public forensic mental health service provider undertakes some forensic disability work, including provision of psychological assessments to the court, and offers outpatient clinical sessions to the forensic disability residential facility [4].

Autism in Forensic Disability Settings in Australia

The effect of autism on an individual's ability to participate in police interviews and court settings has been considered by Freckleton, who emphasises the autistic person's capacity to understand and communicate, and the effect of the autistic individual's observed behaviour during interview and in court. He suggests explanatory evidence should be given in cases involving autistic people [21].

The profile and needs of autistic adults within the Australian forensic system, including in the criminal justice system, are only recently beginning to be considered in the literature. A recent New South Wales study followed eight prisoners and explored themes relating to their experiences in prison These centred around themes of coping with the unpredictability of the environment, being deprived of the ability to control their situation, being in an environment of what at times are illogical rules and routines and the challenges of negotiating the social world of prison, coping through self-isolation and avoidance [22]. Another New South Wales study used consultation groups to consider the service development needs of incarcerated autistic adults. This revealed two main themes: first, the challenges of identifying autistic adults within the prison system, as many have not been diagnosed and there are no publicly available diagnostic services for Australian adults at this time; and secondly the need for development of autism-specific support services for this group [23].

A Focus on Aotearoa New Zealand

Aotearoa New Zealand, a country consisting of North and South Islands (see Figure 23.3), has a population of approximately five million people, who are predominantly (70%) of European origin, followed by 16.5% Māori, the First Nations People of Aotearoa New Zealand, and then 8.1% Pacific peoples (Pasifika) and 15.1% Asian ethnic groups. From a historical perspective, de-institutionalisation in Aotearoa New Zealand was marked in 1992 by the closure of the first large institution, Cherry Farm, near Dunedin on the South Island. The last major institution closed in 2007. Alongside this process, progressive changes to the mental health legislation were made in relation to promoting and protecting the rights of those who accessed the mainstream mental health service.

Healthcare System in Aotearoa New Zealand

Healthcare has been delivered regionally through 20 district health boards (DHBs) across Aotearoa New Zealand's North and South Islands but, in recent years, the Aotearoa New Zealand government has reviewed both the health and disability system and has committed to major reform, prompted by lack of equity and consistency across the different geographical areas of Aotearoa New Zealand. This review has led to a federally administrative national health system known as Health New Zealand with the development of a Māori Health Authority which came into effect in July 2022, which will work with the federal system to directly commission services in order to improve outcomes for Māori people [24].

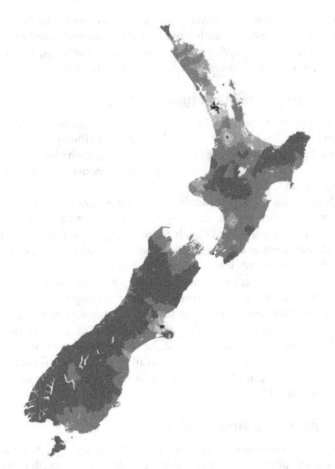

Figure 23.3 Map of New Zealand showing population density (2006). Lighter areas show the greatest density. Source: https://upload.wikimedia.org/wikipedia/commons/5/56/NewZealandPopulationDensity.png.

Mental Healthcare for People with Neurodevelopmental Disorders

Broadly, there is a significant lack of specialised services for people with neurodevelopmental disorders and mental health problems and those that do exist suffer from under-resourcing. People with neurodevelopmental disorders and comorbid mental health problems are expected to access mainstream mental health services in most areas. Some districts do have small specialised neurodevelopmental disorders mental health teams, as described in Table 23.3. All of these teams, covering 10 of the nation's 20 DHB areas, are delivered as part of each respective DHB area's mental health services. This leaves approximately 1.2 of New Zealand's 5 million population without access to specialised ID mental healthcare.

This lack of specialised services for people with neurodevelopmental disorders means that there is a lack of capacity in mainstream services to work with people with such disabilities. This manifests in practical terms as reduced detection of neurodevelopmental disorders and poorer outcomes for those with these disabilities and comorbid health and

Table 23.3 Examples of specialist neurodevelopmental disorder mental healthcare services in Aotearoa New Zealand

New Zealand Island	Administering DHB	DHB area	Total population (million)[a]	Māori population (%)	Pasifika population (%)	Community team	Community team services	Dedicated specialist inpatient beds
North	Counties-Manukau[b]	Counties-Manukau Auckland Waitemata Northern	1.9	15.8	10.5	Regional dual disability mental health service: small multidisciplinary team	Clinics Home visits Education	–
North	Waikato[c]	Waikato (mainly Hamilton)	0.44	24.0	3.0	ID Dual Disorder Service One part-time psychiatrist, two full-time nurses	Community-based, specialised service	–
North	Capital and Coast	Capital and Coast Lakes Hutt Valley	0.6	18.3	6.3	Community mental health ID multidisciplinary team		–
South	Canterbury[d]	Canterbury	0.6	9.8	2.8	Outpatient mental health ID team	Comprehensive mental health assessment and treatment	15 beds for ID + mental health, includes a multidisciplinary team for assessments and intervention

Table 23.3 (cont.)

New Zealand Island	Administering DHB	DHB area	Total population (million)[a]	Māori population (%)	Pasifika population (%)	Community team	Community team services	Dedicated specialist inpatient beds
South	Southern[e]	Southern	0.3	10.8	2.3	Dual diagnosis mental health and ID community services	Range of specialist mental health services	Only beds are secure and primarily for forensic ID clients

[a] www.stats.govt.nz/topics/population; [b] www.countiesmanukau.health.nz/our-services/a-z/dual-disability-regional-mental-health-service/; [c] www.waikatodhb.health.nz/about-us/a-z-of-services/mental-health-and-addictions/intellectual-disability/; [d] https://mherc.org.nz/directory/cdhb-hospital-services/intellectually-disabled-persons-health-service; [e] www.southernhealth.nz/services.

mental health problems. Table 23.3 gives representative view of the current state of services, although of course the specifics of such services continue to change over time.

Māori People

The Treaty of Waitangi was signed in 1840 and gave Māori people the same rights and privileges as pakeha (White/European New Zealanders). However, since that time there has been debate over whether the terms of the Treaty have been adhered to. Māori men are more likely to be treated in a forensic care setting, to be diagnosed with schizophrenia, but to spend less than half the time in hospital than non-Māori men. They are also more likely to have poorer physical health and, as a result of multiple areas of disadvantage, suffer poorer outcomes. It is also important to understand that while 'disability' is a pakeha construct used to describe impairment, for Māori people it may relate more to a loss of land, culture, identity, values, practice and language [25]. The presentation of mental health problems in the Māori is often similar to presentation in the pakeha, but there can be more culturally bound physical and spiritual expressions of distress [26]. There are also several typical presentations that are specific to the Māori, which can mimic mental illness, for example experiencing the presence of ancestors [26].

Diagnosis and Rates of Neurodevelopmental Disorders in Maori People

Māori models of health and disability tend to be more holistic and to focus on spiritual and emotional development, in contrast to the medical illness/disorder-based phenomenology used in medical models [27]. For some Māori, the differences of autism are considered gifts to be nurtured whereas, for others, autism is seen as a consequence or punishment for something the family may have previously done. Until recently, there was no Māori word for autism, the term 'Takiwātanga' has now been proposed and is derived from a term that means my/his/her own time and space [28].

The Māori have higher prevalence rates for disability in general (20%) than non-Māori people (14%), but obtaining accurate data to better understand this finding is difficult. The rates of ID appear to be higher (3% vs 2%) [29] but no statistically significant difference in a parent-reported data set of autism diagnoses in children [30].

Principles to Consider When Interviewing a Maori Person

The Medical Council of New Zealand (Te Kaunihera Rata o Aotearoa) now requires all doctors to meet cultural safety standards. An independent report was published in 2020, which explored the current state of cultural safety and health equity in New Zealand medical practice. Its first point was that it is vital that the systemic racism and privilege that exists in the healthcare sector is acknowledged in order to begin to effect change [31]. Understanding and addressing systemic barriers, spending extra time to understand the person and their context and the importance of whakawhanaungatanga, that is, the understanding and developing of relationships, is highlighted.

Legislative Framework for People with Neurodevelopmental Disorders in Aotearoa New Zealand Who Commit Offences

The introduction of the Mental Health Compulsory Assessment and Treatment Act in 1992 specifically excluded people who had ID in the absence of co-occurring mental illness [32]. This left the court with the only options of sending people with ID to prison, leaving them in the community or, if there were very high levels of risk, admitting them to a forensic hospital as a special patient [33]. There was no legislation pertinent to this group until significant changes were made to legislation in 2004, with the introduction of two Acts of Parliament that provided alternative pathways for people charged with an imprisonable offence who may have ID. These are the Criminal Procedure (Mentally Impaired Persons) (CMPIP) Act 2003 [34] and the Intellectual Disability (Compulsory Care and Rehabilitation) (IDCCR) Act 2003 [35]. In practice, these Acts allow for a concern to be raised with the court in relation to a person's ability to undergo standard court processes. The court than then approach court liaison staff to complete a screen in relation to fitness to stand trial. This can proceed to a 'fitness to stand trial' assessment, under the CPMIP Act and is referred to the local forensic mental health services to be completed by a health assessor. If deemed necessary by the court, further assessment is then arranged through referral to the forensic coordination services (intellectual disability) and an assessment is completed by a specialist assessor [36].

If ID is confirmed through this process, and if there is a significant risk of reoffending, where legal compulsion and specialist residential service provision is required, then the person can be made a 'care recipient' under the IDDCR Act for up to three years. If the person does not have ID, or does have ID but does not require the conditions of the IDCCR Act, they can still proceed through usual correction processes.

Based on at least two reports, the Court will decide whether the person is 'responsible' for the alleged events and if they are unfit to stand trial and if so, then a Specialist Assessment is required. This assessment will add to the previous assessment, which assessed for presence of ID, to provide information to the Court on risk of reoffending and management recommendations. If there are significant risk-related issues, then the person may be made a Care Recipient under the IDCCR Act. If there are no significant risk concerns then the charges may be discharged and no further processes are necessary [36].

Forensic Services for People with Neurodevelopmental Disorders in New Zealand

Concerns regarding inappropriate placement of people with neurodevelopmental disorders who commit offences led to the development of specialised inpatient facilities in the early 2000s. While the advances in legislation have been welcomed and felt to be long overdue, there are significant levels of concern that services are inadequate and inadequately funded for the level of need for people with neurodevelopmental disorders and subject to the IDCCR Act [37]; see Table 23.4 for specific examples of facilities. A particular focus of concern was around the lack of secure care and rehabilitation, and conditions in which some people were being detained, including vulnerability of females on mixed-sex wards. Another concern is that the number of beds has not increased since 2014, despite significant increases in the population. This lack of services adds to the existing lack of capacity in mainstream mental health services for people with neurodevelopmental disorders.

The Chief Ombudsman's report in 2021 detailed that between 200 and 250 people are supported under the Framework developed for this group at any one time. The demographics of this group reveal an over-representation of males (85%) and Maori (37%), compared to general population distribution [37]. Table 23.4 gives an overview of the provision of inpatient beds for people with neurodevelopmental disorders who are subject to the IDCCR Act. Certainly, these figures suggest that it is the minority who are inpatients and that most

Table 23.4 Examples of forensic neurodevelopmental disorder inpatient facilities in Aotearoa New Zealand

New Zealand Island	Region	DHB	Population (million)[a]	Maori (% of total population)	Pasifika (% of total population)	Location of service	Total beds	Type of beds
North	Northern	Northland Auckland Waitemata Counties Manukau	1.9	15.8	10.5	Auckland	12	10 care and rehabilitation beds 2 assessment beds
North	Midland	Waikato Bay of Plenty Hawkes Bay Tairawhiti Taranaki	1.1	25.3	5.5	Hamilton	3	2 secure hospital beds 1 assessment bed
North	Central	Lakes Hutt Valley Capital and Coast MidCentral Wairarapa Whanganui	0.9	15.4	6.0	Kenepuru, Porirua	24 (National + Central region) 8 (National Youth)	14 secure hospital beds 2 assessment beds 8 step-down beds 8 secure hospital beds
South	Upper South	Nelson-Marlborough Canterbury Sth Canterbury West Coast	0.8	10.1	2.5	Christchurch	8	7 secure hospital beds 1 assessment bed

Table 23.4 (cont.)

New Zealand Island	Region	DHB	Population (million)[a]	Maori (% of total population)	Pasifika (% of total population)	Location of service	Total beds	Type of beds
South	Lower South	Southern	0.3	10.8	2.3	Dunedin	11	6 secure hospital beds, 1 assessment bed 4 step-down beds

[a] www.stats.govt.nz/topics/population.

of this group are in the community. There are regional ID liaison community teams (Northern Region, Midland, Central and Southern), but again these are insufficient for the number and geographic spread of clients.

Conclusion

There have been significant advances in some areas of forensic disability legislation, healthcare and services across Australia and Aotearoa New Zealand in recent years, but there remain significant gaps in services and lack of capacity in the health workforce. Overall, there are still major deficits in community and inpatient forensic neurodevelopmental disorder services for this population. It is to be hoped that the improvements in neurodevelopmental disorder healthcare and legislation have follow-on effects to improve capacity in forensic neurodevelopmental disorder services and workforce across Australia and Aotearoa New Zealand.

References

1. Trollor JN, Eagleson C, Ruffell B, Tracy J, Torr JJ, Durvasula S, et al. Has teaching about intellectual disability healthcare in Australian medical schools improved? A 20-year comparison of curricula audits. *BMC Medical Education* 2020; 20(1): 321.

2. Trollor JN, Eagleson C, Turner B, Salomon C, Cashin A, Iacono T, et al. Intellectual disability health content within nursing curriculum: an audit of what our future nurses are taught. *Nurse Education Today* 2016; 45: 72–9.

3. Howlett S, Florio T, Xu H, Trollor J. Ambulatory mental health data demonstrates the high needs of people with an intellectual disability: results from the New South Wales intellectual disability and mental health data linkage project. *Australian and New Zealand Journal of Psychiatry* 2015; 49(2): 137–44.

4. Ogloff JRP, Ruffles J, Sullivan D. Review of the operation of the Forensic Disability Act 2011. Available at: https://documents .parliament.qld.gov.au/tableOffice/TabledP apers/2018/5618T1581.pdf.

5. The Royal Australian and New Zealand College of Psychiatrists. Submission to the Health and Disability System Review Panel New Zealand Health and Disability System Review. 2019. Available at: www.ranzcp.org /files/resources/submissions/submission- to-health-_-disability-system-review- fi.aspx.

6. Royal Commission into Violence, Abuse, Neglect and Exploitation of People with Disability. Interim report. 2020. Available at: https://disability.royalcommission.gov.au/p ublications/interim-report.

7. Royal Australian and New Zealand College of Psychiatrists. Position statement: principles for the treatment of persons found unfit to stand trial. 2020. Available at: www.ranzcp.org/news-policy/policy- and-advocacy/position-statements/per sons-found-unfit-to-stand-trial.

8. Lilley R, Sedgwick M, Pellicano E. Inclusion, acceptance, shame and isolation: attitudes to autism in Aboriginal and Torres Striat islander communities in Australia. *Autism* 2020; 24(7): 1860–73.

9. Glasson EJ, Sullivan SG, Hussain R, Bittles AH. An assessment of intellectual disability among Aboriginal Australians. *Journal of Intellectual Disability Research* 2005; 49(Pt 8): 626–34.

10. Bailey B, Arciuli J. Indigenous Australians with autism: a scoping review. *Autism* 2020; 24(5): 1031–46.

11. Roy M, Balaratnasingam S. Missed diagnosis of autism in an Australian indigenous psychiatric population. *Australasian Psychiatry* 2010; 18(6): 534–7.

12. Dingwall K, Pinkerton J, Lindeman MA. 'People like numbers': a descriptive study of cognitive assessment methods in clinical

practice for Aboriginal Australians in the Northern Territory. *BMC Psychiatry* 2013; 13: 42.

13. LoGiudice D, Smith K, Thomas J. Kimberley Indigenous Cognitive Assessment tool (KICA): development of a cognitive assessment tool for older Indigenous Australians. *International Psychogeriatrics* 2006; 18: 269–80.

14. McIntyre M, Townsend C, Cullen J. Responding to the needs of homeless Aboriginal and Torres Strait Islander young people with complex disability: the Guddi for young people. *Journal of Social Inclusion* 2017; 8(2): 81–9.

15. Shepherd SM, Ogloff JR, Shea D, Pfeifer JE, Paradies Y. Aboriginal prisoners and cognitive impairment: the impact of dual disadvantage on social and emotional wellbeing. *Journal of Intellectual Disability Research* 2017; 61(4): 385–97.

16. Coghlan S, Harden S. The Queensland mental health court: a unique model. *BJPsych International* 2019; 16(4): 86–9.

17. Council of Attorneys-General. National Statement of Principles Relating to Persons Unfit to Plead or Not Guilty by Reason of Cognitive or Mental Health Impairment. Available at: www.ag.gov.au/rights-and-protections/human-rights-and-anti-discrimination/national-statement-principles-relating-persons-unfit-plead-or-not-guilty-reason-cognitive-or-mental-health-impairment.

18. Australian Bureau of Statistics. Estimates of Aboriginal and Torres Strait Islander Australians. Available at: www.abs.gov.au/statistics/people/aboriginal-and-torres-strait-islander-peoples/estimates-aboriginal-and-torres-strait-islander-australians/latest-release.

19. Carter HJW. Challenging behaviour and disability: a targeted response. The State of Queensland, 2006. Available at: https://asksource.info/resources/challenging-behaviours-and-disability-a-targeted-response. See also https://documents.parliament.qld.gov.au/tableoffice/tabledpapers/2014/5414T4214.pdf.

20. Mental Health Act 2016 (Queensland). Available at: www.health.qld.gov.au/clinical-practice/guidelines-procedures/clinical-staff/mental-health/act.

21. Freckleton I. Autism spectrum disorder: forensic issues and challenges for mental health professionals and courts. *Journal of Applied Research in Intellectual Disabilities* 2013; 26: 420–34.

22. Newman C, Cashin A, Waters C. A hermeneutic phenomenological examination of the lived experience of incarceration for those with autism. *Issues in Mental Health Nursing* 2015; 36(8): 632–40.

23. Newman C, Cashin A, Graham I. Identification of service development needs for incarcerated adults with autism spectrum disorders in an Australian prison system. *International Journal of Prisoner Health* 2019; 15(1): 24–36.

24. New Zealand Government. Health and disability system review. Available at: https://systemreview.health.govt.nz/final-report

25. Bevan-Brown J. Including people with disabilities: an indigenous perspective. *International Journal of Inclusive Education* 2013; 17(6): 571–83.

26. Todd FC. Te Ariari o te Oranga: the assessment and management of people with co-existing mental health and substance use problems. 2010. Available at: www.health.govt.nz/system/files/documents/publications/te-ariari-o-te-orang-teariari-13-04-10.pdf.

27. Tupou J, Curtis S, Taare-Smith D, Glasgow A, Waddington H. Maori and autism: a scoping review. *Autism* 2021: 25 (7): 1844–58.

28. Te Pou o te Whakaaro Nui. Determining the workforce development needs of New Zealand's autism workforce. 2015. Available at: www.tepou.co.nz/resources/determining-the-workforce-development-needs-of-new-zealands-autism-workforce.

29. Ministry of Justice, Wellington. Māori health disability statistical report. Available at: https://forms.justice.govt.nz/search/Do

cuments/WT/wt_DOC_151847905/Wai%202575%2C%20B024.pdf.

30. Ministry of Health. Annual data explorer 2018/19: New Zealand health survey. Available at: www.health.govt.nz/publication/annual-update-key-results-2018-19-new-zealand-health-survey.

31. Allen+Clarke. Baseline data capture: cultural safety, partnership and health equity initiatives. 2020. Available at: https://statsnz.contentdm.oclc.org/digital/collection/p20045coll17/id/1129/.

32. Mental Health (Compulsory Assessment and Treatment) Act 1992. Available at: www.legislation.govt.nz/act/public/1992/0046/latest/DLM262176.html.

33. McCarthy J, Duff M. Services for adults with intellectual disability in Aotearoa New Zealand. *BJPsych International* 2019; 16(3): 71–3.

34. Criminal Procedure (Mentally Impaired Persons) Act 2003. Available at: www.legislation.govt.nz/act/public/2003/0115/latest/DLM223818.html.

35. Intellectual Disability (Compulsory Care and Rehabilitation) Act 2003. Available at: www.legislation.govt.nz/act/public/2003/0116/latest/DLM224578.html.

36. Brief overview of the pathway to the IDCCR Act. Available at: www.benchmark.org.nz/assets/Uploads/Brief-overview-of-the-pathway-to-the-IDCCR-Act3.pdf.

37. Boshier P. Oversight: investigation report – an investigation into the Ministry of Health's stewardship of hospital-level secure services for people with an intellectual disability. Available at: www.ombudsman.parliament.nz/sites/default/files/2021-12/OMB%20-%20Oversight%20-%20Final%20opinion.pdf.

Concluding Comments

Chapter 24

Jane M. McCarthy and Eddie Chaplin

This is the first book to bring together the evidence base from leading researchers and clinicians at international level on the forensic needs of people with neurodevelopmental disorders. We hope the readers will find the evidence presented in this book not only informative but a useful reference source for their day-to-day clinical practice. There are many themes running throughout the book but one key one is that people with neurodevelopmental disorders present to the forensic system as complex, with more than one health and social care need. Another theme is the challenge of how best to recognise people with neurodevelopmental disorders across the different parts of the criminal justice system, ensuring there is expertise to provide assessments early on in the journey of defendants. The availability of evidence-based treatments needs to be embedded across forensic settings including correctional settings, health facilities and community-based services. The importance of early intervention is highlighted in the chapters on young people, and we need a robust response to supporting young people with neurodevelopmental disorders, making sure they do not continue within the criminal justice and correctional systems well into their adult life.

The book also provides a framework to aid clinicians and policy makers to identify the key gaps in knowledge and how to use the current evidence to improve outcomes for those with neurodevelopmental disorders within forensic services and the criminal justice system. It indicates that advances in neurosciences and genetic research will change clinical practice in the coming decades. Many countries have been through the process of de-instutionalisation, closing the large institutions, and this to some extent will impact on what services are available in both hospital and community settings. At an individual country level, the impact of these changes will be influenced by national policy, if in existence, and to the subsequent delivery of services for those with neurodevelopmental disorders. It will be difficult to predict policy in many countries as this is determined not only by the evidence base but by the current political and governance systems and, to some extent, by the culture and attitudes within each country to vulnerable groups within the criminal justice system.

The financial challenges for many countries around the world after the coronavirus pandemic and the rising cost of living will be an important influence on service developments, which will need to show they are cost-effective and efficient in their delivery. Therefore, it is important the interventions that are provided are evidence based and there are good measures to show robust outcomes. The whole field of clinical practice is moving in a direction of being person centred and this needs to be also reflected in our professional approach to working with people with neurodevelopmental disorders who offend. In many countries there will also be a workforce issue in developing professionals and practitioners within forensic services and legal systems with the expertise to work with people with neurodevelopmental disorders. Over time, it may be that more developed countries will be able to define care pathways to improve outcomes for people with such disorders so they can access the care and treatment they require.

We hope also that the book not only impacts on clinical practice and service development but also encourages reflection by individual clinicians and practitioners, leading to improvement in practice and research in the future. However, what the book also shows is that the study of neurodevelopmental disorders is still an emerging area, which has not attracted the same kind of funding as general forensic services, often aimed at specific groups such as the seriously mentally ill. As well as providing an up-to-date evidence base and guidance to inform everyday decision making by clinicians, the book showcases innovation in thought and clinical practice, for example an introduction to the concept of subthreshold neurodevelopmental disorders and the development of the Framework for the Assessment of Risk and protection in offenders on the Autistic Spectrum (FARAS). It also examines areas where there is relatively little evidence, and so misinterpretation may occur within the media such as serious crime linked to autistic people. Other areas that require more research include a greater understanding of discrepancies in gender, ethnicity and individual cultural needs across services. By offering a better understanding of these conditions, this book also helps to inform clinical research targets such as screening, therapeutic interventions and positive approaches to risk management.

Finally, there is a need for more service research and evaluation to examine the effectiveness of current and proposed models and pathways through the health and criminal justice system, from police to court to disposal, including probation and health services. This research must include people with neurodevelopmental disorders. To do this we also need to address specific areas such as fitness to plead and effective participation in the legal process for those with neurodevelopmental disorders within the UK and internationally.

Index

Printed in the United States
by Baker & Taylor Publisher Services

Printed in the United States
by Baker & Taylor Publisher Services